Immunobiology of Natural Killer Cells

Volume II

Editor

Eva Lotzová, Ph.D.
Department of General Surgery
University of Texas System Cancer Center
M.D. Anderson Hospital and Tumor Institute
Houston, Texas

Associate Editor

Ronald B. Herberman, M.D.
Pittsburgh Cancer Institute
Pittsburgh, Pennsylvania

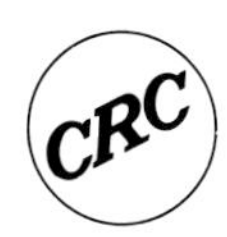

CRC Press, Inc.
Boca Raton, Florida

Library of Congress Cataloging in Publication Data
Main entry under title:

Immunobiology of natural killer cells.

Includes bibliographies and index.
1. Killer cells. 2. Cell-mediated cytotoxicity.
I. Lotzova, Evá, 1936- . II. Herberman, Ronald, B.,
1940- . [DNLM: 1. Immunity, Cellular. 2. Killer
Cells-immunology. QW 568 I317]
QR185.8K54I46 1986 599'.029 85-12744
ISBN 0-8493-6542-2 (v. 1)
ISBN 0-8493-6543-0 (v. 2)

Direct all inquiries to CRC Press, Inc., 2000 Corporate Blvd., N.W., Boca Raton, Florida, 33431.

Second Printing, 1989

International Standard Book Number 0-8493-6542-2 (Volume I)
International Standard Book Number 0-8493-6543-0 (Volume II)

Library of Congress Card Number 85-12744
Printed in the United States

This book is dedicated to the memory of my Mother

Eva Lotzová

PREFACE

It has become increasingly evident that natural killer (NK) cells may play an important role in defense against neoplasias and against exogenous intruders, such as viruses, bacteria, and parasites. More recent evidence also indicates involvement of NK cells in several other biological phenomena. For instance, NK cells were demonstrated to regulate growth and functions of lymphocytes, and to control proliferation and differentiation of myeloid and erythroid series of hemopoietic cells as well as pluripotential stem cells. Even though the mechanism of the effects of NK cells on hemopoiesis and lymphopoiesis has as yet not been elucidated, such regulation may be mediated by various soluble biological substances which are produced by NK cells. These are exemplified by different species of interferon, T cell and B cell growth factors, and colony-stimulating factor. It is quite plausible that NK cells, via their ability to regulate this wide array of biological functions, may represent a major component sustaining homeostasis of the organism. The early appearance of NK cells in phylogenetic development and their conservation through evolution to man, certainly supports this postulation.

Importantly, NK cells may have also a clinical relevance in cancer, nonmalignant diseases, and in the field of bone marrow transplantation. Available evidence indicates that the level of activity of these cells could be of prognostic value in relapse of leukemia or in assessing the severity of graft-vs.-host disease after allogeneic bone marrow transplantation, and perhaps these cells also may play a role in bone marrow graft rejection, benign hemopathies, and regulation of autoimmunity. There are also suggestions that NK cells may be therapeutically effective in cancer after their propagation in vitro.

The possible importance of NK cells in biology and medicine led us to review for the first time comprehensively various aspects of NK cells in a form of a book. This book will be composed of two volumes, and will include the techniques for NK cell quantification and characterization; the phylogeny and ontogeny of NK cells; the genetics of NK cell activity and the mechanisms of their functions; down- and up-regulation of NK cell activity; NK cell-suppressor cell relationships; and propagation and cloning of NK cells in vitro. We have also reviewed the cytotoxic profile of NK cells in cancer patients and its modulation by biological response modifying agents.

We hope that this book will contribute to the advancing knowledge of readers in the field of NK cells, and will be helpful as a teaching device. Furthermore, we trust that this publication will stimulate further research in this interesting and important field.

Eva Lotzová, Editor
Ronald B. Herberman, Associate Editor

THE EDITORS

Dr. Eva Lotzová is Professor of Immunology, Chief of the Division of Immunogenetics at the University of Texas System Cancer Center, M.D. Anderson Hospital and Tumor Institute, Houston. She is also Professor at the Graduate School of Biomedical Sciences, The University of Texas, Houston. Dr. Lotzová received her M.S. and Ph.D. degrees from Charles University, Prague, Czechoslovakia. She has been on the editorial boards of several scientific journals and is Editor-in-Chief of the journal *Natural Immunity and Cell Growth Regulation.* Furthermore, she is a contributing author to CRC Press and Academic Press Scientific Book Series. She has been a consultant to several governmental and private institutions in the area of biological response modification. Dr. Lotzová has been internationally recognized through her contributions to the fields of experimental bone marrow transplantation, natural cell-mediated immunity, and immunomodulation. She has contributed more than 150 publications to the scientific literature and is a member of several scientific organizations including the American Association of Immunologists, American Association for Cancer Research, Transplantation Society, and International Society for Experimental Hematology.

Dr. Ronald B. Herberman, formerly Chief of the Biological Therapeutics Branch, and Acting Associate Director for the Biological Response Modifiers Program, Division of Cancer Treatment, National Cancer Institute, Frederick, Maryland, has recently moved to Pittsburgh to become the first Director of the Pittsburgh Cancer Institute. Dr. Herberman received B.A. and M.D. degrees from New York University, graduating summa cum laude. After internship and residency in internal medicine at the Massachusetts General Hospital, Boston, Dr. Herberman joined the National Cancer Institute as a clinical associate in the Immunology Branch in 1966. He then held a series of positions at the National Cancer Institute, including Chief of the Laboratory of Immunodiagnosis. Dr. Herberman is a Diplomate of the American Board of Internal Medicine and is past president of the Reticuloendothelial Society. He has been or is currently on the editorial boards of a wide variety of oncology and immunology journals, including *Journal of Immunology, Cancer Research, Cellular Immunology, Journal of the National Cancer Institute,* and *Natural Immunity and Cell Growth Regulation.* He has published more than 600 papers in the fields of oncology and immunology and is the author of books on *Immunodiagnosis of Cancer, Natural Cell-Mediated Immunity Against Tumors,* and *NK Cells and Other Natural Effector Cells.*

CONTRIBUTORS

Paola Allavena
Istituto "Mario Negri"
Milan, Italy

Colin G. Brooks
Associate
Program in Basic Immunology
Fred Hutchinson Cancer Research Center
Seattle, Washington

J. Y. Djeu
Department of Medical Microbiology
College of Medicine
University of South Florida
Tampa, Florida

Patricia A. Fitzgerald
Assistant Professor
Department of Pathology
University of Medicine and Dentistry of New Jersey—New Jersey Medical School
Newark, New Jersey

Sidney H. Golub
Professor
Department of Surgery/Oncology
UCLA School of Medicine
Los Angeles, California

Nabil Hanna
Director
Department of Immunology and Antiinfectives Therapy
Smith Kline and French Laboratories
Philadelphia, Pennsylvania

Ronald B. Herberman
Director
Pittsburgh Cancer Institute
Pittsburgh, Pennsylvania

T. Kasahara
Department of Medical Biology and Parasitology
Jichi Medical School
Tochigi-Ken, Japan

Carlos Lopez
Chief, Viral Exanthems and Herpesvirus Branch
Division of Virus Diseases
Center for Infectious Diseases
Centers for Disease Control
Atlanta, Georgia

Eva Lotzová
Professor of Immunology
Department of General Surgery
Section of Immunogenetics
The University of Texas System Cancer Center
M. D. Anderson Hospital and Tumor Institute
Houston, Texas

Jean E. Merrill
Assistant Professor
Department of Neurology
UCLA School of Medicine
Los Angeles, California

Peter M. Moy
Surgical Oncology Fellow
John Wayne Cancer Clinic
Division of Surgical Oncology
Department of Surgery
UCLA School of Medicine
Los Angeles, California

Andrew V. Muchmore
Senior Investigator
Metabolism Branch
National Cancer Institute
Frederick Cancer Research Facility
Frederick, Maryland

Joost J. Oppenheim
Laboratory of Molecular Immunoregulation
Biological Response Modifiers Program
National Cancer Institute
Frederick Cancer Research Facility
Frederick, Maryland

John R. Ortaldo
Acting Chief
Biological Therapeutics Branch
National Cancer Institute
Frederick Cancer Research Facility
Frederick, Maryland

Hugh F. Pross
Professor
Departments of Radiation Oncology and Microbiology and Immunology
Queen's University
Kingston, Ontario, Canada

Cherylyn A. Savary
Research Associate
Department of General Surgery
Section of Immunogenetics
The University of Texas System Cancer Center
M. D. Anderson Hospital and Tumor Institute
Houston, Texas

Giuseppe Scala
I Istituto di Scienze Biochimiche
II Facolta di Medicina, Napoli
Naples, Italy

IMMUNOBIOLOGY OF NATURAL KILLER CELLS

Volume I

Assays for NK Cell Cytotoxicity; Their Values and Pitfalls
Separation and Characterization of Phenotypically Distinct Subsets of NK Cells
Ultrastructure and Cytochemistry of the Human Large Granular Lymphocytes
Phylogeny and Ontogeny of NK Cells
Tissue and Organ Distribution of NK Cells
Genetic Control of NK Cell Activity in Rodents
Phenotype, Functional Heterogeneity, and Lineage of Natural Killer Cells
Target Cell Structures, Recognition Sites, and the Mechanism of NK Cytotoxicity
Natural Killer Cytotoxic Factors (NKCF) Role in Cell-Mediated Cytotoxicity
Characteristics of Cultured NK Cells
Lectin-Dependent Killer Cells
MLC-Induced Cytotoxicity as a Model for the Development and Regulation of NK Cytotoxicity
LGL Lymphoproliferative Diseases in Man and Experimental Animals: The Characteristics of These Cells and Their Potential Experimental Uses

Volume II

In Vivo Activities of NK Cells Against Primary and Metastatic Tumors in Experimental Animals
The Involvement of Natural Killer Cells in Human Malignant Disease
Impaired NK Cell Profile in Leukemia Patients
In Vivo Modulation of NK Activity in Cancer Patients
The Implications of Aberrant Natural Killer (MK) Cell Activity in Nonmalignant Chronic Diseases
NK Cell Role in Regulation of the Growth and Functions of Hemopoietic and Lymphoid Cells
Natural Killer Cells Active Against Viral, Bacterial, Protozoan, and Fungal Infections
Cytokine Secretion and Noncytotoxic Functions of Human Large Granular Lymphocytes
Augmentation of Natural Killer Activity
Regulation of NK Cell Activity by Suppressor Cells
NK Cell Cloning Technology and Characteristics of NK Cell Clones
A Comparison of Antibody-Dependent Cellular Cytotoxicity (ADCC) and NK Activity

TABLE OF CONTENTS

Volume II

Chapter 1

IN VIVO ACTIVITIES OF NK CELLS AGAINST PRIMARY AND METASTATIC TUMORS IN EXPERIMENTAL ANIMALS

Nabil Hanna

TABLE OF CONTENTS

I. INTRODUCTION

To assess the possible role of natural killer (NK) cells in host defenses against tumor growth and metastasis, investigators have studied the in vivo growth characteristics of NK-sensitive or NK-resistant tumor cells in hosts that exhibit low or high levels of NK cell-mediated cytotoxicity (NK CMC). The results of these studies have clearly shown that a correlation exists between the levels of NK CMC as measured in vitro and host resistance against the growth and metastasis of NK-sensitive malignant tumors in vivo. Most studies, however, were carried out with transplantable syngeneic tumors and therefore do not necessarily imply that NK cells play a similar role in resistance against autochthonous primary neoplasms or in surveillance against spontaneous tumors. These issues, however, were addressed recently by several investigators.[1-3] For example, the incidence of spontaneous malignant lymphomas is increased in NK-deficient mice carrying the beige (bg^+/bg^+) mutation.[4] Also, a higher frequency of spontaneous lymphoproliferative disorders was found in NK-deficient patients with Chediak-Higashi syndrome.[5] A similar increase in lymphoproliferative disease was described in cases of severe combined and X-linked immunodeficiencies in which the level of NK cells is markedly depressed.[6] In studying the role of NK cells in the inhibition of carcinogen-induced tumors, several investigators have failed to detect significant differences in the frequency or latency of virally, chemically, or X-irradiation-induced tumors between bg/bg and $bg/^+$ mice.[7] The interpretation of these results is difficult since carcinogens such as dimethylbenzanthracene (DMBA)[7,8] or urethane[9] may suppress NK cells in susceptible strains whereas infection of bg/bg with viruses may activate NK cells to levels comparable to those of uninfected normal controls.

Although the evidence in support of a role of NK cells in immunosurveillance is inconclusive, a large body of data strongly suggest that NK cells play a significant role in the in vivo destruction of transplanted syngeneic tumor cells.

II. IN VIVO ROLE OF NK CELLS IN HOST RESISTANCE AGAINST TUMOR GROWTH

The evidence for the involvement of NK cells in host resistance against tumor growth in vivo is primarily based on the correlation between the levels of NK CMC in vitro and the inhibition of the growth of small inocula of NK-sensitive tumor cells. Thus, in mice of various genotypes, ages, and F_1 hybrid combinations, the resistance against the growth of YAC and other lymphoma cells correlated with the levels of NK cell activity of the host.[10,11] The resistance was expressed only when small numbers of tumor cells were used. Also, beige (bg^+/bg^+) mice with a selective deficit in NK cell activity develop progressively growing tumors faster and at a higher frequency than normal C57BL/6 mice when challenged with low doses of syngeneic NK-sensitive leukemias[12,13] or solid tumors.[14] In contrast, nude mice with high levels of NK CMC exhibit marked resistance against the growth of transplanted syngeneic, allogeneic, and xenogeneic lymphomas and leukemias.[15] However, only tumor cells sensitive to in vitro lysis by NK cells exhibited a reduced growth rate in nude mice compared to nu/+ littermates. NK-resistant tumors grew equally well in both nude and normal syngeneic mice. Thus, both tumor cell sensitivity to NK cell-mediated killing and the level of NK cell activity in the host influence tumor growth in vivo. Recently, an NK-resistant fibrosarcoma cell line was selected in vitro from the NK-sensitive UV-2237 tumor cells.[16] Both cell lines exhibited the same antigenicity, immunogenicity, and sensitivity to killing by specifically sensitized T lymphocytes and by activated macrophages. However, they differed in their ability to bind NK cells, being markedly decreased in the NK-resistant cells. When injected into the footpad of syngeneic mice, the NK-resistant cells developed into a palpable tumor in a significantly shorter time than cells of the NK-sensitive parent tumor. However, no differences in the slopes of the growth curves of the two tumors were observed. Together with the finding that the two cell lines were similar in their growth rate and generation doubling time in vitro, these results strongly suggest that NK cells play a role in the early destruction of transplanted tumor cells and thus may influence the percent take and the time of appearance of palpable tumors. However, the similar slopes of the growth curves of the NK-sensitive and -resistant tumor cells indicate that endogenous NK cells are not effective in controlling tumor growth at later stages of tumor progression.

Further support of the role of NK cells in in vivo resistance against tumor growth was provided by studies in which depletion of NK cells in vivo by treatment with antiasialo-GM1 antibodies resulted in increased tumorigenicity and percent takes of NK-sensitive tumor cells transplanted into syngeneic and nude mice.[17,18] NK cell depletion did not affect the in vivo growth properties of NK-resistant tumor cell lines. Further studies have demonstrated that xenogeneic cell lines which are highly tumorigenic in nude mice were rejected when infected with RNA viruses.[19] Unlike the parent cells, the virus-infected cells were susceptible to NK cell-mediated lysis in vitro. In a subsequent study, it was found that the rejection of virus-infected cells transplanted into nude mice could be overcome by treatment of the recipient mice with anti-interferon (anti-IFN) antibodies which presumably inhibit NK cell activation in vivo.[20]

Studies using T cell-deficient chimeras provided further evidence for the protective role of NK cells against tumor progression.[21] Adult A/Sn hybrid mice were lethally irradiated and reconstituted with bone marrow cells from H-2 compatible donors that exhibit high or low NK cell levels. The repopulated recipients were either high or low NK cell responders according to the genotype of the bone marrow donors. When low doses of YAC lymphoma cells were transplanted subcutaneously in such recipients, the high NK responder hybrid mice exhibited higher resistance against tumor growth than the low NK hybrids. Similar results were obtained with NK-sensitive AKR T lymphoma cells which grew well in the low, but not high, NK responder mice. In contrast, NK-resistant cells grew equally well in chimeras that exhibited either high or low NK cell activity.

Another approach that proved useful in evaluating the in vivo antitumor activity of NK cells utilized the Winn tumor neutralization assay.[22] Positively selected NK cells were mixed with YAC lymphoma cells and injected locally into syngeneic mice. Tumor growth was markedly inhibited in recipients of the tumor-NK cell mixtures. However, the artifactual nature of this experimental design does not allow extrapolation as to the potential role of NK cells in the destruction of primary autochthonous tumor cells that arise in tissues not necessarily accessible to high levels of NK cells.

In most of the above-mentioned studies, the endpoints used for evaluation of tumor resistance were either tumor take and growth rate or percent survival. A precise assessment of such protocols, however, requires monitoring of the indicated parameters for long periods of time, during which multiple effector mechanisms unrelated to NK cells become involved. Therefore, a more rapid assay which measures NK cell-mediated destruction of i.v.-injected, radiolabeled tumor cells was established.[23,24] A close correlation between tumor resistance in this in vivo model and the levels and kinetics of NK CMC was observed.The rapidity of this in vivo reactivity supports the belief that NK cells may represent a first line of defense mechanism against the hematogenous dissemination of tumor metastasis.

III. INHIBITION OF TUMOR METASTASIS BY NK CELLS

The multiplicity of host effector mechanisms involved in resistance against tumor growth and metastasis already suggests that no single mechanism could be identified as being solely responsible for the antimetastatic activity in vivo. Also, considering the complex nature of the metastatic process,[25] certain defense mechanisms may prove effective in destroying circulating tumor cells and inhibiting hematogenous tumor metastasis, even though they are ineffective against established extravascular neoplastic foci. Indeed, most tumor cells that enter the circulation are destroyed during the first 4 to 24 hr and only a few cells survive and develop into distant organ metastases.[24,26]

A large body of evidence implicates NK cells in the destruction of circulating tumor cells and host resistance against tumor metastasis. This is primarily based upon the close correlation found between the levels of NK cell activity in the host and the capacity to eliminate blood-borne NK-sensitive tumor cells, and on the antimetastatic potency of NK cell activation and of NK cells or NK cell lines adoptively transferred into NK-depleted hosts.

The correlation between levels of NK cell activity and resistance against tumor metastasis was established by studying the incidence of tumor metastasis of NK-sensitive and -resistant tumor cells in hosts that exhibit low or high NK CMC. Such studies were facilitated by (1) the identification of animal models that naturally exhibit low (beige mice, young 3-week-old mice) or high (nude mice) NK CMC; (2) the definition of antigenic markers (NK-1 and asialo-GM1) and sensitivity to chemical and hormonal treatments (β-estradiol and cyclophosphamide) which allowed for selective depletion or enrichment of NK cells; (3) the establishment of NK-like cell lines and their use for in vivo reconstitution studies; (4) the definition of crucial steps in the metastatic process which are sensitive to NK cell manipulation; (5) the identification of in vivo assays that detect NK cell-mediated antitumor activity with minimal involvement of other immune cells such as T cells and macrophages; (6) the availability of tumor cell lines and clones selected for high or low metastatic potential that exhibit different degrees of sensitivity or resistance to NK cell-mediated killing.

Initial studies have shown that the incidence of spontaneous and experimental metastasis of NK-sensitive B16 melanoma and 3LL carcinoma in beige mice, that exhibit naturally depressed NK cell activity,[27] was higher than that observed in heterozygous controls.[14,16] NK-resistant tumor cell lines, on the other hand, did not show differential growth or metastasis when inoculated into beige or control mice. The reduced elimination of blood-borne B16 melanoma cells correlated with the low levels of NK cell activity in beige mice which, however, could be reconstituted to normal levels by adoptive transfer of spleen cells from syngeneic control C57BL/6 mice.

Further support for the observation that the in vivo expression of tumor metastatic potential is inversely correlated with the levels of NK cell activity was provided by studies using young 3-week-old mice that exhibit low levels of natural cytotoxicity in vitro against lymphoma and solid tumor target cells.[24] The i.v. injection of tumor cell lines and clones of UV-2237 fibrosarcoma, K-1735, and B16 melanomas produced more lung colonies in 3-week-old than in 8-week-old mice with high NK CMC. This result correlated well with the enhanced survival of radiolabeled NK-sensitive tumor cells inoculated i.v. into young, as compared to adult, syngeneic mice. On the other hand, NK cell activation by IFN inducers enhanced the destruction of i.v.-injected tumor cells and inhibited metastasis formation equally well in both age groups. The antimetastatic activity was most marked when NK cell stimulants were administered shortly before, but not after, i.v. tumor cell inoculation. These results suggest that NK cells are most effective in destroying circulating tumor cells in the vascular capillary bed, whereas they are less effective against tumor cells that already have extravasated and lodged in the organ parenchyma.

The close correlation between the levels of NK cell activity and host resistance against hematogenous metastasis suggested that NK cells may be the effector mechanism responsible for the marked resistance of adult athymic nude mice to spontaneous or experimental tumor metastasis.[28—30] However, unlike adult mice, pathogen-free 3-week-old nude mice were found to exhibit low levels of NK CMC as measured in vitro against lymphomas and solid tumor cells.[31,32] Thus, the in vivo metastatic behavior of malignant tumor cells injected into young and adult nude mice was evaluated. The i.v. injection of metastatic allogeneic or xenogeneic tumor cells into 3-week-old mice resulted in enhanced survival of circulating tumor cells and increased incidence of lung tumor colonies as compared to those observed in adult 6-to-8-week old nude mice.[31,32] Moreover, activation of NK cells by bacterial adjuvants and IFN inducers 1 to 3 days before tumor cell inoculation inhibited the formation of lung tumor colonies in young nude mice. These results, in addition to providing evidence for the in vivo relevance of NK cells in controlling tumor metastasis, have significant implications for studies of metastasis of human malignant neoplasms in NK-deficient nude mice.

The most direct evidence in support of the role of NK cells in the destruction of circulating tumor cells and the inhibition of hematogenous tumor metastasis was provided by studies using experimental depletion and reconstitution of NK cells. Initial studies have shown that a single injection of cyclophosphamide (Cy) 4 days before i.v. tumor cell inoculation markedly enhanced pulmonary and extrapulmonary experimental tumor metastasis.[24] Also, the survival of i.v.-injected radiolabeled tumor cells was markedly enhanced in Cy-treated mice. Most significant, however, is the finding that Cy-induced enhancement of experimental metastasis is reversed by adoptive transfer of normal spleen cells given 24 hr before, but not after, tumor cell injection. The kinetics of effective reconstitution suggested that the effector cells responsible for abrogating the Cy effect are active during a limited period (12 to 14 hr) after i.v. tumor cell inoculation, a period that coincides with the presence of tumor cells in the circulation and before their extravasation into the lung parenchyma.[26] The effector cells active in the Cy reconstitution experiments were non-T, non-B, nonmacrophage cells that express NK 1 and asialo-GM1 antigens.[33,34] Thus, selective depletion of NK cells by anti-NK 1 serum and complement abolished the in vivo reconstitutive antimetastatic activity of normal spleen cells adoptively transferred to Cy-treated mice. Using this system, it was found that cloned NK cells adoptively transferred into Cy-treated mice decreased the survival and lung colonization of B16 melanoma tumor cells.[35] In these studies, only those cell clones endowed with NK cell activity were effective in inhibiting lung colonization. It is noteworthy that in lymphoid adoptive transfer experiments, the effector cells are effective only when injected prior to tumor challenge.

Selective in vivo depletion of NK cells could be achieved by treatment with antiasialo-GM1 antibodies.[22] Treatment of syngeneic mice or allogeneic nude mice with antiasialo-GM1 serum significantly enhanced the survival in the circulation and lung colonization potential of several NK-sensitive solid tumor cells.[36—38] Extrapulmonary metastases were also detected in the NK-depleted recipients. Also, spontaneous metastases from a subcutaneous tumor were enhanced following in vivo depletion of NK cells by repeated injections of antiasialo-GM1.[36] In these studies, NK cell depletion did not influence the size of the primary tumors, which was comparable in both normal and treated mice. Similar studies in rats have demonstrated that adoptive transfer of highly enriched populations of large granular lymphocytes (LGLs) 2 hr before i.v. tumor challenge restored the ability of antiasialo-GM1-treated animals to eliminate radiolabeled tumor cells from the vascular bed of the lungs.[37]

Selective depletion of NK cells in vivo was demonstrated also following systemic treatment of mice with anti-NK 1.1 alloantiserum.[39] Maximal depletion was observed 4 to 6 hr after injection of the antibody and gradually returned to control levels within the next 2 to 3 days. As a result of NK cell depletion in vivo, the survival of radiolabeled NK-sensitive lymphoma cells injected i.v. into mice pretreated with anti-NK 1.1 antibodies was markedly enhanced as compared to untreated control mice.

A more prolonged decreased in NK cell activity may be attained following treatment with the estrogen 17-β-estradiol.;[40—42] Between 6 and 8 weeks after initiation of estrogen treatment a marked reduction in NK CMC in vitro against lymphoma and solid tumor target cells was observed. The depression of NK cell activity was associated with enhanced survival of i.v.-injected tumor cells, as well as increased incidence of experimental and spontaneous metastasis of murine fibrosarcomas (UV-2237) and melanomas.[42] As observed following Cy treatment, β-estradiol-induced enhancement of metastasis could be reversed by adoptive transfer of normal spleen cells from syngeneic mice. The increased susceptibility of estrogen-treated mice to spontaneous metastasis from a s.c. tumor could not be attributed to differential growth of the primary tumors since the growth rate and tumor size were comparable in estrogen-treated and control mice. It is noteworthy that under the experimental conditions employed, T cell-mediated responses and macrophage activation were not affected by estrogen treatment.

Studies from our laboratory have demonstrated that selective depletion of NK cells in adult nude mice is also associated with an increased frequency of experimental and spontaneous tumor metastasis.[38,42] Thus, treatment of nude mice with Cy, β-estradiol, and antiasialo-GM1 antibodies reduced NK CMC and enhanced the incidence of pulmonary metastasis of allogeneic and xenogeneic tumors, including human neoplasms. In these studies, treatment with antiasialo-GM1 antibodies has proven to be the least toxic and best tolerated of the three treatment protocols and appears to be more suitable for long-term studies.

Studies on the antimetastatic effects of NK cell activation by biological response modifying agents (BRMs) also provided evidence in support of the in vivo role of NK cells in the prevention and perhaps therapy of tumor metastasis. As discussed previously, prophylactic treatment with BRMs that stimulate NK cell activity prevents the development of tumor metastasis. Such BRMs however, exhibit weak antimetastatic activity in hosts whose NK cells were depleted by Cy or β-estradiol treatment.[24,42] The BRM-mediated antimetastatic activity could be regained in such recipients by lymphoid reconstitution. Although most BRMs activated both NK cells and macrophages, the different kinetics of activation provided bases for designing short-term experiments in which the antimetastatic effect could be attributed to NK cell and not to macrophage activation. Indeed, the kinetics of BRM-induced destruction of circulating tumor cells and inhibition of lung colonization coincided with the kinetics of NK cell and not macrophage activation.[43] In these studies, it was shown that selective activation of NK cells is sufficient to inhibit hematogenous tumor dissemination. For example, periodate-oxidized *Corynebacterium parvum,* which had lost the ability to activate tumoricidal macrophages but retained the capacity to stimulate NK cell activity, was as effective as untreated *C. parvum* in enhancing the destruction of circulating tumor cells and in preventing the development of pulmonary metastasis. Both vaccines were less effective against tumor cells given 2 weeks after treatment at a time when NK cell activity had subsided. These findings further substantiate the role of NK cells in the early destruction of circulating tumor cells and the prevention of metastasis in normal as well as in BRM-treated hosts.

Another common site for spontaneous metastasis is the lymph nodes draining the primary tumor site. Previous studies have demonstrated that very early after tumor cell implantation, tumor cells could be detected in the draining lymph nodes.[44] In most cases, however, these cells do not lead to the establishment of lymph node metastasis. This may be explained by the rapid destruction of the early infiltrating tumor cells in the popliteal lymph nodes draining the tumor-injected site.[52] However, only after a vascularized local tumor is established does a steady influx of tumor cells into the regional lymph nodes result in metastasis development. Under such conditions, selective activation of NK cells in the regional draining lymph nodes markedly reduced the frequency of metastasis and the tumor burden in the lymph nodes. It should be emphasized, however, that the kinetics and organ distribution pattern of NK cell activation varied according to the type, dose, and route of administration of BRMs.[45] Also from these studies it became apparent that activated NK cells present in the peripheral blood or spleen do not migrate freely into unstimulated lymph nodes and therefore may not necessarily reflect the state of NK cell activation at such sites. Indeed, only BRM treatment protocols that activate NK cells in the relevant lymph nodes containing tumor cells were effective in controlling lymph node metastasis.

Based on the above discussion, the possibility exists that tumor cells able to survive natural host defense mechanisms and able to develop into metastatic foci are resistant to NK cell-mediated lysis. In support of this possibility is the finding that cells obtained from a spontaneous pulmonary metastasis of 3LL carcinoma were more resistant to killing by NK cells than cells isolated from the primary tumor.[46] However, in view of the fact that surviving the natural defense mechanisms is only one step among many required for successful tumor metastasis, it is difficult to assume that resistance to NK cell-mediated lysis alone could account for the metastatic behavior of tumor cells in vivo. In a large series of experiments using cell lines and clones isolated from three different murine solid tumors, no uniform correlation was found between resistance to killing by NK cells in vitro and metastatic potential in vivo.[16] However, one may add that resistance to NK CMC may enhance the expression of the metastatic potential of malignant tumor cells in hosts that exhibit high NK cell activity. This is supported by the finding that cell lines selected under defined condition in vitro for NK resistance exhibited a greater survival rate in the circulation and produced more lung colonies adult syngeneic recipients than the metastatic NK-sensitive parent UV-2237 fibrosarcoma cells.[16] The NK-resistant cells readily metastasized also in adult nude mice shown to exhibit high NK cell levels and increased resistance to tumor metastasis.

Resistance to NK CMC may develop also as a result of adaptation of tumor cells to growth in vivo.[47] This resistance is lost after 2 to 3 weeks of in vitro maintenance in tissue culture. Cloned cell populations derived from the heterogeneous parental tumor display similar behavior, which supports the notion that this is an adaptive rather than selective process. Studies of the metastatic behavior in vitro-grown NK-sensitive and -resistant tumor cells revealed that the latter survived better in the circulation and expressed higher metastatic potential in adult syngeneic hosts than the NK-sensitive cell counterparts maintained in tissue culture.[48]

The resistance of tumor cells to NK cell-mediated lysis acquired by adaptation to in vivo growth or by selection during the metastatic process may impact the potential utility of NK cell activation in the prevention and therapy of metastasis. Recent studies, however, have demonstrated that freshly excised tumor cells resistant to killing by endogeneous NK cells were sensitive to killing by BRM-activated NK cells in vitro and their metastases were markedly inhibited by in vivo administration of NK cell activators.[48] Thus, the emergence of resistance to NK cell-mediated killing does not necessarily interfere with the efficacy of NK cell activation in the control of hematogenous tumor metastasis. Moreover, these findings suggest that the inefficiency of activated NK cells to destroy extravascular tumor cells could not be explained by the development of NK cell resistance, but perhaps by the inaccessibility of tumor cells sequestered in the organ parenchyma to activated NK cells that display a restricted homing pattern. It should be emphasized, however, that in the above-described studies, the antimetastatic effect of NK cell activation was evaluated following a single injection of BRMs. Considering the short duration and transient nature of NK cell activation, effective therapeutic protocols should achieve a persistently high level of activated NK cells without the generation of negative feedback suppression.[48,49]Such a prolonged augmentation of NK CMC and enhanced clearance of i.v.-injected radiolabeled tumor cells were observed in lymphocytic choriomeningitis (LCMV) carrier mice in which low levels of IFN were detected during the observation period of several months.[50] By using a multiple dosing regimen of BRMs it became clear that complex cellular interactions are involved in the regulation of NK cell activation and that the induction of nonspecific suppressor macrophages may interfere with the further activation of NK cells.[48] Therefore, BRMs that selectively stimulate NK without subsequent activation of suppressor macrophages may prove effective in achieving prolonged activation of NK cells and in controlling the growth of established extravascular tumor micrometastasis.

The above-described efficacy of activated NK cells in destroying circulating tumor cells and in preventing tumor metastasis is not without clinical utility. Even though metastasis may have already occurred by the time of diagnosis, activation of NK cells may inhibit further hematogenous dissemination from the primary tumor or from other organ metastatic foci. Increased incidence of widespread metastasis was observed after surgical excision of the primary tumor, which could have resulted from the introduction of tumor cells into the circulation caused by surgical manipulation of the primary neoplasms.[51] Therefore, activation of NK cells by low doses of IFN or other BRMs shortly before and after surgical excision of the primary neoplasm may serve as a powerful tool for preventing the secondary spread of metastatic tumor cells.

REFERENCES

1. **Herberman, R. B., Ed.,** *NK Cells and Other Natural Effector Cells,* Academic Press, New York, 1982.
2. **Oldham, R. K.,** Natural killer cells: artifact to reality, *Cancer Metastasis Rev.,* 2, 323, 1983.
3. **Roder, J. C. and Haliotis, T.,** Do NK cells play a role in anti-tumor surveillance?, *Immunol. Today,* November, 96, 1980.
4. **Loutit, J. F., Towsend, K. M. S., and Knowles, J. F.,** Tumor surveillance in beige mice, *Nature (London),* 285, 66, 1980.
5. **Blume, R. S. and Wolff, S. M.,** The Chediak-Higashi syndrome: studies in four patients and a review of the literature, *Medicine,* 51, 247, 1972.
6. **Kersey, J. H., Spector, B. D., and Good, R. A.,** Primary immunodeficiency diseases and cancer: the immunodeficiency-cancer registry, *Int. J. Cancer,* 12, 333, 1973.
7. **Argov, S., Cochran, A. J., Kärre, K., Klein, G. O., and Klein, G.,** Incidence and type of tumors induced in C57BL bg/bg mice and +/bg littermates by oral administration of DMBA, *Int. J. Cancer,* 28, 739, 1981.
8. **Ehrlick, R., Efrati, M., Bar-Eyal, A., Wollberg, M., Schiby, G., Ran, M., and Witz, I. P.,** Natural cellular reactivities mediated by splenocytes from mice bearing three types of primary tumor, *Int. J. Cancer,* 26, 315, 1980.
9. **Gorelik, E. and Herberman, R. B.,** Inhibition of the activity of mouse natural killer cells by urethane, *J. Natl. Cancer Inst.,* 66, 543, 1981.
10. **Riesenfeld, I., Orn, A., Gidlund, M., Axberg, I., Alm, G. U., and Wigzell, H.,** Positive correlation between *in vitro* NK activity and *in vivo* resistance towards AKR lymphoma cells, *Int. J. Cancer,* 25, 399, 1980.
11. **Kiessling, R., Petranyi, G., Klein, G., and Wigzell, H.,** Genetic variation of *in vitro* cytolytic activity and *in vivo* rejection potential of nonimmunized semi-syngeneic mice against a mouse lymphoma line, *Int. J. Cancer,* 15, 933, 1975.
12. **Kärre, K., Lein, G. O., Kiessling, R., Klein, G., and Roder, J. C.,** Low natural *in vivo* resistance to syngeneic leukemias in natural killer-deficient mice, *Nature (London),* 284, 624, 1980.
13. **Kärre, K., Klein, G. O., Kiessling, R., Klein, G., and Roder, J. C.,** *In vitro* NK-activity and *in vivo* resistance to leukemia: studies of beige, beige/nude and wild-type hosts on C57BL background, *Int. J. Cancer,* 26, 789, 1980.
14. **Talmadge, J. E., Meyers, K. M., Prieur, D. J., and Starkey, J. R.,** Role of NK cells in tumor growth and metastasis in beige mice, *Nature (London),* 284, 622, 1980.
15. **Warner, N. L., Woodruff, M. F. A., and Burton, R. C.,** Inhibition of the growth of lymphoid tumors in syngeneic athymic (nude) mice, *Int. J. Cancer,* 20, 146, 1977.
16. **Hanna, N. and Fidler, I. J.,** Relationship between metastatic potential and resistance to natural killer cell-mediated cytotoxicity in three murine tumor systems, *J. Natl. Cancer Inst.,* 66, 1183, 1981.
17. **Habu, S. and Okumura, K.,** Evidence for *in vivo* reactivity against transplantable and primary tumors, in *NK Cells and Other Natural Effector Cells,* Herberman, R. B., Ed., Academic Press, New York, 1982, 1323.
18. **Kawase, I., Urdal, D. L., Brooks, C. G., and Henney, C. S.,** Selective depletion of NK cell activity *in vivo* and its effect on the growth of NK-sensitive and NK-resistor tumor cell variants, *Int. J. Cancer,* 29, 567, 1982.
19. **Minato, N., Bloom, B. R., Jones, C., Holland, J., and Reid, L. M.,** Mechanisms of rejection of virus persistently infected tumor cells by athymic nude mice, *J. Exp. Med.,* 149, 1117, 1979.

20. **Reid, L. M., Minato, N., Gresser, I., Holland, J., Kadish, A., and Bloom, B. R.,** Influence of anti-mouse interferon serum on the growth and metastasis of tumor cells persistently infected with virus and of human prostatic tumors in athymic nude mice, *Proc. Natl. Acad. Sci., U.S.A.,* 78, 1171, 1981.
21. **Häller, O., Örn, A., Gidlund, M., and Wigzell, H.,** *In vivo* activity of murine NK cells, in *Natural Cell-Mediated Immunity Against Tumors,* Herberman, R. B., Ed., Academic Press, New York, 1980, 1105.
22. **Kasai, M., Yoneda, T., Habu, S., Moruyama, Y., Okumura, K., and Tokunaga, T.,** *In vivo* effect of anti-asialo-GM1 antibody on natural killer activity, *Nature (London),* 291, 334, 1981.
23. **Riccardi, C., Santoni, A., Barlozzari, T., Puccetti, P., and Herberman, R. B.,** *In vivo* natural reactivity of mice against tumor cells, *Int. J. Cancer, 25, 475, 1980.*
24. **Hanna, N. and Fidler, I. J.,** The role of natural killer cells in the destruction of circulating tumor emboli, *J. Natl. Cancer Inst.,* 65, 801, 1980.
25. **Poste, G. and Fidler, I. J.,** The pathogenesis of cancer metastasis, *Nature (London),* 283, 139, 1980.
26. **Fidler, I. J.,** Metastasis: quantitative analysis of distribution and fate of tumor emboli labeled with ^{125}I-51 iodo-2′deoxyuridine, *J. Natl. Cancer Inst.,* 45, 733, 1970.
27. **Roder, J. and Duwe, A.,** The beige mutation in the mouse selectively impairs natural killer cell function, *Nature (London),* 278, 451, 1979.
28. **Fidler, I. J., Caines, G., and Dolan, Z.,** Survival of hematogenously disseminated allogeneic tumor cells in athymic nude mice, *Transplantation,* 22, 208, 1976.
29. **Skov, C. B., Holland, J. M., and Perkins, E. H.,** Development of fewer tumor colonies in lungs of athymic nude mice after intravenous injection of tumor cells, *J. Natl. Cancer Inst.,* 56, 193, 1976.
30. **Povlsen, C. O., Fialkow, P. J., Klein, G., Rygaard, J., and Wiener, F.,** Growth and antigenic properties of a biopsy-derived Burkitt's lymphoma in thymus-less (nude) mice, *Int. J. Cancer,* 11, 30, 1973.
31. **Hanna, N.,** Expression of metastatic potential of tumor cells in young nude mice is correlated with low levels of natural killer cell-mediated cytotoxicity, *Int. J. Cancer,* 26, 675, 1980.
32. **Hanna, N., Davis, T. W., and Fidler, I. J.,** Environmental and genetic factors determine the level of NK activity of nude mice and affect their suitability as models for experimental metastasis, *Int. J. Cancer,* 30, 371, 1982.
33. **Riccardi, C., Barlozzari, T., Santoni, A., Herberman, R. B., and Cesarini, C.,** Transfer to cyclophosphamide-treated mice of natural killer (NK) cells and *in vivo* natural reactivity against tumors, *J. Immunol.,* 126, 1284, 1981.
34. **Hanna, N. and Burton, R. C.,** Definitive evidence that natural killer (NK) cells inhibit experimental tumor metastasis *in vivo, J. Immunol.,* 127, 1754, 1981.
35. **Warner, J. and Dennart, G.,** *In vivo* function of a cloned cell line with NK activity: effects on bone marrow transplants, tumor development and metastases, *Nature (London),* 300, 31, 1982.
36. **Gorelik, E., Wiltrout, R., Okumura, K., Habu, S., and Herberman, R. B.,** Acceleration of metastatic growth in anti-asialo-GM1-treated mice, in *NK Cells and Other Natural Effector Cells,* Herberman, R. B., Ed., Academic Press, New York, 1982, 1331.
37. **Barlozzari, T., Reynolds, C. W., and Herberman, R. B.,** *In vivo* role of natural killer cells: involvement of large granular lymphocytes in the clearance of tumor cells in anti-asialo-GM_1-treated rats, *J. Immunol.,* 131(2), 1024, 1983.
38. **Hanna, N.,** Natural killer cell-mediated inhibition of tumor metastasis *in vivo, Surv. Synth. Pathol. Res.,* 2, 68, 1983.
39. **Pollack, S. B. and Hallenbeck, L. A.,** *In vivo* reduction of NK activity with anti-NK 1 serum: direct evaluation of NK cells in tumor clearance, *Int. J. Cancer,* 29, 203, 1982.
40. **Seaman, W. E., Blackman, M. A., Gindhart, T. D., Roubinia, J. R., Loeb, J. M., and Talal, N.,** β-Estradiol reduces natural killer cells in mice, *J. Immunol.,* 121, 2193, 1978.
41. **Kalland, T. and Forsberg, J.-G.,** Natural killer cell activity and tumor susceptibility in female mice treated neonatally with diethylstilbestrol, *Cancer Res.,* 41, 5134, 1981.
42. **Hanna, N. and Schneider, M.,** Enhancement of tumor metastasis and suppression of natural killer cell activity by β-estradiol treatment, *J. Immunol.,* 130, 974, 1983.
43. **Hanna, N.,** Inhibition of experimental tumor metastasis by selective activation of natural killer cells, *Cancer Res.,* 42, 1337, 1982.
44. **Wood, P. and Carr, I.,** The quantitation of experimental lymph node metastasis, *J. Pathol.,* 114, 85, 1974.
45. **Hisano, G. and Hanna, N.,** Murine lymph node natural killer cells: regulatory mechanisms of activation or suppression, *J. Natl. Cancer Inst.,* 69, 665, 1982.
46. **Gorelik, E., Fogel, M., Feldman, M., and Segal, S.,** Differences in resistance of metastatic tumor cells and cells from local tumor growth to cytotoxicity of natural killer cells, *J. Natl. Cancer Inst.,* 63, 1397, 1979.
47. **Becker, S., Kiessling, R.,, Lee, N., and Klein, G.,** Modulation of sensitivity to natural killer cell lysis after *in vitro* explantation of a mouse lymphoma, *J. Natl. Cancer Inst.,* 61, 1495, 1978.

48. **Hanna, N.,** Role of natural killer cells in control of cancer metastasis, *Cancer Metastasis Rev.*, 1, 45, 1982.
49. **Lotzová, E.,** *C. parvum*-mediated suppression of the phenomenon of natural killing and its analysis, in *Natural Cell-Mediated Immunity Against Tumors,* Herberman, R. B., Ed., Academic Press, New York, 1980, 735.
50. **Bukowski, J. F., Biron, C. A., and Welsh, R. M.,** Elevated natural killer cell-mediated cytotoxicity, plasma interferon, and tumor cell rejection in mice persistently infected with lymphocytic choriomeningitis virus, *J. Immunol.*, 131(2), 991, 1983.
51. **Sugarbaker, E. V. and Ketcham, A. S.,** Mechanism and prevention of cancer dissemination: an overview, *Semin. Oncol.*, 4, 19, 1977.
52. **Hisano, G. and Hanna, N.,** unpublished observation.

Chapter 2

THE INVOLVEMENT OF NATURAL KILLER CELLS IN HUMAN MALIGNANT DISEASE

Hugh F. Pross

TABLE OF CONTENTS

I. INTRODUCTION

Natural killer (NK) cells were "discovered" by investigators attempting to demonstrate the presence of peripheral blood cells with antitumor cytotoxic activity. When it was found that normal donor lymphocytes were also cytotoxic, the research efforts of many tumor immunologists were turned to determining the role of these cells in tumor formation and rejection and, conversely, the effect of malignant disease on their activity.[1,2] In this chapter, the results of studies on human NK cells in patients with solid tumors will be reviewed. The reader is referred to recent reviews[1—3] and other chapters in this book for a description of murine systems. Similarly, other chapters have dealt with NK function in patients with leukemia, NK activity against human primary tumors, the in vivo modulation of NK cell activity in cancer patients, and the characteristics of large granular lymphocyte (LGL) tumors. As far as possible, the discussion in this chapter will be limited to studies using cells which fit the "conventional" definition of the NK cell — a lymphocyte, present in normal donors, capable of lysing tumor target cells in the apparent absence of previous disease or prior immunization of the donor. In the majority of studies, the definition is a functional one based on the level of lysis against K562, as has been discussed in another chapter in Volume I.[4] Cytotoxicity against K562, an HLA-negative, Epstein-Barr virus nuclear antigen negative,[5] highly NK-susceptible erythroleukemia cell line,[6,7] is a consistent property of human NK cells[8,9] and, in contrast to T lymphocyte functions such as phytohemagglutinin responsiveness or E-rosette formation, is comparatively age independent in adulthood.[9] It is generally accepted that cytotoxicity against this line by lymphocytes from cancer patients is due to NK cells.

It is well established from murine studies that if a tumor cell is sensitive to NK cells in vitro, then the ability of an experimental animal to resist tumor take and metastasis formation is usually directly proportional to the NK function of an animal.[1] The question, therefore, is not whether NK cells *can* perform the function of tumor surveillance, but whether in fact they do. There are several points in tumor development at which NK cells could affect the ultimate course of disease, from the donor's genetic susceptibility to tumor formation, to the prevention of metastases in patients with established cancer. The involvement of NK cells in human malignant disease will be discussed from this point of view.

II. NK CELL ACTIVITY IN PEOPLE "AT RISK" FOR CANCER

Patients with genetic deficiencies in NK function, such as those with the Chediak-Higashi syndrome[10] or X-linked lymphoproliferative syndrome,[11] have an increased incidence of a fatal lymphoma-like disorder, and it has been postulated that the defect in NK function is responsible for the failure of surveillance in these patients. Other severe congenital immunodeficiencies are also associated with an increased incidence of cancer, mostly lymphoreticular in origin.[12] NK activity in these patients is frequently within the normal range, however, depending on the severity of the defect and where it occurs in lymphocyte development.[13—17] Furthermore, the presence or absence of an NK defect is not invariable within the same type of immunodeficiency. In a recent review, Peter[16] described NK heterogeneity within patients diagnosed as having severe combined immunodeficiency disease (SCID); some were classified as being B cell negative, NK cell positive SCID, while other were B cell positive, NK cell negative. It is not known whether "heterogeneity" or methodological differences account for the conflicting results seen with other immunodeficiencies, such as ataxia-telangiectasia, which has been described as being associated with normal function by Peter,[16] and severely depressed NK function which has been described by Lipinski et al.[17]

The difficulty in using these studies to support the role of NK cells in surveillance against tumors lies in the fact that the patient populations are abnormal in many other respects besides NK function. The type of study which is needed to answer this question is one in which selectively NK-“deficient” normal donors are followed for long periods of time to determine the incidence of malignancy compared to that observed in a similar group of high NK donors. This type of study is technically possible but economically unfeasible, and most studies attempting to implicate NK cells in surveillance against tumors have dealt with the assessment of patients “at risk” of developing cancer because of various conditions less severe and considerably more common than the congenital immunodeficiencies, but with an expected incidence of cancer higher than the normal population.

There are comparatively few studies on the NK function of normal people at increased risk for tumor development. Strayer et al.[18] reported lower NK in families of patients with a higher incidence of tumors and observed that NK activity varied inversely with the number of family members with cancer. This was significant when assessed by several different methods of data calculation although the differences were small. We recently completed a large study of 155 women[19] at high relative risk (RR) for breast cancer for reasons such as family history (one or more close female relatives with breast cancer, RR = 1.2 to 9), personal gynecological history (early menarche, late first pregnancy, late menopause, RR = 1.3 to 3) or local or diffuse benign breast syndrome (BBS) (RR = 2 to 4), or combinations of all of these factors.[20] BBS refers to a hormonal-related condition characterized by pain and lumpiness in the breast which may be cyclical in nature. At its most severe, biopsy may be required to rule out carcinoma and these biopsies show ductal hyperplasia, fibrocystic disease, and adenomata.[21] The highest RR for subsequent breast cancer appears to be atypical lobular hyperplasia.[21] The syndrome has been the subject of considerable debate recently concerning whether or not it should be classified as “disease” since it is so common.[20] In our study, we observed significantly elevated relative NK (RNK) in the high risk for breast cancer group as a whole (1.21 ± 0.06 vs. 1.00 ± 0.06) ($p<0.02$). When the group was subdivided into the various component risk groups described above, it was found that the entire elevation in NK was attributable to the BBS group, with the highest mean relative NK being shown by patients with diffuse BBS (1.67 ± 0.05, n = 32) compared with the “no BBS” groups of high-risk women (1.07 ± 0.07, n = 102) ($p<0.025$). Of the 155 “patients”, 7 had clinically detectable BBS on one visit and were BBS-free on another. In six of the seven, relative NK activity was higher when BBS was detectable. This was significant at a level of $p<0.001$ (paired “*t*”-test). One interpretation of these results is that the systemic hormonal changes causing BBS[22] were stimulating high NK and that the increased NK activity had no bearing on the risk status of these patients. Conversely, it is possible that NK hyperactivity is in reaction to a stimulus which itself results in malignant transformation in a low proportion of patients, perhaps a viral agent related to murine mammary tumor virus.[23] The mechanism is obviously highly complex, however, since *depressed* NK activity was reported by Cunningham-Rundles et al.[24] in a group of patients who were biopsy-proven to have benign fibrocystic disease. The discrepancy between these results and our own data is most likely due to differences in the patient populations studied and, possibly, factors such as stress, premedication, and the severity of disease in the hospitalized patients.

Several other studies involving risk groups have been reported. Familial melanoma and multiple primary melanoma are two comparatively unusual forms of the disease in which it is possible to identify people at risk for developing primary melanoma. Hersey et al.[25] reported low NK activity in the disease-free members of families with a high incidence of melanoma, while Mukherji and Dajal[26] found no correlation with NK activity and subsequent melanoma development in a group of six patients suffering from multiple primary melanoma. In a study of patients with carcinoma of the cervix, cervical dysplasia, and carcinoma *in situ*, Seltzer et al.[27] found that patients with severe cervical dysplasia and carcinoma *in situ* had significantly lower NK activity than other normal females. While these studies were done on people who were relatively healthy at the time of testing, other risk groups are more difficult to analyze because the disease process which places the patient at risk, or its causative agent, may depress NK function coincidentally. Examples of this are the NK depression which is observed in patients with acquired immunodeficiency syndrome (AIDS)[28] and inflammatory bowel disease,[29] both of which cause profound systemic disease affecting many aspects of the immune response. Thus, despite many years of research, it is still unknown whether NK cells really have any role in tumor surveillance as judged by the relationship between low vs. high NK and the probability of developing primary tumors. It should be pointed out that extremely large numbers of patients would have to be studied to arrive at significant correlations between low NK activity and tumor development because of the wide range of activity which is within normal limits and the comparatively low frequency of tumors in normal "at risk" groups in most cases.

III. NK FUNCTION AND CARCINOGENESIS

Relatively little has been written which might indicate the involvement of NK cells at the level of carcinogenesis and cell transformation. It is implicitly assumed that the NK cell recognizes some target structure (TS) on sensitive targets as being "foreign". At the level of carcinogenesis, therefore, several alternatives are possible: the aberrant cells may never display the relevant TS, the TS may modulate off in the presence of NK cells, or TS positive cells may be destroyed with only NK-resistant populations being able to survive. It is also possible that carcinogens directly inhibit NK activity, allowing sensitive cells to escape. In animal models, carcinogens do inhibit NK activity,[30,31] but this is obviously less easily proven in man. Ferson et al.[32] have demonstrated reduced NK activity in smokers and in individuals exposed to UV light in commercial solaria.[33] In an attempt to correlate NK activity with exposure to UV irradiation in the form of natural sunlight, Hersey et al. also studied 15 normal subjects exposed for 1 hr a day for 12 days over 2 weeks, and compared them to age- and sex-matched controls. An increase in functioning suppressor cells and OKT8 cells was observed in parallel with a slight depression of NK activity. The effects on NK cell function were not significant and were not as marked as those observed in normal donors exposed to higher doses of UV irradiation in solaria.[33] However, NK function can be inhibited by UV irradiation in vitro at doses which could be relevant to in vivo exposure. Shacter et al.[35] compared NK activity and responsiveness to phytohemagglutinin (PHA) of human peripheral blood leukocytes (PBLs) exposed to different doses of UV irradiation. Maximal NK sensitivity was seen at wavelengths of 260 to 280 nm, but inhibition also occurred at 300 nm at doses comparable to those capable of penetrating the epidermis to the capillaries.[36] A dose of approximately 3 mJ/cm^2 resulted in 50% inhibition of NK-mediated Cr-release from K562 at an effector to target (E:T) ratio of 30:1. According to the authors, 4 hr of sunlight "in a temperate clime" would provide 60 to 72 mJ/cm^2 at 300 nm, 10% of which would penetrate to the capillary level. These observations suggest that the NK suppression by natural sunlight observed by Hersey et al.[34] would have been more profound if the subjects had been exposed for longer than 1 hr. The UV light data are interesting in that they indicate that NK cells are potentially susceptible to doses and wavelengths of UV irradiation which are easily experienced by many individuals in the normal course of life. However, it is unknown whether this is relevant to the ultimate development of skin cancer. Our only experience with NK activity in patients with nonmelanoma skin cancer comes from a renal transplant patient with multiple recurrent basal cell carcinomas following long-term prednisone-azathioprine therapy.[37] This patient had virtually no detectable NK activity overall and a markedly suppressed frequency of actively lytic cells in the single cell assay. Hersey et al. also reported reduced NK activity in a patient with multiple skin cancers.[38] In this case, the tumors were squamous cell carcinomas in a patient with Fanconi's syndrome. The NK defect was associated with a defect in interferon (IFN) release from stimulated lymphocytes. A simple hypothesis to explain these data would postulate that the final common pathway in the process of tumor development in these patients is the failure of NK surveillance against UV irradiation -induced transformed cells, the actual NK-inhibiting agent being different in each case.

Limited studies have also been reported on the effect of tumor promoters on NK activity.[39-42] Tumor promoters stimulate the outgrowth of transformed cells without directly inducing transformation themselves. In addition, they also act on host defense mechanisms (reviewed by Keller[39]), including NK cells, either directly or by affecting regulatory functions. Seaman et al.[40] have suggested that monocytes or polymorphonuclear leukocytes release reactive forms of molecular oxygen when exposed to tumor promotors such as phorbol-12-myristate-13-acetate (PMA) and this in turn inhibits NK function. Other studies,[41—43] however, have shown inhibition by PMA to be independent of monocytes. Whether these observations are relevant to in vivo tumor formation is unknown.

IV. NK FUNCTION IN TREATED AND UNTREATED PATIENTS WITH SOLID TUMORS

There are many reports showing normal NK in patients with Stage I cancer[24,27,44—50] and these have been cited as evidence against NK suppression as being a mechanism in tumorigenesis. Furthermore, the tumors which are resected from these patients are comparatively resistant to NK lysis.[51—53] This resistance is not necessarily evidence against a role for NK cell activity in destroying early tumor cells; in fact, it may be the opposite. The strongest argument against NK cells being functional against tumors in vivo would be if active NK cells and sensitive tumor cells coexisted.

To some extent, the resistance of tumor cells to autologous NK cells may reflect the effects of separation procedures and/or the adverse effects of the microenvironment of the solid tumor on NK cells. For this reason, ascites or pleural effusions are an ideal system to study.[54—60] Uchida and Micksche[54] have done extensive work on the NK-tumor interaction using tumor cells from pleural effusions in combination with effusion-derived lymphocytes or PBLs. Lymphocytes from approximately 25% of patients were capable of lysis of autologous tumor cells.[54] When the cells were enriched for LGLs the proportions increased to 75% and, conversely, if lymphocytes forming conjugates with K562 were removed, NK lysis of autologous tumor was also decreased. This work does not necessarily prove that the killer cells were identical to "normal" fresh NK cells, since they may have been activated in vitro, in effect becoming NK-like.[61] NK-like cells differ phenotypically from fresh NK cells and have a broader target repertoire. It is well established, however, that they are (or can be) derived from cells included in the LGL-enriched Percoll light density fraction and that they are capable of lysis of both K562 and autologous tumor targets.[62]

For all intents and purposes, however, the established primary tumor or malignant effusion is NK resistant. This overall resistance is a combination of a low frequency of NK cells at the site,[52,58,59] resistance of the tumor cell itself to lysis,[51—53] and the presence of suppressor cells[55,60,63—65] and/or factors[66,67] such as prostaglandins in the tumor microenvironment.[67]

The fact that the presence of tumor is associated with reduced PBL NK function in in vitro assays is well established and, generally speaking, the higher the stage of disease the greater likelihood that NK function will be lower than normal.[44—49] Cytoreductive therapy by irradiation[68—70] or chemotherapy[46,71—73] also causes a transient decrease in NK, which recovers when the patient comes off therapy. The following section will deal with the more recent studies on NK function in patients with malignant disease.

It has been shown by Balch et al.[74] that patients with colon, lung, breast, and head and neck cancer have significantly depressed levels of HNK-1 positive (LGLs) in the circulation compared with age- and sex-matched normal donors. A study of 66 patients with melanoma and 9 patients with sarcomas showed they had normal frequencies of HNK-1 cells. This population of cells includes most NK cells, even though the proportions observed in normal donors (13.5 to 27.0%) in this study make it obvious that most of the lymphocytes are not active NK cells as judged by the frequency of lytic cells observed in single cell cytotoxicity assays.

Cunningham-Rundles et al.[24] studied the PBLs and lymph node NK activity vs. K562 in 83 women with primary untreated breast cancer. More than one third of these women had low NK activity but as discussed above, a similar result was also seen in women with fibrocystic breast disease. In contrast to the results seen with normal lymph node cells (LNCs), which have low or negative activity, 25% of the patients had evidence of LNC NK activity. The low NK preparations were unresponsive to IFN in vitro. A simultaneous report by Kadish et al.[49] also documented abnormally low NK activity in 31% of the patients, who were all suffering from solid epithelial tumors of various types. The NK abnormality was greater in patients with advanced disease, and lymphocytes from virtually all of these patients were also unresponsive to IFN in vitro. Kadish et al.[49] included in their study an analysis of the ability of the PBLs from the patients to respond to stimulation in vitro with Newcastle Disease Virus by IFN production and found that it was normal. Later studies on these and similar patients[75] using kinetic analysis and single cell cytotoxic assay techniques demonstrated that although the patients' NK cells were present in normal frequency and killed at the normal rate, the maximum killing potential (V_{max}) was reduced, suggesting a defect in recycling capacity. Low NK activity in patients with breast cancer has also been reported by Garam et al.,[76] who studied NK activity in 79 women with breast cancer compared with 70 healthy women, and evaluated cytolytic potential by measuring the maximum possible cell killing (of K562) by PBLs. Even though 75 of 79 patients had Stage I or II disease, a significant suppression of NK activity was observed using this method.

The inverse relationship between NK activity and extent of disease does not apply to all solid tumor systems.[17,77] Lipinski et al.[17] studied a group of 59 patients with malignant lymphoma and found depressed NK levels independent of disease extent and histology. Similar results were obtained by Hawrylowicz et al.[77] In the study by Lipinski et al., the reduced NK in lymphoma was in contrast to the normal NK they observed in 75 patients with localized and metastatic nonlymphoid tumors.[17]

In addition to malignant non-Hodgkin's lymphoma, NK activity is also affected in Hodgkin's disease. Gupta and Fernandes[78] studied a series of 28 patients with Hodgkin's disease with respect to their spleen and PBL NK activity. In contrast to most NK studies, the authors separated the lymphocytes into T and non-T fractions (by E-rosette depletion). No significant differences were observed between the NK activity of either T or non-T lymphocytes from Stage I and II patients compared with III and IV. The group as a whole, however, had lower than normal NK activity in the T cell subpopulation. Splenic NK function, which has rarely been studied, was significantly suppressed compared to PBLs in the non-T NK compartment in these patients, and reduction in activity was unrelated to whether or not the spleen was involved with disease. Their data suggest that there may be regional or subpopulation-selective suppression of NK activity in patients with solid tumors. They also indicate the need for more information on differences in NK activity between PBLs and various lymphoid organs in normal healthy people.

Not all studies have recorded a correlation between advanced disease and reduced NK activity. Forbes et al.[46] concluded that NK activity in treated patients with lung cancer and melanoma varied in *direct* proportion to tumor extent. Thus, while NK activity in untreated patients was depressed compared to age-matched controls, and aggressive chemotherapy further reduced these levels, patients with small cell lung cancer (SCC) in remission had lower NK on average than those in relapse. This observation was not attributable to the presence or absence of chemotherapy in these patients. The authors suggest that changes in NK activity may be a sensitive index of recurrent disease. Our experience in this regard indicates that, even with accurate lytic unit and relative NK quantification, NK activity is influenced by too many factors unrelated to malignancy to be useful for monitoring purposes.

The mechanism of peripheral blood NK cell inhibition in patients with solid tumors is still unknown. As discussed above, a number of mechanisms have been postulated to account for the inhibition of tumor-infiltrating lymphocytes (TILs), and these may affect PBLs also. Golub et al.[79] assessed the frequency and function of NK cells in TILs compared with those in the peripheral blood. They observed extremely low infiltrating lymphocyte NK activity, but the frequency, as judged by the single cell cytotoxic assay, was similar to that in PBLs. The TILs themselves were not suppressive of PBL NK. It was interesting, however, that lymph node cells proximal to the tumor suppressed PBL NK activity, in contrast to a total lack of effect by cells from more distal nodes. These studies support the hypothesis that lymphocyte-mediated suppression of NK function takes place in tumor-bearing patients and suggest that the suppression may be regional in nature, and not necessarily at the tumor site.

A possible candidate for the suppressor cell of peripheral blood NK activity has recently been described by Tarkannen et al.[80] Small lymphocyte, high-density Fc receptor (FcR)-positive suppressor cells were reported by these investigators to inhibit NK cytolysis of K562 by lymphocytes from normal donors and cancer patients. Although the frequency of preparations with suppressor cells could be increased by FcR-positive cell enrichment, the proportion of suppressor cell-positive unfractionated cell preparations was low (9 of 55 normals and 1 of 25 cancer patients). de Boer et al.[48] have also reported regulatory effects of adherent cells on the NK activity of patients with solid tumors. These observations differ from those previously reported by others in that the suppressor of NK activity was a peripheral blood cell, as opposed to being a TIL or ascitic fluid-derived cell.

The therapy used to treat solid tumors may also lead to alterations in NK activity. A number of investigators have reported inhibitory effects of chemotherapy and this usually ceases when the chemotherapy is withdrawn.[46,71—73] Saijo et al.[71] have suggested that NK levels in patients with cancer are more closely related to performance status than tumor burden, and that the failure of NK cells to return to normal after chemotherapy is a bad prognostic sign.

Kadish and Ghossein[70] studied 42 patients undergoing radiotherapy (40 to 70 Gy) for various solid tumors and found no effect on mean NK activity of the group as a whole (vs. K562). This observation is in contrast to those of Blomgren et al.,[68] who found elevated NK activity in patients irradiated for the treatment of breast cancer. NK vs. K562 was significantly reduced after 45.0 Gy, with a return to normal values by 3 to 4 months. This was in contrast to the slight suppression of NK vs. Chang cells, which was followed by an overshoot at 3 to 4 months. The discrepancy between these studies may be explainable on the basis of differences in the patient population studied, the irradiation fields used, and the timing of the assays after irradiation. It is well documented that in vitro γ-irradiation with doses of up to 15 Gy actually enhances NK activity before NK suppression is observed at higher doses.[81] Suppression of NK activity by localized high-dose irradiation in cancer patients implies (1) that circulating lymphocytes are within the field long enough to be exposed to greater than 15 Gy, (2) that tumor destruction results in the release of NK-inhibitory substances, and/or (3) that NK cells localize to the irradiated areas at the expense of the peripheral blood NK pool.

Depressed NK activity in response to therapy is not limited to radiotherapy and chemotherapy. Lukomska et al.[73] examined NK activity in 15 patients with advanced (Stage III and IV) ovarian carcinoma before and after surgery. NK activity was found to be depressed somewhat 24 hr after surgery, with a gradual return to normal values by 7 to 9 days. This occurred in parallel with a reduction in peripheral blood mononuclear cells, but was unrelated to whether or not tumor was removed at laparotomy. In these studies, no evidence of a correlation between reduced NK activity and disease progression was observed.

A transient depression of NK activity after surgery has also been reported by Tønnesen et al.[83] who serially followed NK activity in eight patients undergoing hip replacement surgery. Diazepam premedication and combined agent anesthesia were associated with elevated NK activity which subsequently fell and remained low for 5 days postoperatively. It is necessary, therefore, to consider these effects in studies of patients with malignant disease.

Experimental therapy with agents such as Bacille Calmette-Guerin (BCG) and IFN also cause alterations in NK activity (see Chapter 4 in Volume II[84]).

Although most authors have postulated that depressed NK activity is attributable to direct inhibition of NK function, Rey et al.[50] have suggested that the low NK activity is secondary to reduced interleukin-2 (IL-2) production by stimulated PBLs. In their studies, a highly significant correlation was observed between IL-2 production in vitro and NK activity. As with other studies of immunological function in cancer patients, the possibility that both NK- and IL-2-producing cells were independently inhibited by the same agent could not be ruled out. The failure of cancer patients' lymphocytes to produce extracellular mediators has also been suggested by Steinhauer et al.,[154] who have observed that lymphocytes from patients with solid tumors were deficient in the production of NK cytotoxic factor (NKCF). These studies suggest a great diversity of mechanisms potentially responsible for NK suppression in malignant disease. It should be noted, however, that a single tumor-derived factor capable of inhibiting the synthesis of extracellular mediators, such as IFN, NKCF, or IL-2, could cause all of these effects.

V. NK SURVEILLANCE AGAINST METASTATIC DISEASE

It is apparent from the foregoing discussion that the NK cell is fighting a losing battle against established tumors in vivo. The fact that primary tumors are relatively NK resistant implies that suppression of NK activity is not a primary factor in tumor progression. It could be argued from this that NK cells are not involved at the primary tumor site. Are they involved in preventing metastatic spread, as has been suggested by animal studies? Again, there are few studies of sufficient size and duration which address this question in man. We and others are currently involved in a long-term evaluation of NK activity vs. time to metastasis, the site of metastasis, and survival; however, at present no conclusions can be drawn from the data because of an inadequate follow-up time. In a recent study, Hersey et al.[85] extended their previous analysis of the correlation between low NK activity (vs. allogeneic melanoma cells and Chang liver target cells) and recurrence-free period and time to death. A study of 212 patients with Stage I melanoma and 85 patients with lymph node metastases (Stage II) was performed. No correlation was found between NK activity and prognosis at 3 to 5 years, and differences which were observed could be accounted for by other established prognostic factors such as tumor thickness. As the author points out, the recurrent tumor has already proven itself to be NK resistant and may still escape NK surveillance even though theoretically the NK to target ratio is in favor of the NK cell. Whether these observations will be confirmed for other tumor systems remains to be seen.

VI. SUMMARY

In this chapter the involvement of NK cells in the development, growth, and metastasis of solid tumors has been discussed. Studies using tumor cell lines and lymphocyte surface markers to define and enumerate naturally occurring cytotoxic lymphocytes in vitro indicate that there is heterogeneity in phenotype, function, and localization of these cells. Recent studies have shown that NK cells are capable of lysing fresh autologous tumor cells, although the level of lysis is considerably lower than that observed using cell line targets such as K562. As with other immunological reactions, NK activity is depressed in patients with advanced malignant disease of most types and cytoreductive therapy may cause further transient NK depression. This reduction in NK activity has been variously ascribed to being due to alterations in NK frequency, recycling capacity or responsiveness to IFN, or combinations of these factors; whether the suppression observed is relevant to the survival of metastasizing cells is unknown. A number of well-established observations mitigate against NK cells as being important in the destruction of *established* tumors: (1) most cancer patients with early disease have normal levels of NK activity, (2) lymphocytes from tumors have low NK activity, (3) fresh tumors are relatively NK resistant, and (4) the prognosis of patients with minimal disease does not correlate well with NK activity, at least in patients with melanoma. Because NK cell levels vary markedly between different normal individuals, on one hand, and because NK activity is enhanced or suppressed by a myriad of factors unrelated to malignant disease, on the other, the role of this cell type in defense against metastatic disease will require precise quantification methods, large numbers of patients and many years of follow-up. The immediate problem in the study of NK cells is to determine why cells from most solid tumors are relatively resistant to NK lysis and how this can be overcome.

A summary of the effects of malignant disease on NK cell function is presented in Table 1.

ACKNOWLEDGMENTS

This research was supported by grants from the National Cancer Institute of Canada and the Ontario Cancer Treatment and Research Foundation. H.F. Pross is a Career Scientist of the O.C.T.R.F. I would like to thank Mrs. Christine Jackson and Ms. Joan Gibson for typing the manuscript, Mrs. Mabel Chau and Mrs. Pamela Bandy-Dafoe for technical assistance, and Mr. Peter Rubin for helpful comments and criticisms.

Table 1
A SUMMARY OF NK FUNCTION IN MALIGNANT DISEASE

	Effect on blood NK cell function		
Tumor type	**No change**	**Decrease**	**Increase**
Miscellaneous solid	(65),[a] (86),[b] (17,87,88),[c]	(44,45,48,49,70,75,89,91),[d] (91),[a] (50)[b]	
Melanoma	(92—94)[a]	(95),[d] (96),[b]	
Familial melanoma		(25)[a]	
Ovary	(73)[b]	(97),[d] (55,58,98,99)[b]	
Cervix		(27,76,100),[d]	
Breast	(65,101—104),[a] (105)[b]	(76,106,107),[d] (24,108)[a]	
Lung, (small cell and nonsmall cell)	(46,109)[a] (110),[b] (111,112)[e]	(95),[d] (63),[a] (60,71)[b]	
Colon	(113)[b] (114,115)[e]	(63),[a] (116)[c]	
Stomach		(117)[e]	
Hepatocellular carcinoma		(118)[c]	
Midgut carcinoid	(119)[b]		
Bladder		(120),[a] (121)[e]	
Prostate	(121)[e]	(122)[e]	
Neuroblastoma		(65)[a]	
Myeloma	(123,124)[e]		
Malignant lymphoma		(17,77,88)[e]	
Hodgkin's disease	(89)[e]	(125,126)[a] (127)[c]	(128)[a]
X-linked lymphoproliferative disease		(11,129,130)	
T_γ-leukemia or lymphoproliferation			(131—136)[f]
Leukemia	(137)[g]	(138—140),[g] (141—146),[h] (147—148),[i] (135—150),[j] (150—152),[k] (151),[l] (153)[m]	(149)[j]

Note: This table includes reports in which there may be duplication in the patients described in two different publications.

[a] Mostly nonmetastatic disease reported.
[b] Mostly metastatic disease reported.
[c] Stage not reported, unclear or not applicable.
[d] Percent change proportional to stage.
[e] No stage relationship.
[f] "Increase" in leukemia or leukocytosis indicates the abnormal cell had NK function, usually a single case report.
[g] Preleukemia.
[h] Chronic B lymphocytic leukemia (BCLL).
[i] Chronic T lymphocytic leukemia (TCLL).
[j] Acute lymphocytic leukemia (ALL).
[k] Acute myeloid leukemia (AML).
[l] Chronic myeloid leukemia (CML).
[m] Hairy cell leukemia.

REFERENCES

1. **Roder, J. C. and Pross, H. F.,** The biology of human natural killer cells, *J. Clin. Immunol.,* 2, 249, 1982.
2. **Herberman, R. B., Ed.,** *NK Cell and Other Natural Effector Cells,* Academic Press, New York, 1982, 1175.
3. **Roder, J. C., Kärre, K., and Kiessling, R.,** Natural killer cells, *Prog. Allergy,* 28, 66, 1981.
4. **Pross, H., Callewaert, D., and Rubin, P.,** Assays for NK cell cytotoxicity; their values and pitfalls, in *Immunobiology of Natural Killer Cells,* Vol 1, Lotzová, E. and Herberman, R., Ed., CRC Press, Boca Raton, Fla., 1986, chap. 1.
5. **Klein, E., Ben Bassat, H., Neumann, H., Ralph, P., Zeuthen, J., Polliak, A., and Vanky, F.,** Properties of the K562 line derived from a patient with chronic myeloid leukemia, *Int. J. Cancer.,* 18, 421, 1976.
6. **Lozzio, C. B. and Lozzio, B. B.,** Cytotoxicity of a factor isolated from human spleen, *J. Natl. Cancer Inst.,* 50, 535, 1973.
7. **Andersson, L. C., Jokinen, M., and Gahmberg, C. G.,** Induction of erythroid differentiation in the human leukemia line, K562, *Nature (London),* 278, 364, 1980.
8. **Jondal, M. and Pross, H.,** Surface markers on human B- and T-lymphocytes. VI. Cytotoxicity against cell lines as a functional marker for lymphocyte subpopulations, *Int. J. Cancer,* 15, 596, 1975.
9. **Pross, H. F. and Baines, M. G.,** Studies of human natural killer cells. I. In vivo parameters affecting normal cytotoxic function, *Int. J. Cancer,* 29, 383, 1982.
10. **Roder, J. C., Haliotis, T., Klein, M., Korec, S., Jett, J., Ortaldo, J., Herberman, R. B., Katz, P., and Fauci, A. S.,** A new immunodeficiency disorder in humans involving NK cells, *Nature (London),* 284, 553, 1980.
11. **Sullivan, J. L., Byron, K. S., Brewster, F. F. and Purtilo, D.,** Deficient natural killer cell activity in X-linked lymphoproliferative syndrome, *Science,* 210, 543, 1980.
12. **Gatti, R. A. and Good, R. A.,** Occurrence of malignancy in immunodeficiency diseases: a literature review, *Cancer,* 28, 89, 1971.
13. **Pross, H. F., Gupta, S., Good, R. A., and Baines, M. G.,** Spontaneous human lymphocyte-mediated cytotoxicity against tumor target cells. VII. The effect of immunodeficiency disease, *Cell. Immunol.,* 43, 16, 1978.
14. **Koren, H. S., Amos, D. B., and Buckley, R. B.,** Natural killing in immunodeficient patients, *J. Immunol.,* 120, 796, 1978.
15. **Lipinski, M., Virelizier, J. L., Tursz, T., and Griscelli, C.,** Natural killer and killer cell activities in patients with primary immunodeficiencies or defects in immune interferon production, *Eur. J. Immunol.,* 10, 246, 1980.
16. **Peter, H. H.,** The origin of human NK cells, an ontogenic model derived from studies in patients with immunodeficiencies, *Blut,* 46, 239, 1983.
17. **Lipinski, M., Dokhelar, M.-C., and Tursz, T.,** NK cell activity in patients with high risk for tumors and in patients with cancer, in *NK Cells and Other Natual Effector Cells,* Herberman, R. B., Ed., Academic Press, New York, 1982, 1183.
18. **Strayer, D. R., Carter, W. A., Mayberry, S. D., Pequignot, E., and Brodsky, I.,** Low natural cytotoxicity of peripheral blood mononuclear cells in individuals with high familial incidences of cancer, *Cancer Res.,* 44, 370, 1984.
19. **Pross, H. F., Sterns, E., and MacGillis, D. R. R.,** Natural killer cell activity in women at "high risk" for breast cancer, with and without benign breast syndrome, *Int. J. Cancer,* 34, 303, 1984.
20. **Love, S. M., Gelman, R. S., and Silen, W.,** Fibrocystic "disease" of the breast — a nondisease?, *N. Eng. J. Med.,* 307, 1010, 1982.
21. **Page, D. L., Vander Zwagg, R., Rogers, L. W., Williams, L. T., Walker, W. E., and Hartmann, W. H.,** Relation between component parts of fibrocystic disease complex and breast cancer, *J. Natl. Cancer Inst.,* 61, 1055, 1978.
22. **Golinger, R. C.,** Hormones and the pathophysiology of fibrocystic mastopathy, *Surg. Gynecol. Obstetr.,* 146, 273, 1978.
23. **Cannon, G. B., Barsky, S. H., Alford, T. C., Jerome, L. F., Tinley, V., McCoy, J. L., and Dean, J. H.,** Cell-mediated immunity to mouse mammary tumor virus antigens by patients with hyperplastic benign breast disease, *J. Natl. Cancer Inst.,* 68, 935, 1982.
24. **Cunningham-Rundles, S., Filippa, D. A., Braun, D. W., Jr., Antonelli, P., and Ashikari, H.,** Natural cytotoxicity of peripheral blood lymphocytes and regional lymph node cells in breast cancer in women, *J. Natl. Cancer Inst.,* 67, 585, 1981.
25. **Hersey, P., Edwards, A., Honeyman, M., and McCarthy, W. H.,** Low natural killer cell activity in familial melanoma patients and their relatives, *Br. J. Cancer,* 40, 113, 1979.
26. **Mukherji, B. and Dayal, Y.,** Lymphocyte cytotoxicity of patients developing multiple primary melanomas, *Cancer,* 46, 1566, 1980.

27. **Seltzer, V., Doyle, A., and Kadish, A. S.,** Natural cytotoxicity in malignant and premalignant cervical neoplasia and enhancement of cytotoxicity with interferon, *Gynecol. Oncol.,* 15, 340, 1983.
28. **Lopez, C., Fitzgerald, P. A., and Siegal, F. P.,** Severe acquired immunodeficiency syndrome in male homosexuals: diminished capacity to make interferon-alpha in vitro is associated with severe opportunistic infections, *J. Infect. Dis.,* 148, 962, 1983.
29. **Ginsburg, C. H., Dambrauskas, J. T., Ault, K. A., and Falchuk, Z. M.,** Impaired natural killer cell activity in patients with inflammatory bowel disease: evidence for a qualitative defect, *Gastroenterology,* 85, 846, 1983.
30. **Gorelik, E. and Herberman, R. B.,** Role of natural-cell-mediated immunity in urethane-induced lung carcinogenesis, in, *NK Cells and Other Natural Effector Cells,* Herberman, R. B., Ed., Academic Press, New York, 1980, 1415.
31. **Ehrlich, R., Efrati, M., Malatzky, E., Shochat, L., Bar Eyal, A., and Witz, I. P.,** Natural host defence during oncogenesis. NK activity and dimethylbenzanthracene carcinogenesis, *Int. J. Cancer,* 31, 67, 1983.
32. **Ferson, F., Edwards, A., Lind, A., Milton, G. W., and Hersey, P.,** Low natural killer cell activity and immunoglobulin levels associated with smoking in human subjects, *Int. J. Cancer,* 23, 603, 1979.
33. **Hersey, P., Bradley, M., Hasic, E., Haran, G., Edwards, A., and McCarthy, W. H.,** Immunological effects of solarium exposure in human subjects, *Lancet,* 1, 545, 1983.
34. **Hersey, P., Haran, G., Hasic, E., and Edwards, A.,** Alteration of T cell subsets and induction of suppressor T cell activity in normal subjects after exposure to sunlight, *J. Immunol.,* 131, 171, 1983.
35. **Schacter, B., Lederman, M. M., LeVine, M. J., and Ellner, J. J.,** Ultraviolet radiation inhibits human natural killer activity and lymphocyte proliferation, *J. Immunol.,* 130, 2484, 1983.
36. **Everett, M. A., Yeargers, R. M., Sayre, R. M., and Olson, R. L.,** Penetration of the epidermis by ultraviolet rays, *Photochem. Photobiol.,* 5, 533, 1966.
37. **Pross, H. F., Rubin, P., and Baines, M. G.,** The assessment of natural killer cell activity in cancer patients, in *NK Cells and Other Natural Effector Cells,* Herberman, R. B., Ed., Academic Press, New York, 1982, 1175.
38. **Hersey, P., Edwards, A., Lewis, R., Kemp, A., and McInnes, J.,** Deficient natural killer cell activity in a patient with Fanconi's anemia and squamous cell carcinoma: association with a defect in interferon release, *Clin. Exp. Immunol.,* 48, 205, 1982.
39. **Keller, R.,** Host defense mechanisms against tumors as the principal targets of tumor promoters, *J. Cancer Res. Clin. Oncol.,* 105, 203, 1983.
40. **Seaman, W. E., Gindhart, T. D., Blackman, M. A., Dalal, B., Talal, N., and Werb, Z.,** Suppression of natural killing in vitro by monocytes and polymorphonuclear leukocytes. Requirement for reactive metabolites of oxygen, *J. Clin. Invest.,* 69, 876, 1982.
41. **Abrams, S. I., Bray, R. A., and Brahmi, Z.,** Mechanism of action of phorbol myristate acetate on human natural killer cell activity, *Cell. Immunol.,* 80, 230, 1983.
42. **Goldfarb, R. H. and Herberman, R. B.,** Natural killer cell reactivity: regulatory interactions among phorbol ester, interferon, cholera toxin, and retinoic acid, *J. Immunol.,* 126, 2129, 1981.
43. **Goldfarb, R. H. and Herberman, R. B.,** Characteristics of natural killer cells and possible mechanisms for their cytotoxic activity, *Adv. Inflam. Res.,* 4, 45, 1982.
44. **Pross, H. F. and Baines, M. G.,** Spontaneous human lymphocyte-mediated cytotoxicity against tumor target cells. I. The effect of malignant disease, *Int. J. Cancer,* 18, 593, 1976.
45. **Takasugi, M., Ramseyer, A., and Takasugi, J.,** Decline of natural nonselective cell-mediated cytotoxicity in patients with tumor progression, *Cancer Res.,* 37, 413, 1977.
46. **Forbes, J. T., Greco, F. A., and Oldham, R. K.,** Human natural cell-mediated cytotoxicity. II. Levels in neoplastic disease, *Cancer Immunol. Immunother.,* 11, 147, 1981.
47. **Hersey, P., Edwards, A., Milton, G. W., and McCarthy, W. H.,** Relationship of cell-mediated cytotoxicity against melanoma cells to prognosis in melanoma patients, *Br. J. Cancer,* 37, 505, 1978.
48. **De Boer, K. P., Braun, D. P., and Harris, J. E.,** Natural cytotoxicity and antibody dependent cytotoxicity in solid tumor cancer patients: regulation by adherent cells, *Clin. Immunol. Immunopathol.,* 23, 133, 1982.
49. **Kadish, A. S., Doyle, A. T., Steinhauer, E. H., and Ghossein, N. A.,** Natural cytotoxicity and interferon production in human cancer: deficient natural killer activity and normal interferon production in patients with advanced disease, *J. Immunol.,* 127, 1817, 1981.
50. **Rey, A., Klein, B., Zagur, D., Thierry, C., and Serrou, B.,** Diminished interleukin-2 activity production in cancer patients bearing solid tumors and its relationship with natural killer cells, *Immunol. Lett.,* 6, 175, 1983.
51. **Werkmeister, J. A., Pihl, E., Nind, A. A. P., Flannery, G. R., and Nairn, R. C.,** Immunoreactivity by intrinsic lymphoid cells in colorectal carcinoma, *Br. J. Cancer,* 40, 839, 1979.
52. **Vose, B. M., Vanky, F., Argov, S., and Klein, E.,** Natural cytotoxicity in man: activity of lymph node and tumor infiltrating lymphocytes, *Eur. J. Immunol.,* 7, 753, 1977.
53. **Vose, B. M. and Moore, M.,** Natural cytotoxicity in humans: susceptibility of freshly isolated tumor cells to lysis, *J. Natl. Cancer Inst.,* 65, 257, 1980.

54. **Uchida, A. and Micksche, M.,** Lysis of fresh human tumor cells by autologous large granular lymphocytes from peripheral blood and pleural effusions, *Int. J. Cancer*, 32, 37, 1983.
55. **Allavena, P., Introna, M., Mangioni, C., and Mantovani, A.,** Inhibition of natural killer activity by tumor-associated lymphoid cells from ascites ovarian carcinomas, *J. Natl. Cancer Inst.*, 67, 319, 1981.
56. **Mantovani, A., Peri, G., Polentarutti, N., Bolis, G., Mangioni, C., and Spreafico, F.,** Effects on in vitro tumor growth of macrophages isolated from human ascitic ovarian tumors, *Int. J. Cancer*, 23, 157, 1979.
57. **Mantovani, A., Allavena, P., Sessa, C., Bolis, G., and Mangioni, C.,** Natural killer activity of lymphoid cells isolated from human ascitic ovarian tumors, *Int. J. Cancer*, 25, 573, 1980.
58. **Introna, M., Allavena, P., Biondi, A., Colombo, N., Villa, A., and Mantovani, A.,** Defective natural killer activity within human ovarian tumors: low numbers of morphologically defined effectors present in situ, *J. Natl. Cancer Inst.*, 70, 21, 1983.
59. **Uchida, A. and Micksche, M.,** Natural killer cells in carcinoma tumor pleural effusions, *Cancer Immunol. Immunother.*, 11, 131, 1981.
60. **Uchida, A. and Micksche, M.,** Suppressor cells for natural killer activity in carcinomatous pleural effusions of cancer patients, *Cancer Immunol. Immunother.*, 11, 255, 1981.
61. **Lopez-Botet, M., Moretta, A., and Moretta, L.,** Natural killer-like cytotoxicity of human T-cell clones against various target cells, *Scand. J. Immunol.*, 17, 95, 1983.
62. **Kedar, E., Ikejiri, B. L., Timonen, T., Bonnard, G. O., Reid, J., Navarro, N. J., Sredni, B., and Herberman, R. B.,** Antitumor reactivity in vitro and in vivo of lymphocytes from normal donors and cancer patients propagated in culture with T cell growth factor (TCGF), *Eur. J. Cancer Clin. Oncol.*, 19, 757, 1983.
63. **Vose, B. M.,** Natural killers in human cancer: activity of tumor-infiltrating and draining lymph node lymphocytes, in *Natural Cell-Mediated Immunity Against Tumors*, Herberman, R. B., Ed., Academic Press, New York, 1980, 1081.
64. **Eremin, O.,** NK cell activity in the blood, tumour-draining lymph nodes and primary tumours of women with mammary carcinoma, in *Natural Cell-Mediated Immunity Against Tumors*, Herberman, R. B., Ed., Academic Press, New York, 1980, 1011.
65. **Gerson, J. M.,** Systemic and in situ natural killer activity in tumor-bearing mice and patients with cancer, in *Natural Cell-Mediated Immunity Against Tumors*, Herberman, R. B., Ed., Academic Press, New York, 1980, 1047.
66. **Shimura, T., Fujimoto, S., Ishigami, H., Amemiya, K., Takahashi, O., and Okui, K.,** Effect of cancerous ascites on natural killer activity, *Gan. No Rinsho.*, 29, 133, 1983.
67. **Bankhurst, A. D.,** The modulation of human natural killer cell activity by prostaglandins, *J. Clin. Lab. Immunol.*, 7, 85, 1982.
68. **Blomgren, H., Baral, E., Edsmyr, F., Strender, L.-E., Petrini, B., and Wasserman, J.,** Natural killer activity in peripheral lymphocyte population following local radiation therapy, *Acta Radiol. Oncol.*, 19, 139, 1980.
69. **Onsrud, M. and Thorsby, E.,** Long-term changes in natural killer activity after external pelvic radiotherpay, *Int. J. Radiat. Oncol. Biol. Phys.*, 7, 609, 1981.
70. **Kadish, A. S. and Ghossein, N. A.,** Natural cytotoxicity in patients undergoing radiation therapy, *Am. J. Clin. Oncol.*, 6, 53, 1983.
71. **Saijo, N., Shimizu, E., et a.,** The effect of chemotherapy on natural killer activity and antibody dependent cell-mediated cytotoxicity in carcinoma of the lung, *Br. J. Cancer*, 46, 180, 1982.
72. **Blomgren, H., Edsmyr, F., and Strender, L.-E.,** Effect of pepleomycin on peripheral lymphocytes, *Acta Radiol. Oncol.*, 20, 113, 1981.
73. **Lukomaska, B., Olszewski, W. L., Engeset, A., and Kolstad, P.,** The effect of surgery and chemotherapy on blood NK cell activity in patients with ovarian cancer, *Cancer*, 51, 465, 1983.
74. **Balch, C. M., Tilden, A. B., Dougherty, P. A., and Cloud, G. A.,** Depressed levels of granular lymphocytes with natural killer (NK) cell function in 247 cancer patients, *Ann. Surg.*, 198, 192, 1983.
75. **Steinhauer, E. H., Doyle, A. T., Reed, J., and Kadish, A. S.,** Defective natural cytotoxicity in patients with cancer: normal number of effector cells but decreased recycling capacity in patients with advanced disease, *J. Immunol.*, 129, 2255, 1982.
76. **Garam, T., Pulay, T., Bakacs, T., Svastits, E., Ringwald, G., Totpal, K., and Petranyi, G.,** NK and K cell activity in mammary patients in relation to radiation therapy and the course of disease, in *NK Cells and Other Natural Effector Cells*, Herberman, R. B., Ed., Academic Press, New York, 1982, 1189.
77. **Hawrylowicz, C. M., Rees, R. C., Hancock, B. W., and Potter, C. W.,** Depressed spontaneous natural killing and interferon augmentation in patients with malignant lymphoma, *Eur. J. Cancer Clin. Oncol.*, 18, 1081, 1982.
78. **Gupta, S. and Fernandes, G.,** Natural killing in patients with Hodgkin's Disease, in *NK Cells and Other Natural Effector Cells*, Herberman, R. B., Ed., Academic Press, New York, 1982, 1201.

79. **Golub, S. H., Niitsuma, M., Kawate, N., Cochran, A. J., and Holmes, E. C.,** NK activity of tumor infiltrating and lymph node lymphocytes in human pulmonary tumors, in *NK Cells and Other Natural Effector Cells*, Herberman, R. B., Ed., Academic Press, New York, 1982, 1113.
80. **Tarkkanen, J., Saksela, E., and Paavolainen, M.,** Suppressor cells of natural killer activity in normal and tumor-bearing individuals, *Clin. Immunol. Immunopathol.*, 28, 29, 1983.
81. **Dean, M. D., Pross, H. F., and Kennedy, J. C.,** Spontaneous human lymphocyte-mediated cytotoxicity against tumor target cells. III, *Int. J. Radiat. Oncol. Biol. Phys.*, 4, 633, 1978.
82. **Brovall, C. and Schacter, B.,** Radiation sensitivity of human natural killer cell acitivty: control by X-linked genes, *J. Immunol.*, 126, 2236, 1981.
83. **Tønnesen, E., Mickley, H., and Grunnet, N.,** Natural killer cell activity during premedication, anaesthesia and surgery, *Acta Anaesthesiol. Scand.*, 27, 238, 1983.
84. **Moy, P. M. and Golub, S.,** In vivo modulation of NK acitivity in cancer patients, in *The Immunology of Natural Killer Cells,* Vol. 1, Lotzová, E. and Herberman, R. B., Eds., CRC Press, Boca Raton, Fla., 1986, chap. 4.
85. **Hersey, P., Edwards, A., Milton, G. W., and McCarthy, W. H.,** No evidence for an association between natural killer cell activity and prognosis in melanoma patients, submitted.
86. **Maluish, A., Ortaldo, J., Conlon, J., Sherwin, S., Leavitt, R., Strong, D., Weirnik, P., Oldham, R., and Herberman, R.,** Depression of natural killer cytotoxicity after in vivo administration of recombinant leukocyte interferon, *J. Immunol.*, 131, 503, 1983.
87. **Einhorn, S., Blomgren, H., Strander, H., and Wasserman, J.,** Influence of human interferon-a therapy on cytotoxic functions of blood lymphocytes. Studies on lectin-dependent cellular cytotoxicity, antibody-dependent cellular cytotoxicity, and natural killer cell activity, *Cancer Immunol. Immunother.*, 16, 77, 1983.
88. **Tursz, T., Dokhelar, M., Lipinski, M., and Amiel, J.,** Low natural killer cell activity in patients with malignant lymphoma, *Cancer,* 50, 2333, 1982.
89. **Oldham, R. K., Djeu, J. Y., Cannon, G. B., Siwarski, D., and Herberman, R. B.,** Cellular micro-cytotoxicity in human tumor systems: analysis of results, *J. Natl. Cancer Inst.*, 55, 1305, 1975.
90. **Catalona, W., Ratliff, T., and McCool, R.,** Discordance among cell-mediated cytolytic mechanisms in cancer patients: importance of the assay system, *J. Immunol.*, 122, 1009, 1979.
91. **Menon, M. and Stefani, S.,** Lymphocyte mediated natural cytotoxicity in neoplasia, *Oncology,* 35, 63, 1978.
92. **Kristensen, E.,** A comparative study of natural cytotoxicity and the leukocyte migration inhibition in human melanoma stages I and II, *J. Cancer Res. Clin. Oncol.*, 96, 181, 1980.
93. **Kristensen, E., Brandslund, I., Nielsen, H., and Svehag, S. -E.,** Prognostic value of assays for circulating immune complexes and natural cytotoxicity in malignant skin melanoma (Stages I and II), *Cancer Immunol. Immunother.*, 9, 31, 1980.
94. **Hersey, P., Hobbs, A., Edwards, A., McCarthy, W., and McGovern, V.,** Relationship between natural killer cell activity and histological features of lymphocyte infiltration and partial regression of the primary tumor in melanoma patients, *Cancer Res.*, 42, 363, 1982.
95. **Sibbitt, W., Bankhurst, A., Jumonville, A., Saiki, J., Saiers, J., and Doberneck, R.,** Defects in natural killer cell activity and interferon response in human lung carcinoma and malignant melanoma, *Cancer Res.*, 44, 852, 1984.
96. **Thatcher, N., Swindell, R., and Drowther, D.,** Effects of *Corynebacterium parvum* and BCG therapy on immune parameters in patients with disseminated melanoma. A sequential study over 28 days. II. Changes in non-specific (NK, K and T cell) lymphocytotoxicity and delayed hypersensitivity skin reactions, *Clin. Exp. Immunol.*, 35, 171, 1979.
97. **Pross, H. and Baines, M.,** Natural killer cells in tumour-bearing patients, in *Natural Cell-Mediated Immunity Against Tumors,* Herberman, R. B., Ed., Academic Press, New York, 1980, 1063.
98. **Allavena, P., Introna, M., Sessa, C., Mangioni, C., and Mantovani, A.,** Interferon effect on cytotoxicity of peripheral blood and tumor-associated lymphocytes against human ovarian carcinoma cells, *J. Natl. Cancer Inst.*, 68, 555, 1982.
99. **Colotta, F., Rambaldi, A., Colombo, N., Tabacchi, L., Introna, M., and Mantovani, A.,** Effect of a streptococcal preparation (OK432) on natural killer activity of tumour-associated lymphoid cells in human ovarian carcinoma on lysis of fresh ovarian tumor cells, *Br. J. Cancer,* 48, 515, 1983.
100. **Pulay, T., Benczur, M., and Varga, M.,** Natural killer lymphocyte function in cervical cancer patients, *Neoplasma,* 29, 237, 1982.
101. **Blomgren, H., Strender, L.-E., Petrini, B., and Wasserman, J.,** Changes of the spontaneous cytotoxicity of the blood lymphocyte population following local radiation therapy for breast cancer, *Eur. J. Cancer Clin. Oncol.*, 18, 637, 1982.
102. **Eremin, O., Coombs, R., and Ashby, J.,** Lymphocytes infiltrating human breast cancers lack K-cell activity and show low levels of NK-cell activity, *Br. J. Cancer,* 44, 166, 1981.

103. **Heidenreich, W., Jagla, K., Schussler, J., Borner, P., Dehnhard, F., Kalden, J., Leibold, W., Peter, H., and Deicher, H.,** Spontaneous cell-mediated cytotoxicity (SCMC) and antibody-dependent cellular cytotoxicity (ADCC) in peripheral blood and draining lymph nodes of patients with mammary carcinoma, *Cancer Immunol. Immunother.*, 7, 65, 1979.
104. **Uchida, A., Kolb, R., and Micksche, M.,** Generation of suppressor cells for natural killer activity in cancer patients after surgery, *J. Natl. Cancer Inst.*, 68, 735, 1982.
105. **Mackay, I., Goodyear, M., Riglar, C., and Penschow, J.,** Effect on natural killer and antibody-dependent cellular cytotoxicity of adjuvant cytotoxic chemotherapy including melphalan in breast cancer, *Cancer Immunol. Immunother.*, 16, 98, 1983.
106. **Garner, W., Minton, J., James, A., and Hoffmann, C.,** Suppressed natural killer cell surveillance in human breast cancer, *Surg. Forum*, 33, 422, 1982.
107. **Garner, W., Minton, J., James, A., and Hoffmann, C.,** Human breast cancer and impaired NK cell function, *J. Surg. Oncol.*, 24, 64, 1983.
108. **White, D., Jones, D., Cooke, T., and Kirkham, N.,** Natural (NK) activity in peripheral blood lymphocytes of patients with benign and malignant breast disease, *Br. J. Cancer*, 46, 611, 1982.
109. **Forbes, J. T., Greco, F. A., and Oldham, R. K.,** Natural cell-mediated cytotoxicity in human tumor patients, in *Natural Cell-Mediated Immunity Against Tumors*, Herberman, R. B., Ed., Academic Press, New York, 1980, 1031.
110. **Moore, M. and Vose, B.,** Extravascular natural cytotoxocity in man: anti-K562 activity of lymph-node and tumour-infiltrating lymphocytes, *Int. J. Cancer*, 27, 265, 1981.
111. **Liberati, A., Voelkel, J., Borden, E., Coates, A., Citrin, D., and Bryan, G.,** Influence of non-specific immunologic factors on prognosis in advanced bronchogenic carcinoma, *Cancer Immunol. Immunother.*, 13, 140, 1982.
112. **Saijo, N., Shimizu, E., Irimajiri, N., Ozaki, A., Kimura, K., Takizawa, T., and Niitani, H.,** Analysis of natural killer activity and antibody-dependent cellular cytotoxicity in healthy volunteers and in patients with primary lung cancer and metastatic pulmonary tumors, *J. Cancer Res. Clin. Oncol.*, 102, 195, 1982.
113. **Balch, C., Tilden, A., Dougherty, P., Cloud, G., and Abo, T.,** Heterogeneity of natural killer lymphocyte abnormalities in colon cancer patients, *Surgery*, 95, 63, 1984.
114. **Waller, C., Gill, P., and MacLennan, I.,** Enhancement of lymphocyte-mediated cytotoxicity after tumor resection in patients with colorectal cancer, *J. Natl. Cancer Inst.*, 65, 223, 1980.
115. **Vose, B., Gallagher, P., Moore, M., and Schofield, P.,** Specific and non-specific lymphocyte cytotoxicity in colon carcinoma, *Br. J. Cancer*, 44, 846, 1981.
116. **Lang, I., Feuer, L., Nekam, K., Szigeti, A., Gergely, P., and Petranyi, G.,** Glutaurine enhances the depressed NK cell activity of tumor patients, *Immunol. Commun.*, 12, 519, 1983.
117. **Tanaka, N., Hashimoto, T., Matsui, T., Ohida, J., Ono, M., and Orita, K.,** Natural cytotoxic reactivity of peripheral blood lymphocytes from digestive tract cancer patients against a colon cancer cell line and virus-infected hela cells, *Gann.*, 74, 419, 1983.
118. **Son, K., Kew, M., and Rabson, A.,** Depressed natural killer cell activity in patients with hepatocellular carcinoma, *Cancer*, 50, 2820, 1982.
119. **Funa, K., Alm, G., Ronnblom, L., and Oberg, K.,** Evaluation of the natural killer cell — interferon system in patients with mid-gut carcinoid tumours treated with leucocyte interferon, *Clin. Exp. Immunol.*, 53, 716, 1983.
120. **Vilien, M., Wolf, H., and Rasmussen, F.,** Titration of natural and disease-related cytotoxicity of lymphocytes from bladder cancer patients, *Cancer Immunol. Immunother.*, 8, 189, 1980.
121. **Ratliff, T., McCool, R., and Catalona, W.,** Antibody-dependent and spontaneous lympholysis in urologic cancer patients, *Br. J. Cancer*, 39, 667, 1979.
122. **Kalland, T. and Haukaas, S.,** Effect of treatment with diethylstilbestrol-polyestradiol phosphate or estramustine phosphate (Estracyt) on natural killer cell activity in patients with prostatic cancer, *Invest. Urol.*, 18, 437, 1981.
123. **Einhorn, S., Ahre, A., Blomgren, H., Johansson, B., Mellstedt, H., and Strander, H.,** Interferon and natural killer activity in multiple myeloma. Lack of correlation between interferon-induced enhancement of natural killer activity and clinical response to human interferon-a, *Int. J. Cancer*, 30, 167, 1982.
124. **Einhorn, S., Blomgren, H., Strander, H., and Wasserman, J.,** Influence of human interferon-a therapy on cytotoxic function of blood lymphocytes. Studies on lectin-dependent cellular cytotoxicity, antibody-dependent cellular cytotoxicity, and natural killer cell activity, *Cancer Immunol. Immunother.*, 16, 77, 1983.
125. **Al Sam, S., Jones, D., Payne, S., and Wright, D.,** Natural killer (NK) activity in the spleen of patients with Hodgkin's disease and controls, *Br. J. Cancer*, 46, 806, 1982.
126. **Gupta, S. and Fernandes, G.,** Spontaneous and antibody-dependent cellular cytotoxicity by lymphocyte subpopulations in peripheral blood and spleen from adult patients with Hodgkin's disease, *Clin. Exp. Immunol.*, 45, 205, 1981.

127. **Gupta, S. and Fernandes, G.,** Natural killing in patients with Hodgkin's Disease, in *NK Cells and Other Natural Effector Cells,* Herberman, R. B., Ed., Academic Press, New York, 1982, 1201.
128. **Rotstein, S., Baral, E., Blomgren, H., and Johansson, B.,** In vitro radiosensitivity of the spontaneous cytotoxicity of blood lymphocytes in patients with untreated Hodgkin's disease, *Eur. J. Cancer Clin. Oncol.,* 19, 1405, 1983.
129. **Seeley, J., Bechtold, T., Purtillo, D., and Lindsten, T.,** NK deficiency in X-linked lymphoproliferative syndrome, in *NK Cells and Other Natural Effector Cells,* Herberman, R. B., Ed., Academic Press, New York, 1982, 1211.
130. **Harada, S., Bechtold, T., Seeley, J., and Putilo, D.,** Cell-mediated immunity to Epstein-Barr Virus (EBV) and natural killer (NK)-cell activity in the X-linked lymphoproliferative syndrome, *Int. J. Cancer,* 30, 739, 1982.
131. **Pross, H., Pater, J., Dwosh, I., Giles, A., Gallinger, L., Rubin, P., Corbett, W., Galbraith, P., and Baines, M.,** Studies of human natural killer cells. III. Neutropenia associated with unusual characteristics of antibody-dependent and natural killer cell-mediated cytotoxicity, *J. Clin. Immunol.,* 2, 126, 1982.
132. **Ferrarini, M., Romagnani, S., Montesoro, E., Zicca, A., Del Prete, G., Nocera, A., Maggi, E., Leprini, A., and Grossi, C.,** A lymphoproliferative disorder of the large granular lymphocytes with natural killer activity, *J. Clin. Immunol.,* 3, 30, 1983.
133. **Gupta, S. and Fernandes, G.,** Natural killer and antibody-dependent cytotoxic activities in T cell chronic lymphocytic leukemia, *J. Clin. Lab. Immunol.,* 12, 155, 1983.
134. **Itoh, K., Tsuchikawa, K., Awatagiuchi, T., Shiiba, K., and Kumagai, K.,** A case of chronic lymphocytic leukemia with properties characteristic of natural killer cells, *Blood,* 61, 940, 1983.
135. **Komiyama, A., Kawai, H., Miyagawa, Y., and Akabane, T.,** Childhood lymphoblastic leukemia with natural killer activity: establishment of the leukemia cell lines retaining the acitivity, *Blood,* 60, 1429, 1982.
136. **Palutke, M., Eisenberg, L., Kaplan, J., Hussain, M., Kithier, K., Tabaczka, P., Mirchandani, I., and Tenenbaum, D.,** Natural killer and suppressor T-cell chronic lymphocytic leukemia, *Blood,* 63, 627, 1983.
137. **Matera, L. and Giancotti, F.,** Natural killer activity and low-affinity E rosettes in acute leukemias, *Acta Haematol.,* 70, 158, 1983.
138. **Anderson, R., Volsky, D., Greenberg, B., Knox, S., Bechtold, T., Kuszynski, C., Haradi, S., and Putilo, D.,** Lymphocyte abnormalities in preleukemia. I. Decreased NK activity, anomalous immunoregulatory cell subsets and deficient EBV receptors, *Leuk. Res.,* 7, 389, 1983.
139. **Porzsolt, F. and Heimpel, H.,** Natural killer cell activity in preleukemia, *Lancet,* 1, 449, 1982.
140. **Takaku, S. and Takaku, F.,** Natural killer cell activity and preleukemia, *Lancet,* 2, 1178, 1981.
141. **Kay, N. and Zarling, J.,** Impaired natural killer activity in patients with chronic lymphocytic leukemia is associated with a deficiency of azurophilic cytoplasmic granules in putative NK cells, *Blood,* 63, 305, 1984.
142. **Platsoucas, C., Gupta, S., Good, R., and Fernandes, G.,** Deficient NK and ADCC mediated by purified E-rosette positive and E-rosette negative cells from patients with B-cell chronic lymphocytic leukemia. Augmentation by in vitro treatment with human leukocyte interferon, in *NK Cells and Other Natural Effector Cells,* Herberman, R. B., Ed., Academic Press, New York, 1982, 1195.
143. **Behelak, Y., Banerjee, D., and Richter, M.,** Immunocompetent cells in patients with malignant disease. I. The lack of naturally occurring killer cell activity in the unfractionated circulating lymphocytes from patients with chronic lymphocytic leukemia (CLL), *Cancer,* 38, 2274, 1976.
144. **Ziegler, H.-W., Kay, N., and Zarling, J.,** Deficiency of natural killer cell activity in patients with chronic lymphocytic leukemia, *Int. J. Cancer,* 27, 321, 1981.
145. **Platsoucas, C., Fernandes, G., Gupta, S., Kempin, S., Clarkson, B., Good, R., and Gupta, S.,** Defective spontaneous and antibody-dependent cytotoxicity mediated by E-rosette positive and E-rosette-negative cells in untreated patients with chronic lymphocytic leukemia: augmentation by in vitro treatment with interferon, *J. Immunol.,* 125, 1216, 1980.
146. **Hokland, P. and Ellegaard, J.,** Immunological studies in chronic lymphocytic leukemia. II. Natural killer- and antibody-dependent cellular cytotoxicity potentials of malignant and non-malignant lymphocyte subsets and the effect of a-interferon, *Leuk. Res.,* 5, 349, 1981.
147. **Pandolfi, F., Strong, D., Slease, R., Smith, M., Ortaldo, J., and Herberman, R.,** Characterization of a suppressor T-cell chronic lymphocytic leukemia with ADCC but not NK activity, *Blood,* 56, 653, 1980.
148. **Hooks, J., Haynes, B., Detrick-Hooks, B., Diehl, L., Gerrard, T., and Fauci, A.,** Gamma (immune) interferon production by leukocytes from a patient with a T_G cell proliferative disease, *Blood,* 59, 198, 1982.
149. **Gupta, S. and Fernandes, G.,** Natural killing and antibody-dependent cytotoxicity by T leukaemic blasts from acute lymphoblastic leukaemia, *Scand. J. Immunol.,* 16, 477, 1982.
150. **Nasrallah, A. and Miale, T.,** Decreased natural killer cell activity in children with untreated acute leukemia, *Cancer Res.,* 43, 5580, 1983.

151. **Lotzova, E., McCredie, K. B., Maroun, J. A., Dicke, K. A., and Freireich, E. J.,** Some studies on natural killer cells in man, *Transplant. Proc.*, 11, 1390, 1979.
152. **Fernandes, G., Garrett, T., Madhavan, N., Straus, D., Good, R., and Gupta, S.,** Studies in acute leukemia. I. Antibody-dependent and spontaneous cellular cytotoxicity by leukemic blasts from patients with acute nonlymphoid leukemia, *Blood*, 54, 573, 1979.
153. **Ruco, L., Procopio, A., Maccallini, V., Calogero, A., Uccini, S., Annino, L., Mandelli, F., and Baroni, C.,** Severe deficiency of natural killer activity in the peripheral blood of patients with hairy cell leukemia, *Blood*, 61, 1132, 1983.
154. **Steinhauer, E. H., Doyle, A. T., Reed, J., and Kadish, A. S.,** Deficient NKCF production in patients with advanced cancer, *J. Natl. Cancer Inst.*, in press.

Chapter 3

IMPAIRED NK CELL PROFILE IN LEUKEMIA PATIENTS

Eva Lotzová, Cherylyn A. Savary, and Ronald B. Herberman

TABLE OF CONTENTS

I. INTRODUCTION

The phenomenon of natural resistance to hemopoietic malignancies was described more than 2 decades ago in the murine experimental model.[1,2] Natural resistance was manifested by lower incidence and reduced growth rate of parental leukemia-lymphoma tumors after transplantation into F_1 hybrid recipients in comparison to the optimal growth of the same tumors upon transplantation into syngeneic mice. Because of its (at that time) obscure immunogenetics,[3] this phenomenon was considered as an exception to the rules of transplantation, and had not received well-deserved attention. The interest in natural resistance was rejuvenated with the discovery of murine natural killer (NK) cells,[4—6] which phenotypically and functionally resembled effector cells involved in antileukemia resistance in vivo.[7] The development of less intricate in vitro cytotoxic assays allowed more precise characterization of NK cells and revealed their close relationship with the effector cells operating in natural resistance against normal and malignant hemopoietic cells.[8—11] These observations, together with the demonstration that strains of mice with low NK cell activity experience a high incidence of leukemias, and that leukemia rarely occurs in high NK cells responding mouse strains,[6] strongly indicated the role of NK cells in defense against leukemia. This premise was further substantiated by the existence of NK cells in man[6,12—14] and several other species,[15] the exquisite sensitivity of tumors of leukemia-lymphoma origin to NK cell killing, and the high risk of the individuals with NK cell defects to malignant diseases, primarily to those of lymphoma-leukemia type. The group of individuals with low NK cell cytotoxic status and high susceptibility to hemopoietic malignancies is exemplified by patients with Chediak-Higashi syndrome,[16] X-linked lymphoproliferative or combined immunodeficiency syndrome,[17] systemic lupus erythematosus,[18] paroxysmal nocturnal hemoglobinuria,[19,20] Sjögren's syndrome,[21] and allogeneic kidney graft recipients with drug induced, long-term NK cell depletion[17] (Table 1). Additionally, NK cell deficiency was detected in patients with various types of leukemia.[22,23] it can be argued that in the leukemic patients, NK cell defect may be a consequence rather than the cause of leukemic disease. However, the observation that patients with preleukemic disorder also display inferior NK cell cytotoxic potential supports the latter possibility.[24] It is interesting to note that patients with chronic lymphocytic leukemia (CLL) who are NK cell deficient experience a high frequency of secondary malignancies, such as histiocytic lymphomas (3 to 10% of CLL patients)[25] and skin cancers (the incidence of the latter cancer is eightfold increased in CLL patients in comparison to the normal population).[26] This suggests that higher tumor incidence in CLL patients may be related to NK cell deficiency.

In the context with the possible role of NK cells in immune surveillance against leukemia, it is important to discern the possible connection between low NK cell cytotoxic activity in bone marrow and origination of leukemia in this tissue. Experimental animal data indicate that NK cells are dependent on bone marrow not only for their origin, but most likely also for their adequate differentiation and maturation.[27] However, the fully mature, cytolytically competent NK cells are present in quite a low frequency in this tissue.[22,27—28] Thus, it is plausible to postulate that the low NK cell activity in bone marrow may be responsible for the failure of the surveillance mechanism against leukemia. As a consequence of the failure of the primary leukemia surveillance mechanism, the metastasis of leukemic cells to the peripheral blood and other organs may occur. Furthermore, leukemia-caused disturbances in bone marrow (the tissue critical for NK cell origin and differentiation) may lead to insufficient NK cell production and improper NK cell differentiation. Such complications may contribute to a suboptimal supply of NK cells to other organs, the phenomenon leading to diminished defense against already-onset leukemic disease. The situation becomes even more complex when the recently demonstrated role of NK cells in the regulation of human

Table 1
ASSOCIATION BETWEEN NK CELL CYTOTOXIC DEFECT AND HIGH-RISK GROUP OF PATIENTS TO HEMOPOIETIC MALIGNANCIES

Primary malignancies
Chediak-Higashi syndrome
X-Linked lymphoproliferative syndrome
Combined immunodeficiency syndrome
Systemic lupus erythematosus
Paroxysmal nocturnal hemoglobinuria
Sjögren's syndrome
Preleukemic disorders
Allogeneic kidney graft recipients
Secondary malignancies
Histiocytic lymphomas
Skin cancers

and animal hemopoiesis and lymphopoiesis,[29—31] is taken into consideration. In this connection, qualitative and/or quantitative changes in NK cells may lead to aberrant control of growth and differentiation of various components of the hemopoietic and lymphoid system, and may directly or indirectly contribute to leukemic disease prior to or after its onset.

The implication of NK cells in defense against leukemia and in regulation of hemopoiesis and lymphopoiesis (the leukemia-related phenomenon) triggered our interest in studies concerning the cytotoxic profile of NK cells in patients with hemopoietic malignancies. This chapter is designed to summarize the current status of NK cell-mediated cytotoxicity (NK CMC) in individuals with various type of leukemia, to analyze the mechanism of NK cell defect(s) in leukemic patients, and finally, to entertain the possible therapeutic role of NK cells in the treatment of leukemic disease.

II. NK CELL CYTOTOXIC PROFILE IN PATIENTS WITH VARIOUS TYPES OF LEUKEMIA

In contrast to the multitude of investigations on NK cell cytotoxicity in patients with solid cancers, studies of the NK cell cytotoxic profile in patients with leukemia are relatively infrequent. We demonstrated in 1979 that patients with acute and chronic myeloid leukemia (AML and CML, respectively) displayed a defect in peripheral blood and bone marrow NK cell activity against the NK cell-sensitive target cell lines, K562 and CEM.[22,28] We have recently expanded our studies to patients with chronic and acute lymphocytic leukemia (CLL and ALL, respectively), and similar to other investigators,[32—35] have found that these groups of leukemia-diseased patients also displayed deficient NK cell activity. In addition to a NK cell defect, leukemic patients were found to display an impairment in antibody dependent cell-mediated cytotoxicity (ADCC),[32—35] which is not surprising in view of the close relationship or identity of effector cells mediating these two phenomena.[36]

As indicated in Figure 1, and as reported previously,[23,37] the majority of the normal donors belong to the high and medium NK cell responder classes (48 and 42%, respectively, out of 77 normal donors tested). Only a minority (10%) of the normal donor population displayed low NK cell responder status. In contrast, the mean percent of NK cell cytotoxicity of patients with all types of leukemia (with the exception of patients with ALL) falls below the cytotoxicity levels displayed by low NK responding normal individuals. Dissection of

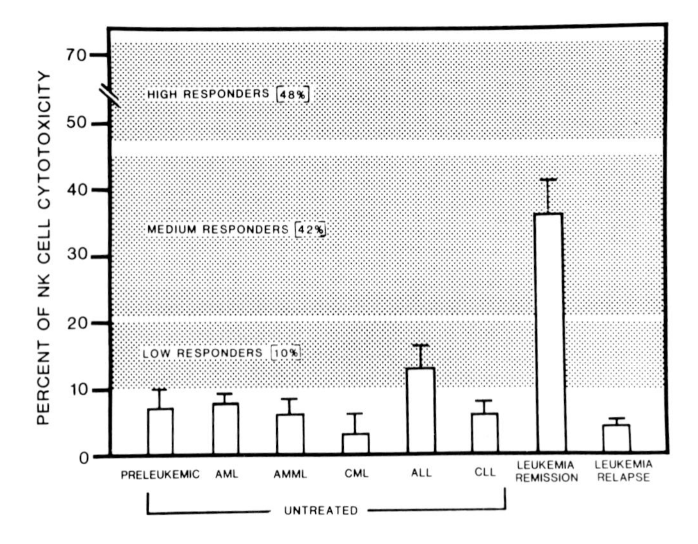

FIGURE 1. NK cell cytotoxic profile of leukemic patients. Shaded area represents the range of NK cell cytotoxicity levels of Ficoll-Hypaque separated peripheral blood mononuclear cells of 77 normal donors. The brackets indicate the percent of normal donors with high, medium, and low NK cell phenotype. The open columns represent the mean percent of cytotoxicity ± standard error (vertical lines) of leukemic patients (5 to 22 patients were tested in each group). NK cell activity was measured in a 3-hr ^{51}Cr-release assay (1:50 T:E cell ratio) against the K562 cell line. All leukemic patients were either untreated or were treatment-free for at least 3 weeks prior to the NK test (remission and relapse). There was a statistically significant difference ($p < 0.005$ to <0.05) between leukemic patients and low-responding normal individuals, with the exception of the ALL group, as determined by Student's *t*-test.

levels of NK cell cytotoxicity of female and male patients with AML showed that even though both of these groups of patients exhibited low NK cell potential, the females' NK cell cytotoxicity against the K562 cell lines was consistently lower (Table 2). This observation is compatible with that in a normal donor population demonstrating a lower NK cell cytotoxicity profile in females than in males.[38] Whether the lower NK cell activity in female patients is related to the levels of estrogen, which has been reported to decrease NK cell cytotoxic potential,[39] remains to be determined.

It is important to mention that NK cell cytotoxic potential is restored in leukemic patients in remission[22,28,40,41] (Figure 1). This observation indicates that the NK cell defect in leukemia-diseased patients is acquired rather than intrinsic. It has to be noted that some of the investigators reported low ADCC and NK cell activity in AML patients in remission.[42,43] However, from these studies it appears that the depression of NK cell and ADCC functions was related to chemotherapy. This statement is based on the observation that progressive recovery of ADCC occurred 3 to 4 weeks following each cycle of chemotherapy.[43]

Figure 1 also illustrates that NK cell cytotoxicity significantly declines in relapse of leukemia. The latter observation raises the clinically relevant question as to whether NK cells could provide a prognostic tool for relapse of leukemic disease prior to its clinical manifestation and diagnosis. It is apparent that such early diagnosis of leukemia relapse might lead to less aggressive treatment of this disease.

Table 2
COMPARISON OF NK ACTIVITY OF FEMALE AND MALE PATIENTS WITH AML

T:E cell ratio	Percent cytotoxicity[a]		
	Females	Males	*p* value[b]
1:6	0.3 ± 0.2	3.1 ± 0.4	<0.02
1:12	1.9 ± 0.9	4.6 ± 0.8	<0.05
1:25	2.3 ± 1.1	8.8 ± 1.7	<0.01
1:50	4.4 ± 2.0	10.8 ± 1.7	<0.02

[a] Cytotoxicity of Ficoll-Hypaqued peripheral blood of 9 female and 12 male patients was tested in a 3-hr ^{51}Cr-release assay against K562 target.

[b] As analyzed by a Student's *t*-test, there was a significant difference between cytotoxicity of male and female patients at all T:E cell ratios.

III. MECHANISM OF DEFECTIVE NK CELL CYTOTOXICITY IN PATIENTS WITH LEUKEMIA

A. Role of Leukemic Cells in Deficient NK Cell Cytotoxicity

Most of the studies on the mechanism of NK cell cytotoxicity are in agreement that the deficient NK cell activity in leukemic patients could not be attributed to the dilution of effector cells by leukemic blasts. For instance, in the studies of Ziegler et al.,[33] the NK cell defect in CLL patients persisted even after separation of effector lymphocytes from malignant B cells by sheep red blood cell (SRBC) rosette formation, and/or by depletion of the leukemic cells with a monoclonal antibody and complement. Moreover, the inability of leukemic cells to prevent the lysis of K562 target cells in cold target competition experiments indicated the failure of leukemic cells to interfere with the cytotoxic mechanism.[33,34] Another argument against dilution of effector cells by leukemic blasts, as a mechanism of low NK cell cytotoxicity of CLL patients, is that an increase in target-to-effector (T:E) cell ratios did not result in an increase in NK and ADCC activities.[32,34]

We have also explored the possibility of dilution of NK cells by leukemic blasts as the factor responsible for impaired cytotoxicity of patients with myelogenous leukemia. First, we correlated NK cell cytotoxicity levels with the content of blast cells and/or lymphocytes in patients' peripheral blood. No direct correlation was detected; the NK cell cytotoxicity was low also in patients with a high content of lymphocytes and virtually no blast cells in peripheral blood (Figure 2). Second, in agreement with the other investigators,[32,34] no significant increase in NK cell cytotoxicity was observed by increasing the T:E cell ratio (Figure 3). Third, the aberrant slopes of the NK cell dose-response curve of leukemic patients (in comparison to the slopes of normal donors) argued against NK cell dilution by leukemic blasts. If NK cell dilution alone was responsible for inferior cytotoxicity, lower but parallel slopes of the dose-response curve of leukemic patients would be expected.

Furthermore, we investigated the putative suppressive effect of allogeneic blasts on NK cell cytotoxicity of normal donors. This possibility was examined in mixing experiments of peripheral blood lymphocytes (PBLs) of leukemic patients and normal donors. Figure 4 illustrates that no inhibition of normal donors' NK cell cytotoxicity was detected under these experimental conditions. However, these experiments, even though suggestive, do not prove unequivocally that blast cells do not inhibit NK cell cytotoxicity in leukemia patients in vivo, since histocompatibility between effector cells and leukemic cells may be required for

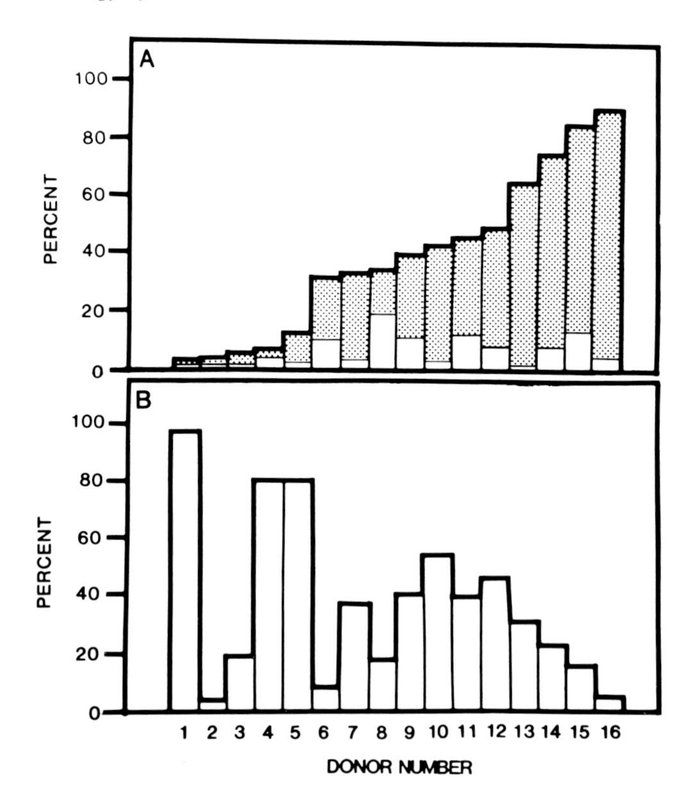

FIGURE 2. Lack of correlation between content of leukemic blasts or lymphocytes and NK cell cytotoxicity in AML patients. NK cell cytotoxicity (□) of Ficoll-Hypaqued peripheral blood of patients with myeloid leukemia was tested in a 3-hr ^{51}Cr-release assay against the K562 cell line at 1:50 T:E cell ratio (A). Blast cell content (▩) was evaluated by morphological analysis of May-Grünwald- and Giemsa-stained cytocentrifuge slides (A). Percentage of lymphocytes in the peripheral blood of leukemic patients is illustrated in (B).

optimal interaction. Similar to our studies, the lack of inhibition of anti-K562-directed cytotoxicity of normal PBLs by cryopreserved blast cells obtained from AML and ALL patients was observed by another group of investigators.[44] Interestingly, in contrast to the cryopreserved leukemic cells, the leukemia cell lines were effective in inhibiting NK cell activity in the latter studies.

B. Characterization of NK Effector Cells in Leukemic Patients

The studies on the characterization of peripheral blood effector cells displaying impaired cytotoxic potential are sporadic and to some degree controversial. One group of investigators reported that whereas both T and non-T effector cells (characterized by their capacity to form rosettes with SRBCs) of normal donors mediated NK cell and ADCC activity, neither of these lymphocyte populations of CLL patients displayed NK cell or ADCC functions.[34] In contrast with this report are the studies of Hokland and Ellegaard[35] reporting the cytotoxic defect of patients with CLL (especially that of ADCC function) primarily in the non-T cell fraction of PBLs. Moreover, correlative studies between the NK cell surface phenotype of PBLs and the NK cell cytotoxic profile of CLL patients indicated an NK cell defect in subpopulations of lymphocytes expressing receptors for the Fc portion of IgG and reactive with OKT11A and OKM1 antibody.[45]

More recently, most of the peripheral blood NK cell activity has been shown to be

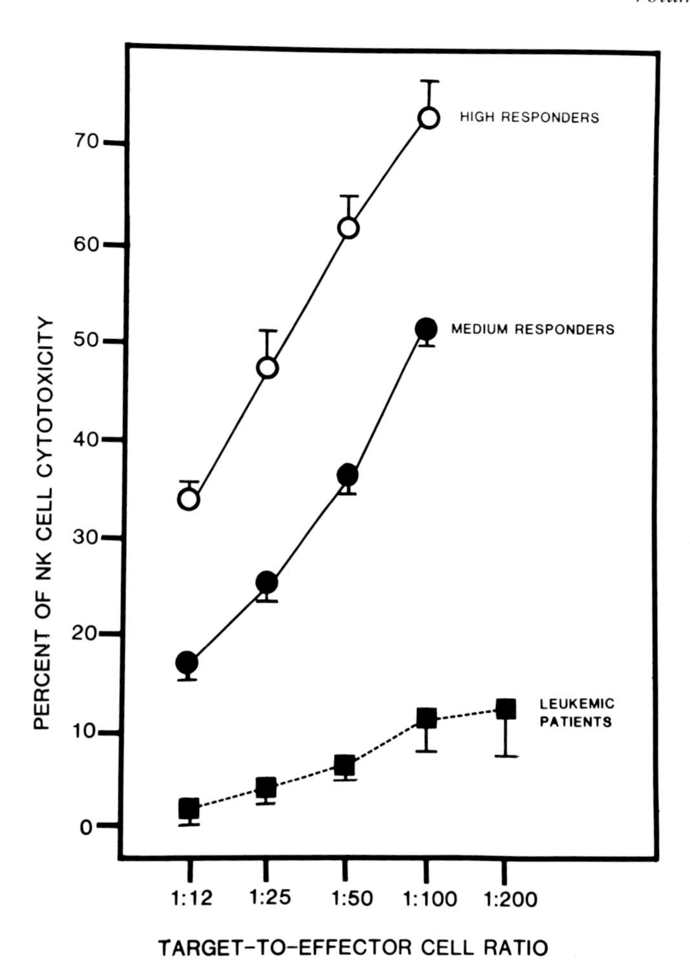

FIGURE 3. NK cell dose-response curves of normal individuals and leukemia-diseased patients. Symbols represent the mean percent of Ficoll-Hypaqued peripheral blood NK cell cytotoxicity ± S.E. of 18 normal individuals (○, 7 high and ●, 11 medium responders), and 20 untreated patients with leukemia (■, 9 AML, 5 ALL, 3 AMML, 2 CML, and 1 CLL). Cytotoxicity to K562 was measured in a 3-hr ^{51}Cr-release assay. As evaluated by the analysis of covariance, the slope of dose-response curve of leukemic patients (13.1) was significantly different ($p<0.001$) from the slopes of high (41.3) and medium (33.8) NK cell responding normal donors. The slopes were calculated by linear regression analysis and the corresponding correlation coefficients (r) were 0.60, 0.67, and 0.78, for leukemic patients and high and medium normal donors, respectively.

associated with a subpopulation of lymphoid cells designated large granular lymphocytes (LGLs), characterized morphologically by a reniform nucleus, a low nucleus to cytoplasm ratio, and cytoplasmic azurophilic granules.[46] It has been shown earlier that the morphological changes in LGL granulation were associated with impaired NK cell activity in Chediak-Higashi patients.[16] Analyses of LGL patterns in patients with CLL also revealed a defect in LGL granulation.[45] Specifically, the effector cells with impaired NK cell activity were found to be phenotypically (FcR positive, and reactive with OKT11A, 9.6, and OKM1 antibody)[45,47] and morphologically similar to normal donors' NK cells; however, they exhibited defective azurophilic granulation.[45] More than 75% of these cells of CLL patients had no obvious

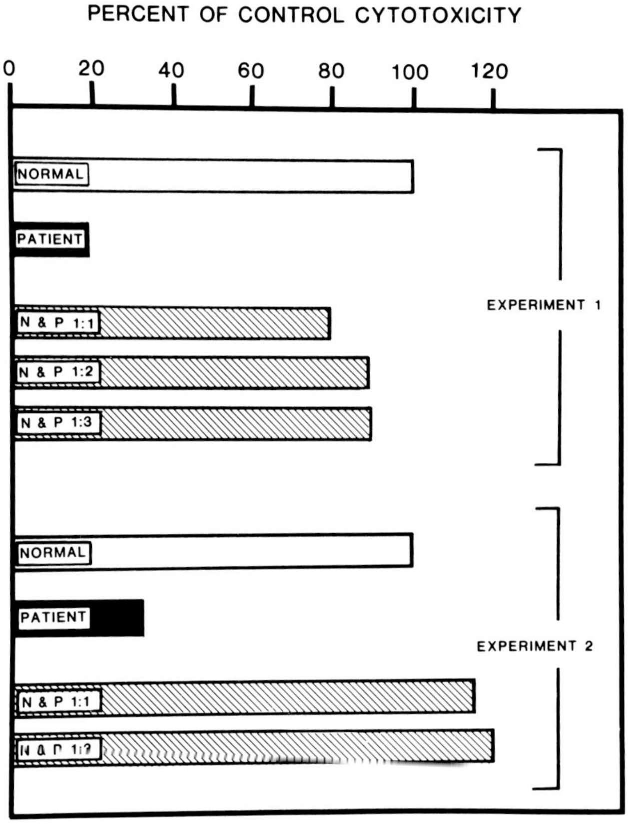

FIGURE 4. Lack of inhibition of NK cell cytotoxicity of normal donors by leukemic blast cells. Ficoll-Hypaqued peripheral blood of one AML (experiment 1) and one ALL (experiment 2) patient and two normal donors were evaluated for NK cell cytotoxicity either alone (1:50 T:E cell ratio) or in mixtures consisting of normal donor and leukemic patients' peripheral blood. The normal donor to leukemia patient effector cell ratio was 1:1, 1:2, and 1:3. Cytotoxicity was measured in a 3-hr ^{51}Cr-release assay against the K562 target cell line, and is expressed as the percent of control cytotoxicity.

azurophilic granules. Since the granules were implicated in NK cell cytolytic function,[48-51] the absence of cytoplasmic azurophilic granules could be responsible for impaired NK cell activity of CLL patients. The role of azurophilic granules in the LGL cytotoxic mechanism is indicated by the observation that degranulation of LGLs by strontium was followed by a loss of NK cell activity and conversely, NK cell activity was regained with reacquisition of azurophilic granules.[48,49]

We also investigated in our laboratory the relationship between NK cell cytotoxicity and LGL characteristics (morphology and content) in patients with myeloid and lymphoid leukemias. In the first series of studies, we examined the correlation between NK cell cytotoxicity and LGL content of Ficoll-Hypaqued and/or nylon wool (NW)-filtered peripheral blood of normal donors and leukemic patients (Figures 5 and 6). Whereas significant differences in NK cell cytotoxicity were observed among low, medium and high NK cell responding normal donors in Ficoll-Hypaqued peripheral blood samples, no differences in LGL content were seen among these three categories of NK cell responders. The ranges of LGLs were 3.5 to 13.5%, 2 to 38.5%, and 5 to 21% in low, medium and high NK cell responding normal donors, respectively (Figure 5). In the majority of normal donors, a slight

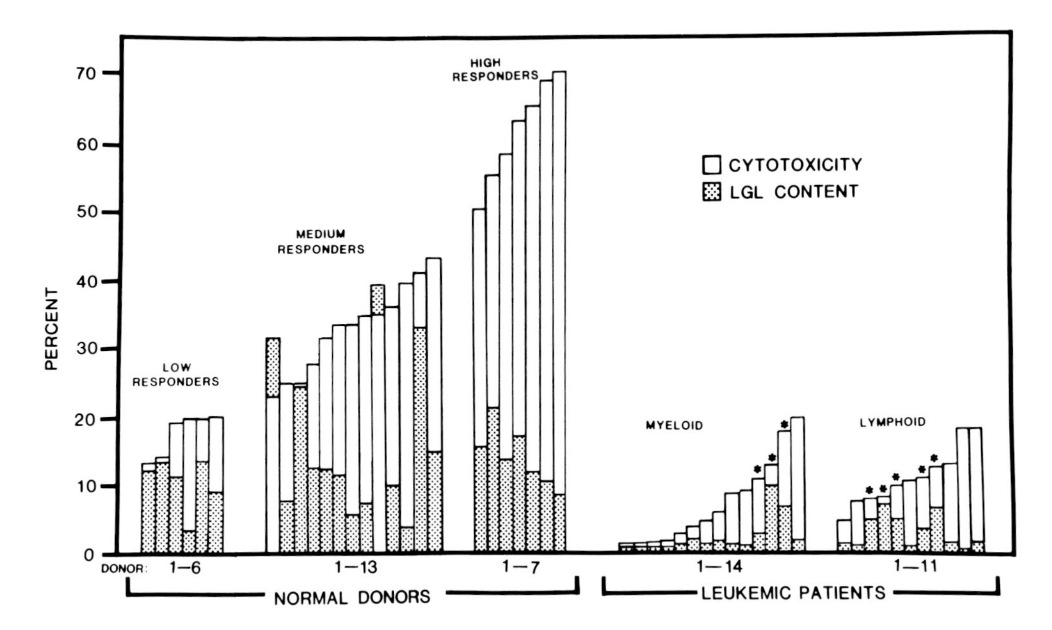

FIGURE 5. Comparison between NK cell cytotoxicity and LGL content of Ficoll-Hypaqued peripheral blood of normal donors and leukemic patients. NK cell cytotoxicity (□) against the K562 was measured in a 3-hr ^{51}Cr-release assay (1:50 T:E cell ratio). The content of LGL (▩) was evaluated by analysis of May-Grünwald- and Giemsa-stained cytocentrifuge slides. Patients with myeloid leukemia included: 2 CML (No. 1 and 3), 1 AMML (No. 7), 1 APL (No. 13), and 10 AML patients (No. 2, 4—6, 8—12, and 14); patients with lymphoid leukemia were composed of 10 ALL (No. 1—5 and 7—11), and 1 CLL (No. 6). Asterisks indicate the leukemic patients with the LGL content within the range of normal donors. As evaluated by Student's *t*-test, there was a significant difference in NK cell cytotoxicity of low, medium, and high NK cell responders (p values <0.001 to <0.02), and between all categories of normal donors and leukemic patients ($p<0.001$ to 0.005). No significant differences were observed in LGL content among normal donor population, however, most of the patients displayed decrease in percent of LGL ($p<0.01$).

(but not statistically significant) increase in NK cell cytotoxicity and LGL content was achieved after NW filtration (Figure 6).

Patients with myeloid and lymphoid leukemia exhibited low levels of NK cell cytotoxicity in Ficoll-Hypaqued peripheral blood (Figure 5). Most of these patients (68%) also had a low LGL content, below that of normal donors; the range of LGLs was <0.1 to 9.2% and <0.1 to 6% in patients with myeloid and lymphoid leukemia, respectively. No changes in NK cell cytotoxicity of leukemic patients were noted after NW filtration; however, a moderate even though statistically significant increase in LGL content was evident in both groups of patients (Figure 6). Hence, neither in the normal donor population nor in patients was a correlation between LGL content and the degree of NK cell cytotoxicity detected.

The results of these studies indicate that the low LGL content found in some (but not in all) patients with leukemia may be responsible for the NK cell cytotoxic defect in a certain proportion of these patients. the fact that 32% of leukemic patients displayed low NK cell cytotoxicity in spite of relatively high levels of LGLs (as high as 18%), however, indicates that in the latter group of patients the defect in LGL lytic machinery may underlie the low NK cell cytotoxic potential.

To further investigate the involvement of LGLs in NK cell cytotoxicity of leukemic patients, we separated LGLs on discontinuous Percoll density gradients and analyzed individual fractions for cytotoxicity and LGL content. Two types of Percoll gradients were used in these studies: the Percoll gradient as described by Timonen et al.[46] and a gradient modified by the addition of two lighter Percoll densities. The lighter gradient was employed in order to remove the majority of leukemic cells from peripheral blood samples. Four

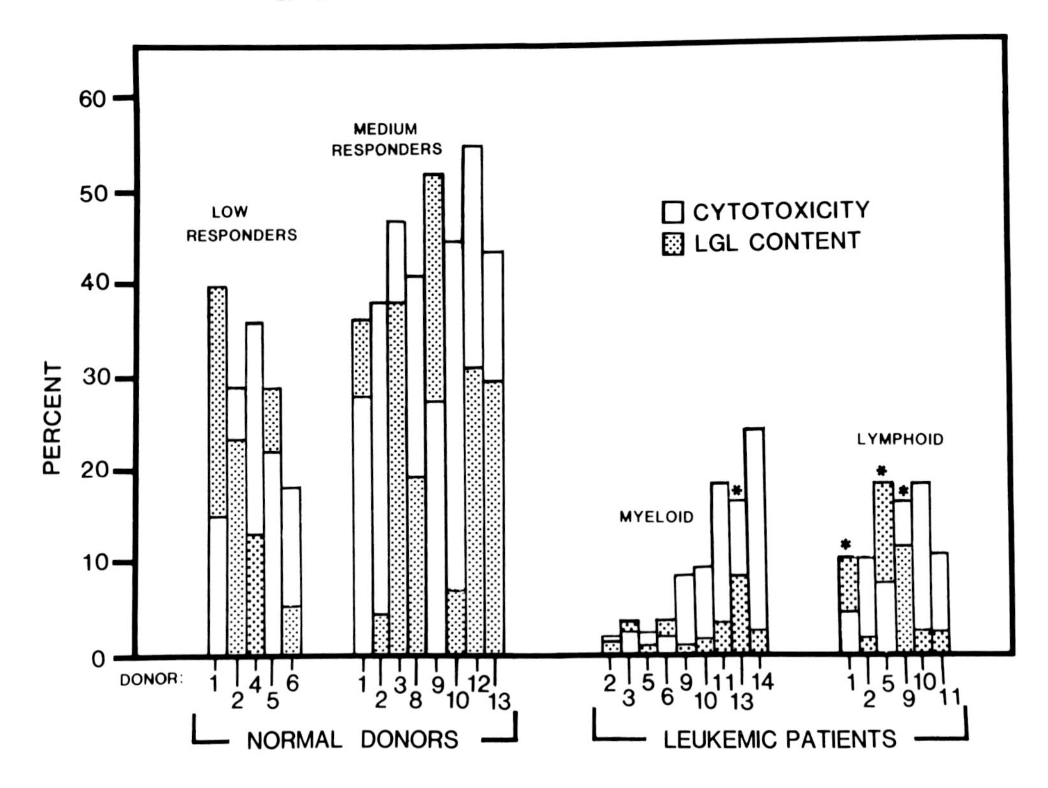

FIGURE 6. Comparison of NK cell cytotoxic potential and LGL content of NW-filtered peripheral blood of normal donors and leukemic patients. NK cell cytotoxicity (□) was measured and the content of LGL (▩) was evaluated as indicated in Figure 5. The numbers of normal donors and patients correspond to those indicated in Figure 5. Asterisks indicate the leukemic patients with LGL content within the range of normal donors. As analyzed by a paired *t*-test, there was a significant increase in the LGL content of peripheral blood effector cells of myeloid ($p<0.02$) and lymphoid ($p<0.05$) leukemic patients, following NW filtration.

patients and three normal donors were analyzed in parallel. The patient population included one patient with hairy cell leukemia (HCL) (Figure 7), one with ALL (Figure 8), and 2 patients with AML (Figure 9). It can be seen from Figure 7 that the maximum enrichment of normal donor peripheral blood NK cell cytotoxicity and LGL content (approximately threefold) was achieved in fraction 3 of the Percoll gradient. A more modest, even though significant, increase in LGL content (from 1.0% to 20%) and NK cell cytotoxicity (from 4 to 15%) was also observed in the same fraction of the HCL patient. This study demonstrates a close relationship between LGL content and NK cell cytotoxicity in both normal donor and HCL patient, and furthermore suggests that the low numbers of LGLs may have been responsible for the defective NK cell cytotoxicity of this patient. The separation of patients' and normal donors' LGLs in the same fraction of the Percoll gradient indicates that the LGLs are of the same (light) density.

A different relationship between LGL content and NK cell cytotoxicity was seen in the ALL patient (Figure 8). The latter patient had a low LGL content in the NW-filtered fraction of peripheral blood (4%). However, after separation of effector cells on the modified Percoll gradient and furthermore, after removal of the population of lymphocytes forming rosettes with SRBC,[46] dramatic enrichment of LGLs (to 60%) was achieved in the pooled sample of fractions 1 and 2. The enrichment of LGLs in this patient was comparable to that of a normal donor studied under the same conditions (Figure 8). However, in contrast to the normal donor, whose LGL enrichment was paralleled by augmentation of NK cell cytotoxicity (two to threefold), virtually no cytotoxic activity (6%) was displayed in the LGL-rich fractions

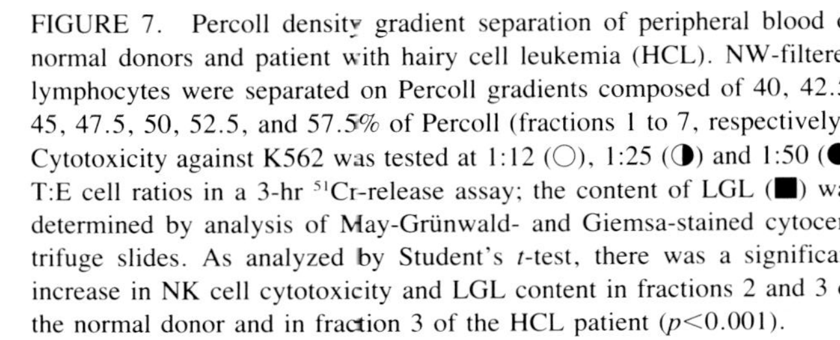

FIGURE 7. Percoll density gradient separation of peripheral blood of normal donors and patient with hairy cell leukemia (HCL). NW-filtered lymphocytes were separated on Percoll gradients composed of 40, 42.5, 45, 47.5, 50, 52.5, and 57.5% of Percoll (fractions 1 to 7, respectively). Cytotoxicity against K562 was tested at 1:12 (○), 1:25 (◑) and 1:50 (●) T:E cell ratios in a 3-hr ^{51}Cr-release assay; the content of LGL (■) was determined by analysis of May-Grünwald- and Giemsa-stained cytocentrifuge slides. As analyzed by Student's *t*-test, there was a significant increase in NK cell cytotoxicity and LGL content in fractions 2 and 3 of the normal donor and in fraction 3 of the HCL patient ($p<0.001$).

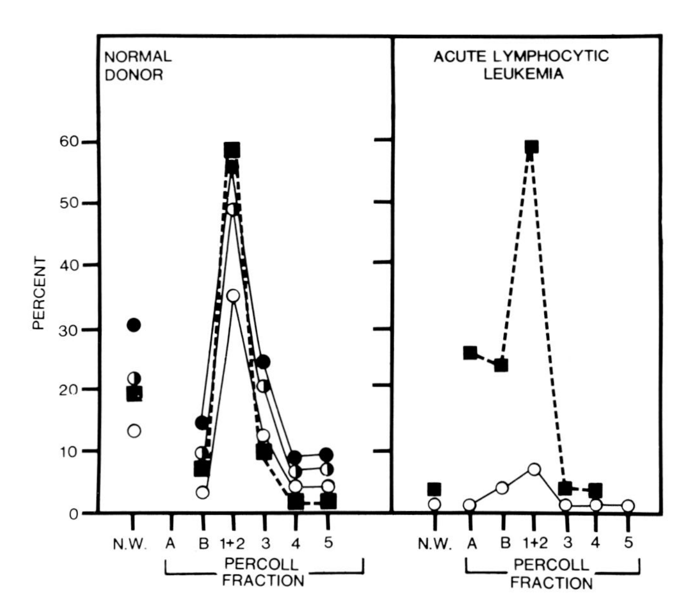

FIGURE 8. Percoll density gradient separation of peripheral blood of normal donor and ALL patient. NW-filtered cells were separated on Percoll gradients composed of 35, 37.5 (fractions A, B), 40, 42.5, 45, 47.5, and 50% of Percoll (fractions 1 to 5). Fractions 1 and 2 were pooled and depleted of high-affinity SRBC-forming rosettes.[46] NK cell cytotoxicity was measured against the K562 target cell line (○ 1:6, ◑ 1:12; ● 1:25 T:E cell ratios), and LGL content (■) was evaluated as indicated in legend of Figure 7. As analyzed by a Student's *t*-test, there was a significant increase in the NK cell cytotoxicity ($p<0.001$) in fractions 1 and 2 of the normal donor, and in the LGL content of both normal donor and ALL patient.

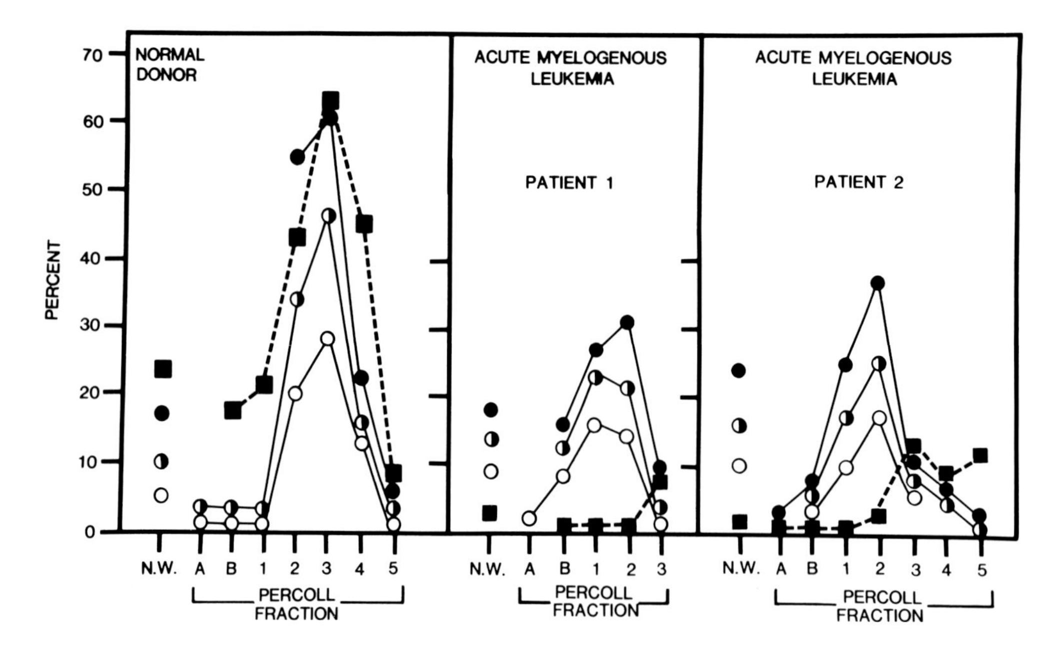

FIGURE 9. Percoll density gradient separation of peripheral blood of normal donor and two AML patients. Separation of NW-filtered lymphocytes on Percoll gradient, and evaluation of NK cell cytotoxicity to K562 (○ 1:12, ◑ 1:25, ● 1:50 T:E cell ratios), and LGL content (■) was performed as indicated in legend of Figure 7. As analyzed by a Student's *t*-test, there was a significant increase in NK cell cytotoxicity in fractions 2 and 3 in the normal donor, in fraction 1 and 2 in patient 1, and in fraction 2 in patient 2 ($p<0.001$).

of the ALL patient. The lack of augmentation of NK cell cytotoxicity in LGL-enriched fractions of the ALL patient could not be explained by interference of the leukemic cells with NK cell cytotoxicity, since fractions 1 and 2 contained only 2% leukemic cells. The results of this study indicate that LGLs of ALL patient are of the same physical characteristics as LGLs of normal donors, but are defective in their lytic machinery.

An inverse relationship between LGL content and NK cell cytotoxic potential was observed in the third group of patients, i.e., those with AML (Figure 9). In these patients a slight enrichment in LGL content was obtained in fractions 3 to 5 of both patients (from 3 to 8% in patient 1, and from 2 to 12% in patient 2), the fractions with low NK cell cytotoxicity. In contrast, cytotoxicity was significantly increased in fractions 1 and 2 of patient 1 and in fraction 2 of patient 2 (1.5- to 1.7-fold in both patients), the fractions containing practically no LGLs. In the normal donor tested in the same experiment, the highest content of LGLs was found in the fraction exhibiting the highest cytotoxicity (Figure 9). As will be discussed below, leukemic cells of some patients may mediate cytotoxicity against K562 target cells. To determine whether leukemic blasts could account for the cytotoxicity by the LGL-poor fraction of the AML patient, we evaluated each Percoll fraction for its content of leukemic blasts. Since only 7.5% of leukemic blasts were found to be present in the NK active fraction (fraction 2) and 75 to 78% of blasts in fractions displaying low NK cell activity (fractions A and B) of AML patients, the leukemic blasts were most likely not involved in the cytotoxicity phenomenon. Thus, in some of the AML patients, NK cell cytotoxicity may be mediated by effector cells morphologically distinct from LGLs. In summary, three different patterns of NK cell cytotoxicity and LGL content were detected in leukemic patients: the first pattern was found in an HCL patient and was manifested by the correlation between low LGL content and low NK cell cytotoxicity in peripheral blood. Furthermore, both LGL content and cytotoxic potential were moderately augmented after Percoll gradient separation. This pattern suggests that the low numbers of LGLs may be responsible for inferior NK cell cytotoxicty in this patient.

The second pattern was exemplified by the lack of correlation between LGL content and NK cell cytotoxicity in the peripheral blood of an ALL patient. This was represented by the lack of NK cell activity in the Percoll fraction highly enriched for LGLs. Additionally, no significant levels of NK cell cytotoxicity were seen in any other fraction of the Percoll gradient in this patient. This pattern indicates that the NK cell defect may reside in the cytotoxic mechanism of the LGLs.

The third pattern was identified in AML patients and consisted of relatively high NK cell activity in Percoll fractions with virtually no LGLs. Moreover, the lowest NK cell activity was noted in moderately LGL-enriched Percoll fractions. This pattern indicates that effector cells other than LGLs may have been involved in the cytotoxicity of these patients. It is evident from these studies that inferior NK cell activity in various groups of patients with leukemia may be mediated by different mechanisms.

We have also analyzed the morphological profile of LGLs on May-Grünwald- and Giemsa-stained cytocentrifuge slides. In general, we observed that the majority of LGLs in normal individuals have large, and the minority have subtle, azurophilic granules. The LGLs of leukemic patients showed two types of granulation: the patients with AML displayed predominantly small numbers of granules which were, however, of quite large size and the patients with ALL and AMML exhibited numerous granules of a subtle type (Plate 1).* Whether these patterns of cytoplasmic azurophilic LGL granulation truly reflect the AML and ALL (AMML) disease category has to be confirmed on a larger panel of leukemic patients. Similarly, the relevance of azurophilic granulation to the lytic process of LGLs remains to be determined. The fact, however, that granules were implicated to play a role in the cytotoxic reaction[48—51] suggests that these differences in granulation between normal and leukemia-diseased patients should not be neglected.

The observation that some of the leukemic patients, in spite of the normal LGL content, displayed negligible NK cell cytotoxicity suggested a defect in the NK cell cytotoxic mechanism. Thus, we investigated in detail the various parameters of the cytotoxic mechanism in patients with leukemia and compared these data with those obtained with normal donors.

C. Relationship Between Duration of Cytotoxicity Assay and Expression of NK Cell Activity in Leukemia Patients

Initially, we questioned whether low NK cell cytotoxicity of leukemic patients could be due to the slow kinetics of the cytotoxic reaction rather than to the inability of effector cells to mediate cytotoxicity. To answer this question, we incubated target and effector cells for short (3-hr) and long (16-hr) time intervals. Figure 10 illustrates that a significant increase in NK cell cytotoxicity against the K562 target cell line was observed after 16 hr of incubation (in comparison to 3 hr of incubation) in normal individuals; no such increase was detected in patients with leukemia. This suggested that the inferior NK cell cytotoxicity of leukemic patients was caused by some defect in the NK cell lytic mechanism rather than by a slow development of cytotoxic reactivity.

* Plate 1 can be found after page 46.

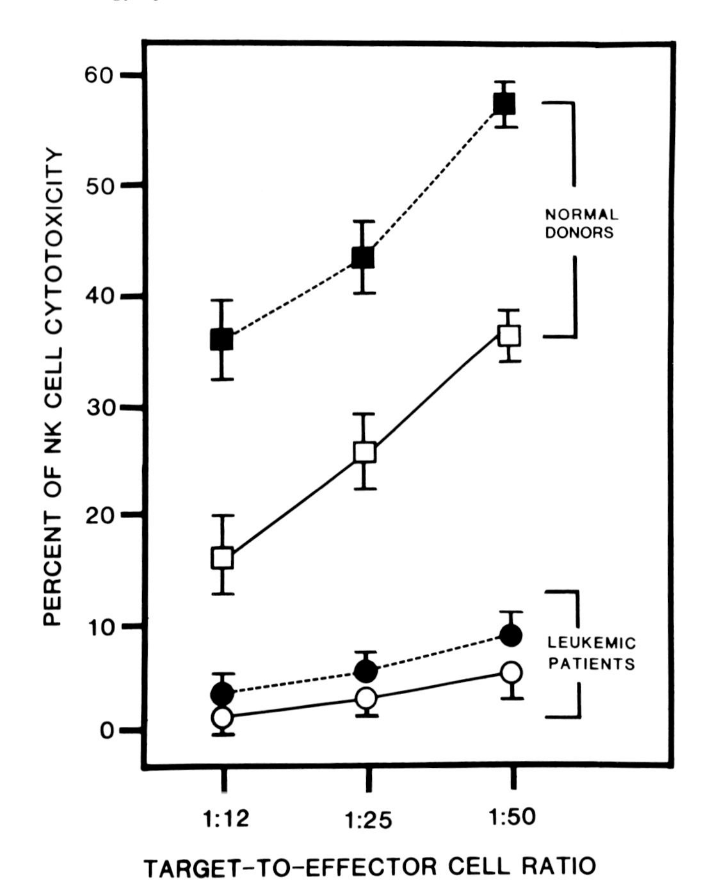

FIGURE 10. Comparison between short- and long-term incubation times and peripheral blood NK cell cytotoxicity of normal donors and leukemic patients. NK cell cytotoxicity against K562 was tested in a 3-hr (—) and 16-hr (---) ^{51}Cr-release assay. Symbols represent the mean percent of cytotoxicity ± S.E. of 11 normal individuals and 19 leukemic patients (9 AML, 3 AMML, 1 CML, 5 ALL, and 1 CLL). There was a statistically significant difference between NK cell cytotoxicity of normal donors tested in 3-hr and 16-hr ^{51}Cr-release assay ($p<0.02$). No difference was found in leukemic patients.

D. Analysis of Maximal Rate of Killing (V_{max}) by NK Cells of Leukemic Patients

It has been shown that the NK cell cytotoxic reaction resembles an enzyme-substrate (NK cell-target cell) interaction, and may be analyzed by the Michaelis-Menten kinetic model.[52] The cytotoxicity under these conditions is expressed as V_{max} and reflects the maximal rate of target cell killing when the system is saturated with target cells, but contains a constant number of effector cells. It is often believed that V_{max} is a more precise expression of NK cell cytotoxic potential than percent lysis. Thus, we used this model to determine V_{max} of peripheral blood NK cells of patients with myeloid and lymphoid leukemia. Normal donors were tested for comparison in these studies.

The results of these experiments showed that the V_{max} of effector cells of all patients with myeloid leukemia and 86% of patients with lymphoid leukemia was significantly lower than that of normal individuals (Table 3). There was no association between V_{max} values and the percent of LGLs or percent of blast cells in the tested peripheral blood samples of leukemia patients (data not shown).

Table 3
MAXIMUM RATE OF LYSIS (V_{max}) BY PBLs OF LEUKEMIC PATIENTS AND NORMAL DONORS

	V_{max} ($\times 10^3$)[a]		
		Leukemic patients[b]	
Donor no.	Normal donors	Myeloid	Lymphoid
1	2.5	0.7	0.2
2	3.0	0.5	1.1
3	3.6	1.3	0.7
4	4.6	0.9	0.4
5	5.9	0.3	3.0
6	7.0	0.1	0.6
7	8.9	0.5	1.4
Mean ± S.E.	5.1 ± 0.9	0.6 ± 0.1[c]	1.1 ± 0.4[c]

[a] NW-filtered effector cells (10^5) were incubated with various concentrations of K562 target cells (ranging from 0.03×10^5 to 1×10^5) for 3 hr in a ^{51}Cr-release assay; V_{max} was determined according to the Michaelis-Menten kinetic model.[52]

[b] Patients with myeloid leukemia included AMML (1), AML (2 to 5), CML (6 and 7), and patients with lymphoid leukemia, hairy cell leukemia (1), and ALL (2 to 7).

[c] As analyzed by a Student's *t*-test, there was a significant decrease in the V_{max} of myeloid ($p<0.001$) and lymphoid ($p<0.002$) leukemic patients.

E. Analysis of NK Cell Lytic Mechanism of Patients with Leukemia

The NK cell cytotoxic mechanism consists of several steps. The first step involves the recognition and binding to the tumor; the second step is the programing for the lysis; the third step is the release of the cytotoxic factor(s) (NKCF); the fourth step is the binding of NKCF to the acceptor site on target cells; the final step is target cell lysis (see Chapter 9, Volume I for more details). Additionally, each NK cell has a recycling capacity, i.e., a capability to kill more than one tumor cell and thus, all of the above-mentioned steps are repeated several times by a single NK cell.

To determine which of the parameters of the effector cell cytotoxic mechanism is impaired in leukemic patients, each step of cytotoxicity was analyzed and compared to normal donors.

1. Evaluation of Tumor Binding Properties, Lytic Capacity, and Frequency of Lytic NK Cells

Using a single cell assay[53] we evaluated the tumor binding capacity (TBC) and tumor lytic capacity (C-TBC) of peripheral blood effector cells from leukemic patients and normal donors. Combining these two assays, the frequency of cytotoxic effector cells was estimated. As indicated in Figure 11, the patients with leukemia exhibited a significantly lower TBC (5.0 ± 0.3 and 3.4 ± 0.4 for myeloid and lymphoid leukemia patients, respectively) and C-TBC (13.8 ± 3.8 and 11.6 ± 2.5 for myeloid and lymphoid leukemia patients, respectively) potential in comparison to TBC (8.4 ± 0.4) and C-TBC (24.8 ± 1.6) of normal donors. Consequently, the frequency of cytotoxic effector cells in the peripheral blood of leukemic patients was three- to fivefold lower than that in the peripheral blood of normal individuals.

To characterize the type of effector cells which bound to K562 target cells, we analyzed

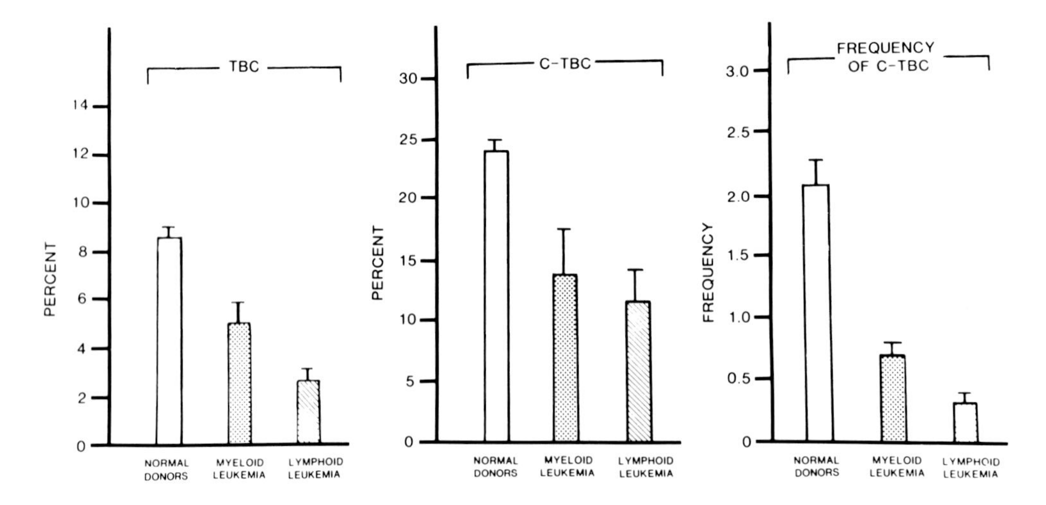

FIGURE 11. Tumor binding and killing capacity, and frequency of peripheral blood NK cells of normal donors and leukemic patients. Percent of TBCs, C-TBCs, and the frequency of C-TBC was tested in a single cell assay.[47] NW-filtered effector cells and the K562 tumor were incubated in 1:1 ratio for 3 hr. Bars represent mean percent of TBC, C-TBC, and frequency of C-TBC ± S.E. of 20 normal donors, 12 patients with myeloid leukemia (7 AML, 2 AMML, 2 APL, and 1 CML), and 9 patients with ALL. As analyzed by a Student's *t*-test, there was a significant decrease in TBC ($p<0.001$ in both groups of patients), C-TBC ($p<0.05$ and $p<0.001$ in myeloid and lymphoid groups, respectively), and frequency of C-TBC ($p<0.001$ in both groups of patients).

the morphology of TBC on Giemsa-stained cytocentrifuge slides as described previously.[46] Figure 12 shows that the percent of TBC was sightly higher using the cytocentrifuge slide technique than in a single cell assay (11.6 ± 1.1 and 7.2 ± 0.7 in normal donors and leukemic patients, respectively). However, both of these techniques showed unequivocally that the TBC potential of leukemic patients was significantly below that of normal donors. Interestingly, in normal donors, most of the TBC (60 to 80%) were of LGL morphology, whereas in leukemic patients only 7 to 33% of TBC were LGLs. Thus, in the leukemic patients the defect in binding is LGL-related. No correlation between blast cells and/or LGL content and TBC potential was observed in the patients' peripheral blood. It is important to note that the non-LGL TBC in normal donor as well as in patient populations was composed of lymphocytes. In some patients (Nos. 2, 3, and 5), however, a significant number of blast cells was found to bind to the tumor.

2. Evaluation of Recycling Capacity of Effector Cells of Patients with Leukemia

As has been indicated above, more than one target cell can be killed by a single NK cell. Such an NK cell recycling property may be analyzed by combining the data obtained from a single cell assay and from a ^{51}Cr-release assay (V_{max}).[54] Using this system, we evaluated the NK cell recycling capacity in the peripheral blood of normal donors and leukemic patients (Table 4). The results of these experiments showed that three out of four patients with myeloid and three out of six patients with lymphoid leukemia exhibited significantly lower recycling capacity than the normal donors. Thus, the inferior NK cell recycling ability illustrates another defect in the cytotoxic mechanism of patients with leukemia.

3. Production of NKCF by Effector Cells of Leukemic Patients

Studies of Bonavida et al.[55] revealed that cytotoxic factor(s) (NKCF) is involved in NK cell-mediated lysis. NKCF is generated after coculture of effector cells with NK cell-sensitive target cells and is effective in destroying the NK cell-susceptible target without any further assistance from effector cells. In contrast, the control supernatant generated after incubation

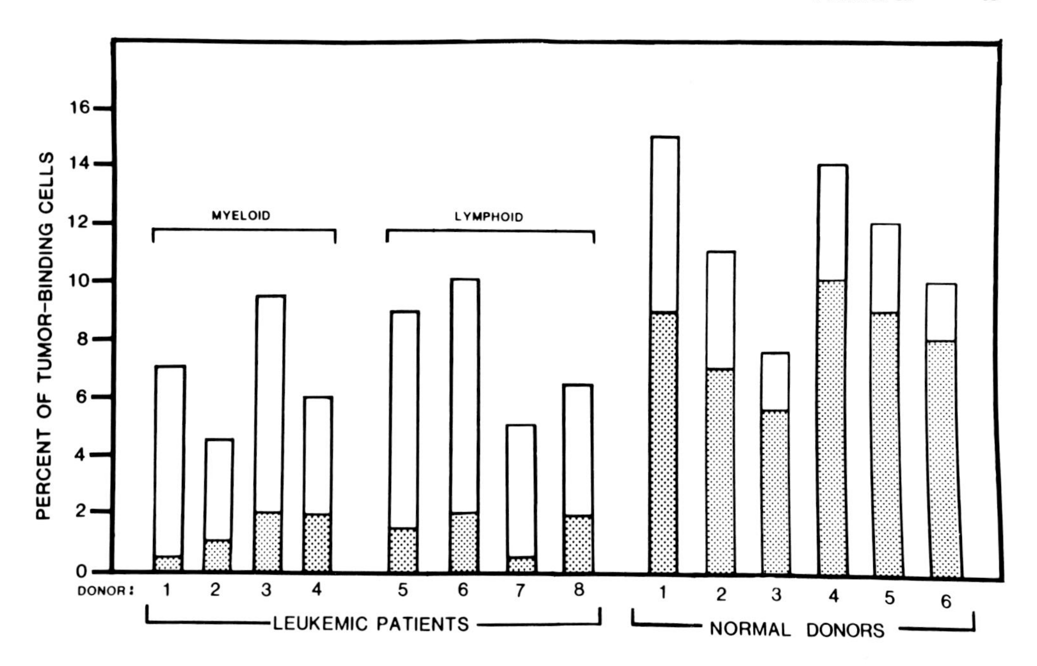

FIGURE 12. Morphological analysis of TBCs in peripheral blood of normal individuals and leukemic patients. NW-filtered effector cells were incubated with the K562 cell line (1:1 ratio), and the morphology of TBCs was evaluated on May-Grünwald- and Giemsa-stained cytocentrifuge slides. Bars represent the percent of entire TBC population (□) and of LGL-TBC (▦). As analyzed by a Student's *t*-test, the leukemic patients demonstrated a significant decrease in both the percentage of entire TBC population ($p<0.005$) and in TBC with LGL morphology ($p<0.001$).

Table 4
MAXIMAL RECYCLING CAPACITY OF NK CELLS OF LEUKEMIA PATIENTS AND NORMAL DONORS

	Maximal recycling capacity[a]		
Donor no.	**Normal donors**	**Leukemic patients[b]**	
1	7.1	0.2	Myeloid leukemia
2	7.0	1.3	Myeloid leukemia
3	6.9	0.5	Myeloid leukemia
4	5.5	0.3	Myeloid leukemia
5	5.0	0.3	Lymphoid leukemia
6	3.3	0.9	Lymphoid leukemia
7	2.6	0.7	Lymphoid leukemia
8	1.9	2.7	Lymphoid leukemia
9	1.5	5.2	Lymphoid leukemia
10	1.2	5.0	Lymphoid leukemia
Mean ± S.E.	4.2 ± 0.7	1.7 ± 0.6[c]	

[a] Maximal recycling capacity was determined by combining the data from single cell assay and ^{51}Cr-release assay, using V_{max}.[52] NW-filtered effector cells and K562 target cell line were used in these studies.

[b] Leukemic patients included AML (1 to 3), CML (4), hairy cell leukemia (5), and ALL (6 to 10) patients.

[c] As analyzed by a Student's *t*-test, there was a significant decrease in the maximal recycling capacity of leukemic patients ($p<0.002$).

Table 5
PRODUCTION OF NKCF BY EFFECTOR CELLS OF LEUKEMIC PATIENTS AND NORMAL DONORS

Donor no.	Percent of cytotoxicity by supernatant from[a,c]	
	Unstimulated cells	Stimulated cells
Leukemic patients[b]		
1	21.4	30.0
2	10.4	12.9
3	−6.4	−8.6
4	−10.9	−18.7
5	10.0	11.6
Normal donors		
1	1.7	70.0
2	20.1	42.3
3	1.0	18.1
4	6.1	76.6
5	8.6	20.2

[a] NKCF was generated by incubating NW-filtered effector cells with unlabeled K562 target cells (1:100 T:E cell ratio) for 24 hr (stimulated cells); K562 cell line was found mycoplasma-free as determined by fluorescent staining.[76] The control group consisted of supernatants from unstimulated cells. The cytotoxicity of supernatants was measured in a microcytotoxicity test (10^3 K562 tumor cells were incubated for 40 hr with 10 $\mu\ell$ of either NKCF or control supernatant).

[b] Leukemic patients included AML (1 and 2), AMML (3), and ALL (4 and 5).

[c] As analyzed by a Student's *t*-test, there was a significant increase in NKCF-mediated cytotoxicity (experimental) in comparison to control group in all normal donors ($p<0.001$). No significant NKCF-mediated cytotoxicity was exhibited by effector cells of leukemic patients.

of effector cells alone displays no or low cytotoxic activity. To obtain information on another parameter of the NK cell cytotoxic reaction, in the next series of studies we investigated the ability of PBLs from normal donors and patients with leukemia to produce NKCF. As shown in Table 5, effector cells from normal donors were effective in generating NKCF with high lytic activity against K562 target cells. In contrast, there was no production of cytotoxic factor above the control levels by the effector cells of leukemic patients. No association between levels of NKCF and LGLs (or blast cells in leukemic patients) was observed in normal donors or patients (data not shown).

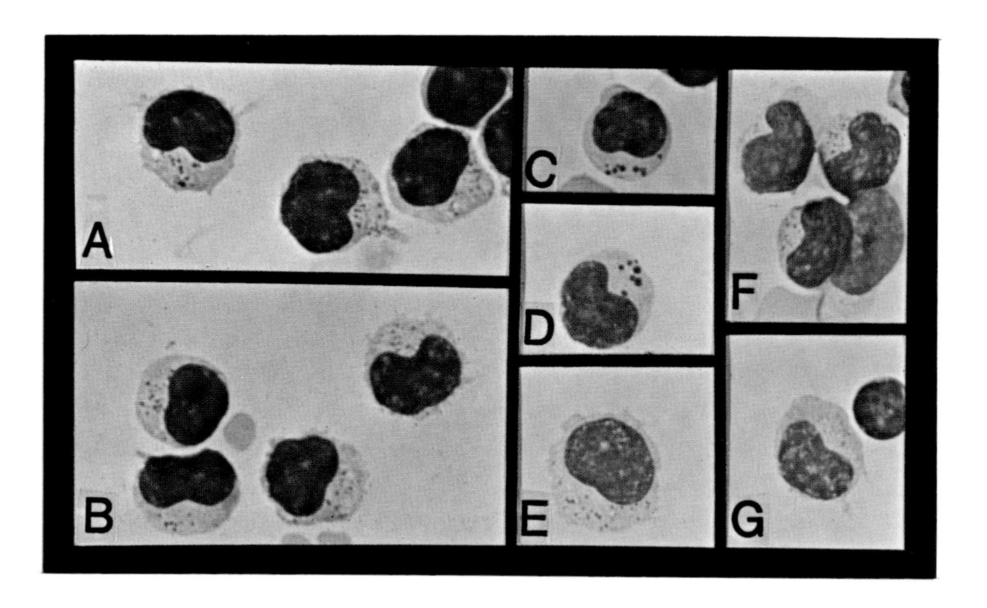

Plate 1. Morphology of LGL from peripheral blood of normal donors and leukemic patients. Two normal donors (panels A and B), 2 AML patients (panels C and D), 1 AMML patient (panel E), and 2 ALL patients (panels F and G).

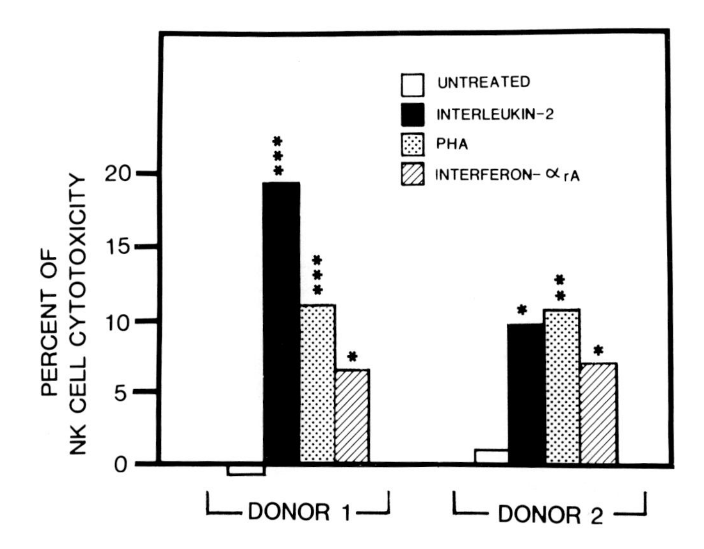

FIGURE 13. Reactivity of peripheral blood NK cells against allogeneic, freshly derived leukemic blasts. Effector cells were incubated with blast cells (1:100 T:E cell ratio) either alone, or in the presence of IL-2 (10% final concentration), phytohemagglutinin-P (2% final concentration), or IFN-αrA (10^3 U/mℓ) for 16 hr. Asterisks indicate a significant increase in NK cell activity following treatment: *$p<0.05$, **$p<0.01$, ***$p<0.001$.

IV. NK CELL REACTIVITY AGAINST FRESH LEUKEMIC CELLS

The critical question which has been raised repeatedly concerns the capacity of NK cells to recognize and lyse fresh leukemic cells. It is obvious that such information is essential for the understanding of the role of NK cells in surveillance and defense against leukemia. The first evidence for the susceptibility of fresh leukemic cells to lymphocyte attack was shown as early as 1972 by Rosenberg et al., who reported that lymphocytes from identical twins, parents, and siblings of leukemia patients as well as lymphocytes from unrelated donors exerted cytotoxic activity against patients' leukemic cells.[12] More recently, several other laboratories have addressed the question of NK cell reactivity against freshly derived leukemic cells. These studies demonstrated the lytic activity of PBLs of normal donors against fresh AML, CML (in blast crisis), and CLL leukemic cells after pretreatment with IFN-α or IFN-β.[56—59] In addition to allogeneic cytotoxicity, in a limited number of patients an autologous antileukemia effect was displayed by IFN-β stimulated effector cells.[57] We have also tested in our laboratory the cytotoxic potential of normal donors' NK cells on leukemic blasts of AML patients. As indicated in Figure 13, no cytotoxicity against freshly derived AML targets was displayed by endogenous PBLs of two normal donors; however, significant cytotoxic levels were observed after treatment of effector cells with interleukin-2 (IL-2) or phytohemagglutinin (PHA). Minimal, even though statistically significant, NK cell augmentation was also seen after treatment with recombinant IFN-α.

The characterization studies showed that the IFN-activated effector cells mediating the antileukemia effect displayed characteristics similar to endogenous NK cells. For example, both cell populations expressed receptors for the Fc portion of IgG (FcR negative cells were not augmented by IFN), were nonadherent to plastic, and were reactive against the NK cell-sensitive target, K562. Furthermore, separation of IFN-β activated PBLs on discontinuous Percoll gradient showed substantial augmentation of reactivity against primary ALL tumors in fractions enriched for LGLs.[57]

Even though a variety of fresh tumors displayed susceptibility to NK cell lysis, it appears that less mature leukemic cells are the primary NK cell targets. This possibility is in concert with two relatively recent observations. First, IFN-α-activated peripheral blood NK cells lysed efficiently leukemic blasts of CML patients in blast crisis, but not those of patients with chronic-phase CML, suggesting that less differentiated leukemic blasts are more sensitive to NK cell lysis than more differentiated granulocytes.[60]

Second, it has been shown that freshly derived leukemic cells of patients with AML, accelerated-phase CML, and chronic myleomonocytic leukemia, (CMoL) displayed less susceptibility to lysis in the ^{51}Cr-release assay than in a clonogenic leukemic cell assay (CFU-L).[61] In contrast to the effectiveness of allogeneic (endogenous or IFN-α-stimulated) PBLs to inhibit substantially the in vitro growth of clonogenic leukemic target cells, no or minimal lysis of the same leukemic targets was observed in the ^{51}Cr-release assay. That the effector cells operating in inhibition of CFU-L were indeed NK cells was indicated by their lack of adherence, their separation in the light-density fractions of Percoll, their high sensitivity to potentiation by IFN, and their lytic activity against the K562 cell line.

The discrepant results between low NK cell killing capacity of allogeneic lymphocytes in ^{51}Cr-release assay and their high activity against clonogenic leukemic cells in CFU-L assay may be explained by the preferential NK cell reactivity against less mature leukemic cells (perhaps leukemic "stem" cells). If this postulation was correct, the lower levels of NK cell cytotoxicity would be expected in ^{51}Cr-release assay where the population of leukemic cells is quite heterogeneous and the NK cell most sensitive (more primitive) leukemic cells are in the minority. On the contrary, in the CFU-L assay, where the more primitive (clonogenic) leukemic cell population represents a target of NK cell attack, high antileukemia reactivity should be detected. In line with the postulation of high susceptibility of less differentiated (as opposed to more differentiated) leukemia targets to NK cell attack is the observation that induced differentiation of highly NK cell-sensitive K562 cell line resulted in the loss of its susceptibility to lysis by NK cells.[62]

Alternatively, the effectiveness of NK cells to inhibit the growth of leukemic cells in clonogenic assay as opposed to their ineffectiveness to mediate a lysis in the cytotoxicity assay may reflect a different mechanism of NK cell reactivity (cytostasis vs. cytolysis) or greater sensitivity of clonogenic assay.

To summarize, the above-reviewed data demonstrate the NK cell activity not only against leukemic cell lines, but also against primary leukemic tumors, and hence, strongly support the postulated NK cell role in immune surveillance against leukemia.

V. MALIGNANT CELLS WITH NK CELL CHARACTERISTICS

It has been shown that some of the T_γ-lymphoproliferative disorders (T_γ-LPDs) exhibit LGL morphological features.[63] In addition to similar morphology, malignant LGLs displayed several other characteristics in common with LGLs from the peripheral blood of normal donors. For instance, these cells were shown to be peroxidase negative, acid phosphatase positive, expressed FcR for IgG, and formed rosettes with SRBCs. Moreover, malignant LGLs expressed markers present on NK cells of normal donors, such as HNK-1, VEP-13, and OKM-1, and were cytotoxic in NK cell and ADCC reaction against NK- and K cell-susceptible targets. Compatible with this observation is the report of another group of investigators.[64] In the latter investigation, the malignant LGLs from patients with abnormal lymphoproliferative syndrome also displayed typical LGL morphology, cell surface phenotype, and exhibited high NK cell and ADCC activity.[64] However, certain differences between normal and malignant LGLs were dissected in this study. In contrast to LGLs from normal donors which are positive for α-naphthyl acetate esterase, LGLs from the patient with lymphoproliferative syndrome were negative for this acid hydrolase. Additionally, ultrastructural studies revealed that malignant LGLs displayed a primarily immature type of granulation, contained less azurophilic granules, and experienced an active process of granulogenesis, the activity infrequently observed in normal LGLs. Since granulogenesis is mostly a feature of early maturational stages of hemopoietic cells,[65,66] it appears that the patient's cells represented less mature LGLs. This suggestion is further supported by the lack of α-naphthyl acetate esterase reaction (the property of lymphocytes at a later stage of differentiation) and the expression of Ia antigens (the characteristic of less mature hemopoietic cells)[67] on malignant LGLs.

Since NK cells may be involved in defense against cancer [68] and in the regulation of various function of the hemopoietic and lymphoid systems (granulocyte, erythrocyte, T cell, and B cell growth),[69] it is possible that their major biological function could be the maintenance of homeostasis of the organism. Consequently, NK cell aberrancy (conversion from normal to malignant state) may lead to disturbances in the equilibrium of the organism and underlie various diseases, such as autoimmunity, immunodeficiency, and secondary cancer. For these reasons it is imperative to study and understand the mechanism of LGL LPDs and the changes in NK cell regulatory functions in these conditions.

It is important to note that malignant LGLs are not the only type of malignant cells mediating spontaneous and ADCC activity. It has been reported that T cell leukemic blasts were efficient mediators of both NK cell and ADCC functions.[70] Similar cytotoxic activity was attributed recently to monoblasts from patients with acute monoblastic leukemia.[71] The relationship between NK cells and malignant hemopoietic cells is currently unknown. However, the better understanding of this relationship may be instrumental in delineating the lineage and differentiation patterns of the NK cell system.

VI. CLINICAL RELEVANCE OF NK CELLS AND POSSIBLE ROLE IN LEUKEMIA THERAPY

As discussed above, NK cells may play a role in the defense against leukemia in man. In addition, NK cells are involved in the regulation of hemopoiesis and lymphopoiesis,[11,69,72] the leukemia-related phenomena. Hence, the qualitative or quantitative changes in NK cell activities may lead to disturbances in the equilibrium of the lymphoid and hemopoietic systems, and may result in aberrant growth kinetics and differentiation patterns, or in suboptimal or superoptimal production of a variety of NK cell (or other lymphocyte) factors. Such violation of the homeostasis within the biological system may lead to various types of benign or malignant diseases of the hemopoietic and lymphoid systems e.g., leukemias and lymphomas. Indeed, the observation that patients with preleukemic disorders experience low NK cell cytotoxic potential strongly suggests that a defective NK cell mechanism may underlie the leukemic disease. Moreover, as shown earlier, all of the leukemic patients maintain a low NK cell level during the active stage of disease. In light of these observations, maximum efficiency of the NK cell system in leukemic patients would be desirable.

There are two possible approaches to the correction of the NK cell defect. The first would involve administration of biologic response modifying agents (BRMs), which are known to potentiate NK cell activity. Such an approach, however, may not be necessarily effective, since most BRMs display rather short-term effects and thus, would have to be administered frequently. However, after prolonged administration in vivo, some of the BRMs (e.g., IFN) were shown to inhibit rather than potentiate NK cell functions.[73]

The second approach could consist of propagation of NK cells in vitro followed by subsequent transplantation of these cells (or infusion of NK cell cytotoxic products) into the patients. That this approach is quite feasible is illustrated by the ability of NK cells from both normal donors and leukemic patients to grow in vitro upon stimulation with IL-2. Moreover, it was shown that the NK cell defect of CML patients can be corrected after in vitro cloning.[74] Under these conditions, NK cell clone(s) became reactive not only against allogeneic, but most importantly, also against autologous leukemic cells.[74]

NK cells may also be of therapeutic value in autologous bone marrow transplantation of leukemic patients. For instance, it may be possible to eradicate residual leukemic cells present in the bone marrow graft prior to bone marrow cell infusion by preincubation with endogenous (or IFN or other BRM-augmented) NK cells in order to abate the recurrence of leukemia. Furthermore, transplantation of NK cells (or infusion of NK cell cytotoxic products) prior to or together with autologous bone marrow transplants may be beneficial in eliminating the residual leukemic cells present in the recipient.

In addition to their therapeutic value in leukemia, NK cells may serve as a prognostic tool of leukemia relapse. We and others observed that the decline in NK cell cytotoxicity precedes clinical manifestation of leukemia relapse.[40,75] Such early diagnosis of leukemia relapse could lead to less aggressive treatment of this disease.

Finally, NK cells may have an importance in allogeneic bone marrow transplantation since these cells have been shown to participate in rejection of histoincompatible bone marrow transplants. Thus, the NK cell assay may be perhaps a potentially useful tool in the selection of donor-recipient pairs for successful allogeneic bone marrow transplantation.

In conclusion, a better understanding of NK cell immunobiology may contribute to the development of new diagnostic tests and protocols for the treatment of cancer.

ACKNOWLEDGMENT

The work from this laboratory was supported by Grants CA 39632 and 31394 from the National Cancer Institute. The authors wish to acknowledge Dr. M. J. Keating for providing patients' blood samples and Ann Childers for assistance in the preparation of this manuscript.

REFERENCES

1. **Hauschka, T. S. and Fürth, J.,** The pathophysiology and immunogenetics of transplantable leukemia, in *The Leukemias: Etiology, Pathophysiology and Treatment,* Rebuck, J. W., Bethel, F. H., and Monto, R. W., Eds., Academic Press, New York, 1957, 87.
2. **Snell, G. D.,** Histocompatibility genes of the mouse. II. Production and analysis of isogeneic resistant lines, *J. Natl. Cancer Inst.*, 21, 843, 1958.
3. **Cudkowicz, G.,** Hybrid resistance to parental grafts of hemopoietic and lymphoma cells, in *The Proliferation and Spread of Neoplastic Cells. XXI. Annual M. D. Anderson Symposium on Fundamental Research,* Williams & Wilkins, Baltimore, 1968, 661.
4. **Herberman, R. B., Nunn, M. E., and Lavrin, D. H.,** Natural cytotoxic reactivity of mouse lymphoid cells against syngeneic and allogeneic tumors. I. Distribution of reactivity and specificity, *Int. J. Cancer,* 16, 216, 1975.
5. **Kiessling, R., Klein, E., and Wigzell, H.,** Natural killer cells in the mouse. I. Cytotoxic cells with specificity for mouse Moloney leukemia cells. Specificity and distribution according to genotype, *Eur. J. Immunol.*, 5, 112, 1975.
6. **Lotzová, E. and McCredie, K. B.,** Natural killer cells in mice and man and their possible biological significance, *Cancer Immunol. Immunother.*, 4, 215, 1978.
7. **Herberman, R. B., Djeu, J. Y., Kay, H. D., Ortaldo, J. R., Riccardi, C., Bonnard, G. D., Holden, H. T., Fagnani, R., Santoni, A. S., and Puccetti, P.,** Natural killer cells: characteristics and regulation of activity, *Immunol. Rev.*, 44, 43, 1979.
8. **Lotzová, E. and Savary, C. A.,** Possible involvement of natural killer cells in bone marrow graft rejection, *Biomedicine,* 27, 341, 1977.
9. **Kiessling, R., Hochman, P. S., Haller, O., Shearer, G. M., Wigzell, H., and Cudkowicz, G.,** Evidence for a similar or common mechanism for natural killer cell activity and resistance to hemopoietic grafts, *Eur. J. Immunol.*, 7, 655, 1977.
10. **Lotzová, E.,** Hemopoietic histocompatibility: genetic and immunological aspects, in *Compendium of Immunology,* Vol. 3, 2nd ed., Schwartz, L. M., Ed., Van Nostrand Reinhold, New York, 1983, 468.
11. **Lotzová, E.,** Natural bone marrow graft rejection phenomenon in mice, *Surv. Immunol. Res.*, 1, 155, 1982.

12. **Rosenberg, E. B., Herberman, R. B., Levine, P. H., Halterman, R. H., McCoy, J. L., and Wunderlich, J. R.,** Lymphocyte cytotoxicity reactions to leukemia-associated antigens in identical twins, *Int. J. Cancer*, 9, 648, 1972.
13. **Kay, H. D. and Sinkovics, J. G.,** Cytotoxic lymphocytes from normal donors, *Lancet*, 2, 296, 1974.
14. **Herberman, R. B. and Holden, H. T.,** Natural cell-mediated immunity, *Adv. Cancer Res.*, 27, 305, 1978.
15. **Savary, C. A. and Lotzová, E.,** Phylogeny and ontogeny of NK cells, in *Immunobiology of Natural Killer Cells*, Vol. 1, Lotzová, E. and Herberman, R. B., Eds., CRC Press, Boca Raton, 1986, chap. 4.
16. **Roder, J. C., Haliotis, T., Klein, M., Korec, S., Jett, J., Ortaldo, J., Herberman, R. B., Katz, P., and Fauci, A. S.,**. A new immunodeficiency disorder in humans involving NK cells, *Nature (London)*, 284, 553, 1980.
17. **Tursz, T., Dokhelar, M. C., Lipinski, M., and Amiel, J. L.,** Low NK cell activity and malignant lymphoma, in *NK Cells: Fundamental Aspects and Role in Cancer. Human Cancer Immunology*, Elsevier, Amsterdam, 1982, 241.
18. **Hoffman, T. and Ferrarini, M.,** A role for natural killer cells in survival: functions of large granular lymphocytes including regulation of cell proliferation, *Clin. Immunol. Immunopathol.*, 29, 323, 1983.
19. **Sirchia, G. and Lewis, S. M.,** Paroxysmal nocturnal hemoglobinuria, *Clin. Haematol.*, 4, 199, 1975.
20. **Yoda, Y., Abe, T., Mitamura, K., Saito, K., Kawada, K., Onozawa, Y., Adachi, Y., and Nomura, T.,** Deficient natural killer (NK) cell activity in paroxysmal nocturnal haemoglobinuria, *Br. J. Haematol.*, 52, 559, 1982.
21. **Minato, N., Takeda, A., Kano, S., and Takaku, F.,** Studies of the functions of natural killer-interferon system in patients with Sjögren syndrome, *J. Clin. Invest.*, 69, 581, 1982.
22. **Lotzová, E., McCredie, K. B., Maroun, J. A., Dicke, K. A., and Freireich, E. J.,** Some studies on natural killer cells in man, *Transplant. Proc.*, 11, 1390, 1979.
23. **Lotzová, E., Savary, C. A., and Keating, M. J.,** Leukemia diseased patients exhibit multiple defects in natural killer cell lytic machinery, *Exp. Hematol.*, 10 (Suppl. 12), 83, 1983.
24. **Anderson, R. W., Volsky, D. J., Greenberg, B., Knox, S. J., Bechtold, T., Kuszynski, C., Harada, S., and Purtilo, D. T.,** Lymphocyte abnormalities in preleukemia. I. Decreased NK activity, anomalous immunoregulatory cell subsets and deficient EBV receptors, *Leuk. Res.*, 7, 389, 1983.
25. **Trump, D. L., Mann, R. B., Phelps, R., Roberts, H., and Conley, L. C.,** Richter's syndrome: diffuse histiocytic lymphoma in patients with chronic lymphocytic leukemia, *Am. J. Med.*, 68, 539, 1980.
26. **Manusow, D. and Weinerman, B. H.,** Subsequent neoplasia in chronic lymphocytic leukemia, *JAMA*, 232, 267, 1975.
27. **Haller, O. and Wigzell, H.,** Suppression of natural killer cell activity with radioactive strontium: effector cells are marrow dependent, *J. Immunol.*, 118, 1503, 1977.
28. **Lotzová, E., McCredie, K. B., Muesse, L., Dicke, K. A., and Freireich, E. J.,** Natural killer cells in man: their possible involvement in leukemia and bone marrow transplantation, in *Experimental Hematology Today*, Baum, S. J. and Ledney, G. D., Eds., Springer-Verlag, New York, 1979, 207.
29. **Hansson, M., Beran, M., Andersson, B., and Kiessling, R.,** Inhibition of in vitro granulopoiesis by autologous and allogeneic human cells, *J. Immunol.*, 129, 126, 1982.
30. **Mangan, K. F., Harnett, M. E., Matis, S. A., Winkelstein, H., and Abo, T.,** Natural killer cells suppress human erythroid stem cell proliferation in vitro, *Blood*, 63, 260, 1984.
31. **Pistoia, V., Nocera, A., Ghio, R., Leprini, A., Perata, A., Pistone, M., and Ferrarini, M.,** PHA-induced human T cell colony formation: enhancing effect of large granular lymphocytes, *Exp. Hematol.*, 11, 249, 1983.
32. **Behalak, Y., Banerjee, D., and Richter, M.,** Immunocompetent cells in patients with malignant disease. I. The lack of naturally occurring killer cell activity in the unfractionated circulating lymphocytes from patients with chronic lymphocytic leukemia (CLL), *Cancer*, 38, 2274, 1976.
33. **Ziegler (Löms), H. W., Kay, N. E., and Zarling, J. M.,** Deficiency of natural killer activity in patients with chronic lymphocytic leukemia, *Int. J. Cancer*, 27, 321, 1981.
34. **Platsoucas, C. D., Fernandes, G., Gupta, S. L., Kempin, S., Clarkson, B., Good, R. A., and Gupta, S.,** Defective spontaneous and antibody-dependent cytotoxicity mediated by E-rosette-positive and E-rosette-negative cells in untreated patients with chronic lymphocytic leukemia: augmentation by in vitro treatment with interferon, *J. Immunol.*, 125, 1216, 1980.
35. **Hokland, P. and Ellegaard, J.,** Immunological studies in chronic lymphocytic leukemia. II. Natural killer- and antibody-dependent cellular cytotoxicity potentials of malignant and non-malignant lymphocyte subsets and the effect of α-interferon, *Leuk. Res.*, 5, 349, 1981.
36. **Herberman, R. B.,** Natural killer cells and cells mediating antibody-dependent cytotoxicity against tumors, *Clin. Immunobiol.*, 4, 73, 1980.
37. **Lotzová, E., Savary, C. A., Gutterman, J. U., and Hersh, E. M.,** Modulation of natural killer cell-mediated cytotoxicity by partially purified and cloned interferon-α, *Cancer Res.*, 42, 2480, 1982.

38. **Pross, H. F. and Baines, M. G.,** Studies of human natural killer cells. I. In vivo parameters affecting normal cytotoxic function, *Int. J. Cancer*, 29, 383, 1982.
39. **Seaman, W. E., Blackman, M. A., Gindhart, T. D., Roubinian, J. R., Loeb, J. M., and Talal, N.,** β-Estradiol reduces natural killer cells in mice, *J. Immunol.*, 121, 2193, 1978.
40. **Stupp, Y., Rosenkovitch, E., and Izak, G.,** Natural killer activity in patients with acute myelocytic leukemia, *Isr. J. Med. Sci.*, 14, 1212, 1978.
41. **Schiliro, G., Musumeci, S., Sciotto, A., Russo, A., and Marino, S.,** K cell activity in acute lymphoblastic leukaemia of childhood, *Acta Haematol.*, 64, 221, 1980.
42. **Zighelboim, J.,** Deficiency of antibody-dependent cellular cytotoxicity and mitogen-induced cellular cytotoxicity effector cell function in patients with acute myelogenous leukemia in remission, *Cancer Res.*, 39, 3357, 1979.
43. **McGeorge, M. B., Russell, E. C., and Mohanakumar, T.,** Immunologic evaluation of long-term effects of childhood ALL chemotherapy: analysis of in vitro NK- and K cell activities of peripheral blood lymphocytes, *Am. J. Hematol.*, 12, 19, 1982.
44. **Ortaldo, J. R., Oldham, R. B., Cannon, G. C., and Herberman, R. B.,** Specificity of natural cytotoxic reactivity of normal human lymphocytes against a myeloid leukemia cell line, *J. Natl. Cancer Inst.*, 59, 77, 1977.
45. **Kay, N. E. and Zarling, J. M.,** Impaired natural killer activity in patients with chronic lymphocytic leukemia is associated with a deficiency of azurophilic cytoplasmic granules in putative NK cells, *Blood*, 63, 305, 1984.
46. **Timonen, T., Ortaldo, J. R., and Herberman, R. B.,** Characteristics of human large granular lymphocytes and relationship to natural killer and K cells, *J. Exp. Med.*, 153, 569, 1981.
47. **Kay, H. D., Bonnard, G. D., West, W. H., and Herberman, R. B.,** A functional comparison of human Fc-receptor-bearing lymphocytes active in natural cytotoxicity and antibody-dependent cellular cytotoxicity, *J. Immunol.*, 188, 2058, 1977.
48. **Neighbour, P. A., Huberman, H. S., and Kress, Y.,** Human large granular lymphocytes and natural killing: ultrastructural studies of strontium-induced degranulation, *Eur. J. Immunol.*, 12, 588, 1982.
49. **Neighbour, P. A. and Huberman, H. S.,** Sr^{++}-induced inhibition of human natural killer (NK) cell mediated cytotoxicity, *J. Immunol.*, 128, 1236, 1982.
50. **Millard, P. J., Henkart, M. P., Reynolds, C. W., and Henkart, P. A.,** Purification and properties of cytoplasmic granules from cytotoxic rat LGL tumors, *J. Immunol.*, 132, 3197, 1984.
51. **Goldfarb, R. H., Timonen, T., and Herberman, R. B.,** Production of plasminogen activator by human natural killer cells. Large granular lymphocytes, *J. Exp. Med.*, 159, 935, 1984.
52. **Callewaert, D. M., Johnson, D. F., and Kearny, J.,** Spontaneous cytotoxicity of cultured human cell lines mediated by normal peripheral blood lymphocytes. III. Kinetic parameters, *J. Immunol.*, 121, 710, 1978.
53. **Grimm, E. and Bonavida, B.,** Mechanism of cell-mediated cytotoxicity at the single-cell level. I. Estimation of cytotoxic T lymphocyte frequency and relative lytic efficiency, *J. Immunol.*, 123, 2861, 1979.
54. **Ullberg, M. and Jondal, M.,** Recycling and target binding capacity of human natural killer cells, *J. Exp. Med.*, 153, 615, 1981.
55. **Bonavida, B. and Wright, S. C.,** Natural killer cytotoxic factors (NKCF) role in cell-mediated cytotoxicity, in *Immunobiology of Natural Killer Cells*, Vol. 1, Lotzová, E. and Herberman, R. B., Eds., CRC Press, Boca Raton, 1986, chap. 9.
56. **Zarling, J. M., Eskra, L., Borden, E. C., Horoszewicz, J., and Carter, W. A.,** Activation of human natural killer cells cytotoxic for human leukemia cells by purified interferon, *J. Immunol.*, 123, 63, 1979.
57. **Oshimi, K., Oshimi, Y., Motoji, T., Kobayashi, S., and Mizoguchi, H.,** Lysis of leukemia and lymphoma cells by autologous and allogeneic interferon-activated blood mononuclear cells, *Blood*, 61, 790, 1983.
58. **Moore, M., Taylor, G. M., and White, W. J.,** Susceptibility of human leukemias to cell-mediated cytotoxicity by interferon-treated allogeneic lymphocytes, *Cancer Immunol. Immunother.*, 13, 56, 1982.
59. **Pattengale, P. K., Gidlund, M., Nilsson, K., Sundström, C., Sällström, J., Simonsson, B., and Wigzell, H.,** Lysis of fresh human B-lymphocyte-derived leukemia cells by interferon-activated natural killer (NK) cells, *Int. J. Cancer*, 29, 1, 1982.
60. **Pattengale, P. K., Sundström, C., Yu, A. L., and Levine, A.,** Lysis of fresh leukemic blasts by interferon-activated human natural killer (NK) cells, *Natl. Immunol. Cell Growth Regul.*, 3, 165, 1984.
61. **Beran, M., Hansson, M., and Kiessling, R.,** Human natural killer cells can inhibit clonogenic growth of fresh leukemic cells, *Blood*, 61, 596, 1983.
62. **Gidlund, M., Örn, A., Pattengale, P. K., Jansson, M., Wigzell, H., and Nilsson, K.,** Natural killer cells will only kill tumor cells at a given stage of differentiation, *Nature (London)*, 292, 848, 1981.
63. **Herrmann, F., Sieber, G., Komischke, B., Schrekenberg, A., Ludwig, A.-D., and Ruhl, H.,** Expanded Tγ cell populations with the morphology of large granular lymphocytes. I. Immunological, clinical, and morphological characterization, *Leuk. Res.*, 7, 667, 1983.

64. **Ferrarini, M., Romagnani, S., Montesoro, E., Zicca, A., Del Prete, G. F., Nocera, A., Maggi, E., Leprini, A., and Grossi, C. E.,** A lymphoproliferative disorder of the large granular lymphocyte with natural killer activity, *J. Clin. Immunol.*, 3, 30, 1983.
65. **Cohn, Z. A. and Benson, B.,** The differentiation of mononuclear phagocytes. Morphology, cytochemistry and biochemistry, *J. Exp. Med.*, 121, 153, 1965.
66. **Bainton, D. F. and Farquhar, M. G.,** Origin of granules in polymorphonuclear leukocytes. Two types derived from opposite faces of the Golgi complex in developing granulocytes, *J. Cell Biol.*, 28, 277, 1966.
67. **Winchester, R. J., Ross, G. D., Jarowski, C. I., Wong, C. Y., Halper, J., and Broxmeyer, H. E.,** Expression of Ia-like antigen molecules on human granulocytes during early phases of differentiation, *Proc. Natl. Acad. Sci., U.S.A.*, 74, 4012, 1977.
68. **Herberman, R. B. and Ortaldo, J. R.,** Natural killer cells: their role in defense against disease, *Science*, 214, 24, 1981.
69. **Lotzová, E.,** Function of natural killer cells in various biological phenomena, *Surv. Synth. Pathol. Res.*, 2, 41, 1983.
70. **Gupta, S. and Fernandes, G.,** Leukemic blasts as effectors in natural killing and antibody dependent cytotoxicity assay, in *NK Cells and Other Natural Effector Cells*, Herberman, R. B., Ed., Academic Press, New York, 1982, 1141.
71. **Hokland, P., Hokland, M., and Ellegaard, J.,** Malignant monoblasts can function as effector cells in natural killer cell and antibody-dependent cellular cytotoxicity, *Blood*, 57, 972, 1981.
72. **Lotzová, E., Savary, C. A., and Pollack, S. B.,** Prevention of rejection of allogeneic bone marrow transplants by NK 1.1 antiserum, *Transplantation*, 35, 490, 1983.
73. **Lotzová, E., Savary, C. A., Gutterman, J. U., Quesada, J. R., and Hersh, E. M.,** Regulation of human natural killer cell cytotoxicity by recombinant leukocyte interferon clone A, *J. Biol. Resp. Modif.*, 2, 482, 1983.
74. **Fujiyama, Y., Linker-Israeli, M., Bakke, A., Horwitz, D., and Pattengale, P.,** Successful cloning and amplification of functionally-defective HNK-1$^+$ mononuclear cells from patients with chronic granulocytic leukemia, in *The Second International Workshop on Natural Killer Cells*, Detroit, Mich., 1984, 64.
75. **Talpaz, M., Bielski, M., and Hersh, E. M.,** Studies on natural killer cell activity and antibody-dependent cell-mediated cytotoxicity among patients with acute leukemia in complete remission, *Cancer Immunol. Immunother.*, 14, 96, 1982.
76. **Chen, T. R.,** In situ detection of mycoplasma contamination in cell cultures by fluorescent Hoechst 33258 stain, *Exp. Cell Res.*, 104, 255, 1977.

Chapter 4

IN VIVO MODULATION OF NK ACTIVITY IN CANCER PATIENTS

Peter M. Moy and Sidney H. Golub

TABLE OF CONTENTS

I. INTRODUCTION

Cell-mediated immunity as a mechanism of host resistance to malignant neoplasms has been the subject of intense interest. Among the various immune components with antitumor activity, natural killer cell-mediated cytotoxicity (NK CMC) is of great current interest as it has been implicated as a possible immune surveillance mechanism in tumor-bearing hosts. In several animal studies, elevated levels of NK activity have been correlated with decreased growth rates of tumor cells introduced into host animals. NK cells have also been shown to inhibit metastatic spread of tumor cells.[1-10] In addition, depressed NK function has been noted in patients with large tumor burdens.[11-14] However, the role of NK cells in modulating the growth of established solid tumors remains unclear.

One approach to the investigation of the role of NK cells in the host-tumor relationship is the use of immunomodulatory agents as probes to examine the events of NK regulation in human cancer patients. Several agents such as interferon (IFN), Bacille Calmette-Guerin (BCG), indomethicin, levamisole, and OK432 have been shown to augment NK activity in vitro and in animal systems.[15-22]

To examine the relationship of immunomodulation by these agents to in vivo NK modulation, we will focus on the studies involving IFN and BCG as prototypes for alteration of immune function. While several other agents are being investigated, these two agents are perhaps the most well known and most intensively studied. Furthermore, our personal experience is limited to these agents. Aspects such as the alteration of cell populations by IFN or BCG, the time course of their effects, and possible mechanisms for their action will be considered.

II. STUDIES WITH IFN

IFN is an agent which has generated considerable interest as a possible clinical antitumor agent.[23-31] In animals, IFN has been shown to inhibit the growth of transplantable tumors as well as chemically and virally induced tumors.[32-34] In addition to its other wide range of biologic activities, its known properties of modulating NK activity has made this agent appealing for the examination of NK regulation in cancer patients.

We sought to determine the regulatory events in the modulation of NK activity in human cancer patients by IFN. Our experience with IFN was part of a multiinstitutional trial sponsored by the American Cancer Society. The clinical study at UCLA was directed by Dr. Martyn Burk and Dr. Donald Morton, who investigated the possible therapeutic benefits of human leukocyte IFN (IFN-α) administration in the treatment of malignant melanoma. While the effects of IFN are diverse, we chose to examine the effects on NK activity as a model system for immune modulation.

Of the 35 evaluable patients treated at UCLA, Memorial Sloan-Kettering, and Yale Cancer Center, 6 had evidence of tumor regression.[35] Toxicity was related to dose and the most frequent side effects included reversible leukopenia, thrombocytopenia, and elevation of liver enzymes. Fever, chills, anorexia, and malaise were also common during treatment.

The UCLA study examined 16 patients with metastatic malignant melanoma. Patients had metastases to s.c. tissues and/or lungs. The patients were randomized as to dosage regimen and all the IFN was administered i.m. The IFN used was a partially purified IFN-α. Patients received daily i.m. doses of 1×10^6 U, 3×10^6 U, or 9×10^6 U of IFN for 42 consecutive days. Serial heparinized blood samples were obtained prior to initiation of therapy and during the course of therapy. Lymphocytes were separated by standard Ficoll-Hypaque discontinuous gradient centrifugation methods and washed. All cytotoxicity assays were performed on freshly obtained and purified peripheral blood lymphocytes (PBLs). Samples were also cryopreserved for additional analyses. A 4-hr ^{51}Cr-release assay against the K562 myeloid

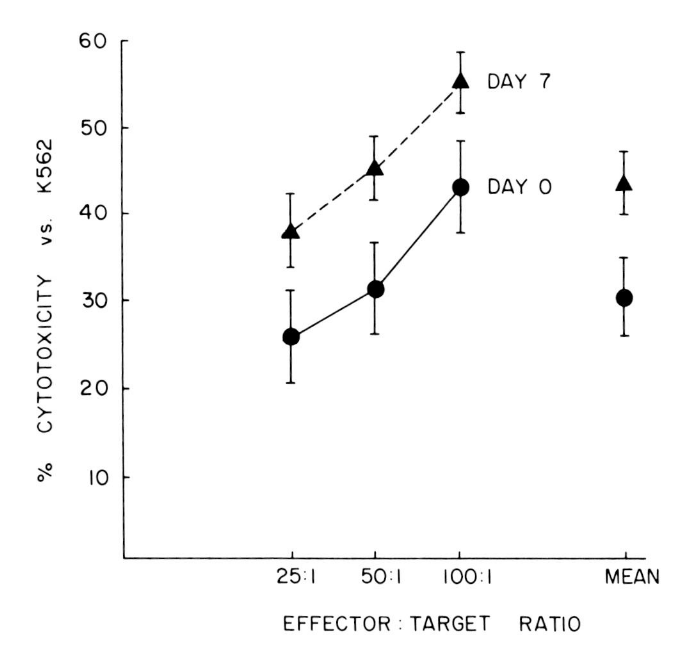

FIGURE 1. NK cytotoxicity vs. K562 targets of 14 IFN-treated melanoma patients at two effector to target ratios. All results are the average percentages of cytotoxicity for the patients tested at each time point. Patients administered partially purified human leukocyte IFN daily for 42 consecutive days. Results combined for all dosages (1 × 10^6 U/day, 3 × 10^6 U/day, and 9 × 10^6 U/day).

leukemia cell line was used for all assays with effector to target ratios of 100:1, 50:1, 25:1, and 12.5:1. Details of these results have been reported.[36]

Typically, the level of cytotoxicity initially declined after 24 hr of treatment then steadily increased until day 7 of treatment (Figure 1). A representative time course of all patients' NK activity is shown in Figure 2. This pattern was seen at all effector to target ratios tested. At day 7, 81% of the patients exhibited higher NK activity than pretreatment levels while only 56% remained elevated at day 21.

We also examined whether IFN-augmented cytotoxicity was restricted to NK-sensitive targets or could encompass other targets as well. One target cell line tested was M14, which was established from a patient with metastatic malignant melanoma. M14 cells are susceptible to natural cytotoxic (NC) cells in long-term assays but are generally resistant in a short-term 4-hr ^{51}Cr-release assay. The L14 cell line is an Epstein-Barr (EB) virus-transformed B cell line derived from the PBLs of the same patient who provided the M14 melanoma line. The L14 targets are moderately sensitive to NK cells in a short-term assay In a preliminary study of three patients, all of whom demonstrated marked increases in lysis of K562 targets, none showed increased cytotoxicity after IFN treatment when tested against the NK-resistant M14 melanoma line. Cytotoxicity both before and after IFN treatment never exceeded 5% lysis. In another experiment, one of the three patients was tested against L14 cell. There was again an augmentation from a value on day 0 of 7% to a peak value of 47% during IFN treatment. These results suggested that IFN can increase cytotoxicity against some less susceptible NK targets such as L14 but not all since untreated M14 cells remained resistant.

We examined whether the augmentation of NK activity was dose-related. While the number of patients treated did not allow adequate statistical analysis, we have observed that the lowest dosage used (1 × 10^6 U/day) was equally effective in augmenting NK activity and perhaps more effective at maintaining elevated NK activity than higher doses (3 × 10^6 or

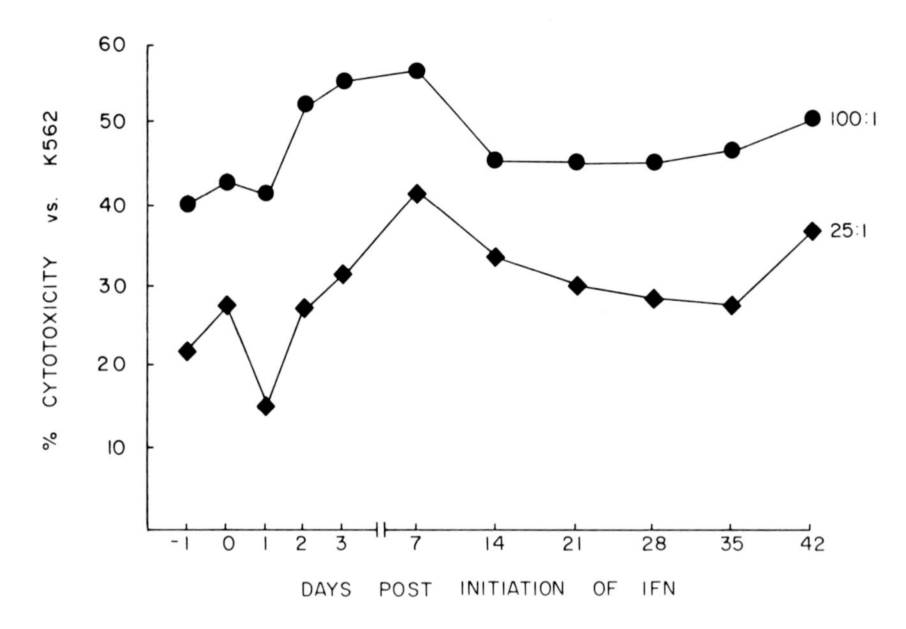

FIGURE 2. Average NK cytotoxicity for all 14 patients at days 0 and 7 of treatment. Horizontal axis shows mean of four ratios. Vertical bars indicate standard error of the mean. Patients administered partially purified human leukocyte IFN daily for 42 consecutive days. Results combined for all dosages (1×10^6 U/day, 3×10^6 U/day, and 9×10^6 U/day).

9×10^6 U/day). Patients receiving the higher doses exhibited a more pronounced leukopenia than those receiving lower doses.

Our major experimental focus was on the regulatory events associated with the initial increase of NK activity by IFN administration and those events associated with the subsequent decline in NK activity.[37] To address these questions, we analyzed the serial PBL specimens from IFN-treated patients using the single cell binding and lysis assay as developed by Grimm and Bonavida.[38] It has been previously shown that a subpopulation of lymphocytes will spontaneously bind to NK-sensitive targets such as K562, and roughly half of the binding cells will mediate target cell lysis. The sequential samples of PBLs from seven patients were incubated with K562 targets and mixed with a warm liquid 1% agarose solution for single cell analysis. The proportions of both the binding and killing cells increased relative to the total numbers of lymphocytes increased early during IFN treatment. The data from the four patients with the most complete available information are summarized in Table 1. The peak activity was found during the 1st week of treatment which paralleled the increased cytotoxic activity assessed by ^{51}Cr-release. The proportions of target binding cells subsequently declined despite continued IFN administration. The proportions of binding and killing cells returned to near pretreatment levels but remained slightly elevated.

To determine whether the augmentation in binding and killing from IFN treatment was restricted to NK-sensitive targets, we also analyzed the NK-resistant M14 cell line in the single cell assay. These targets have been previously described to be resistant to lysis by either normal or IFN-activated NK cells. Although the proportions of cells binding the M14 cells were equivalent to those binding K562, the proportion of M14 killers was low prior to and during IFN treatment and the proportion of binders was unaffected by IFN treatment. Thus, the enhanced cytotoxic capabilities appeared to be restricted to NK-sensitive targets only.

Passage of PBLs over EAγ monolayers to deplete Fc_γ receptor cells resulted in marked reduction in the proportion of cells mediating lysis while reducing the proportion of binding cells by about half. Passage of PBLs over a nylon fiber column to deplete B cells and

Table 1
BINDING AND LYSIS OF K562 TARGETS BY PBLs OF FOUR IFN-TREATED MELANOMA PATIENTS[a]

Day of treatment	Percent binding[b]	Percent NK[c]
−1	9.0 ± 1.6	3.4 ± 2.7
0	11.1 ± 2.0	6.0 ± 2.7
1	16.3 ± 3.0	8.0 ± 2.3
2	21.0 ± 2.9	9.8 ± 1.5
3	24.5 ± 6.5	12.5 ± 2.2
7	30.0 ± 2.2	13.3 ± 2.5
14	40.4 ± 21.0	13.3 ± 1.9
21	23.8 ± 2.5	12.0 ± 1.4
28	16.8 ± 2.9	11.0 ± 1.2
35	15.0 ± 2.4	9.7 ± 1.2
42	13.7 ± 2.0	9.0 ± 1.4

[a] Patients administered partially purified human leukocyte IFN i.m. daily. Two patients received 9 × 10^6 U/day, one patient received 3 × 10^6 U/day, and one received 1 × 10^6 U/day.
[b] Percent of PBL binding to targets; 200 lymphocytes scored.
[c] Percent of NK among all PBLs. (Product of a × percent of binders mediating target lysis.)

monocytes augmented binding as well as lytic capabilities. Thus, the cells mediating the augmented anti-K562 cytotoxicity have the characteristics of NK cells.

Since the single cell assay data showed an increase in the number of target binding and lytic cells following IFN treatment, we addressed the question as to whether IFN treatment increases the number or activity of NK cell precursors in the peripheral blood. To do this we attempted to generate NK-like activity in vitro. Cryopreserved PBLs from blood specimens obtained from various days of treatment were utilized. While cryopreserved lymphocytes express lower NK activity than freshly prepared PBLs, we were only interested in generating NK-like activity from a potential precursor population. Thus, cryopreserved PBLs were passed over EA_γ monolayers to deplete remaining NK activity, and nonadherent cells were then stimulated with allogeneic lymphoblastoid cells. After 6 days of incubation in the mixed lymphocyte cultures (MLCs), the cells were then tested for cytotoxic activity against K562 targets. The ability to generate NK-like activity in MLCs paralleled the original NK activity seen in the native PBLs. Nonstimulated control PBLs showed no cytotoxicity. This suggested that the IFN treatment was associated with an increase in the number of NK cell precursors. This result is in agreement with the increase in target binders and suggests that IFN can recruit precursor cells into the NK pathway.

We then sought to explain the possible mechanisms for the decline in NK activity with continued IFN injections. One possibility was that the mature NK cells were maximally stimulated by IFN and were then refractory to additional stimulation by IFN. This possibility was examined by comparing PBLs obtained at varying time points during the course of IFN therapy with or without a 60-min in vitro preincubation with 100 U of IFN. In ten patients examined in this manner, the PBLs obtained in the pretreatment, early treatment (days 1 to 3), and PBLs from control subjects, exhibited augmented NK activity response to exogenous IFN. Pretreatment NK cytotoxicity was augmented by an average of 8.4% and the activity of PBLs obtained from the early treatment period rose by an average of 7.7%. However, PBLs obtained during later treatment periods when in vivo NK activity was either at peak (day 7) or had returned to baseline levels (days 21 to 42) had less than 1% augmentation.

Table 2
PROPORTIONS OF E, EAC, AND LEU-1 POSITIVE CELLS IN PBLs OF IFN-TREATED MELANOMA PATIENTS[a]

Day	No. samples	Percent E	Percent EAC	Percent Leu-1
−1	8	57 ± 6	10 ± 2	NT[b]
0	9	62 ± 6	11 ± 3	68
1	9	55 ± 5	10 ± 1	NT
2	7	59 ± 6	9 ± 6	70
3	9	54 ± 4	9 ± 2	68
7	9	60 ± 4	10 ± 2	70
14	9	53 ± 3	10 ± 2	NT
21	9	64 ± 3	8 ± 2	69
35	9	62 ± 4	10 ± 1	NT

[a] Patients received partially purified human leukocyte IFN i.m. daily over 42 days. Results combined for all dosage levels (1×10^6 U/day, 3×10^6 U/day, and 9×10^6 U/day). Percentage positive rosetting cells ± S.E.M.

[b] NT = Not tested.

Post-treatment PBLs showed a return of augmentation of NK activity by IFN incubation. These results showed that PBLs obtained from the period of peak NK cytotoxicity through the subsequent decline in NK cytotoxicity were less responsive to in vitro IFN stimulation.

We next examined whether an adherent suppressor cell population accounted for the decline in NK activity. G-10 adherent suppressor cells have been described in murine systems with exposure to carageenan or *Corynebacterium parvum*.[39,40] Adherent suppressor cells have also been shown to inhibit NK activity against human tumor target cells in vitro. Thus, PBLs were tested before and after passage over a Sephadex G-10 column. After the depletion of G-10 adherent cells, most PBL samples from normal donors had a moderate increase in cytotoxicity, but this treatment failed to augment the low NK activity in patient PBL samples drawn past the peak of in vivo NK activity.

Prostaglandins, a known secretory product of macrophages, has been demonstrated as a mechanism for depression of NK activity.[41] To determine whether a suppressor cell effect was due to prostaglandins, 10^{-5} *M* indomethicin was incubated with control lymphocytes or IFN-treated patient lymphocytes. Treatment in this manner, with or without the additional incubation with IFN, failed to restore depressed postpeak NK activity although moderate increases were observed in control samples. Thus, there was no evidence to suggest that there was an activation of a G-10 adherent, prostaglandin-secreting suppressor cell population to account for the depressed NK activity in the latter periods of IFN treatment.

Since intercellular interactions may play a role in modulation of NK activity by IFN, we also sought to find the changes in PBL subpopulations as assessed by the ability to form sheep red blood cells (SRBCs), EA_γ, and EAC rosettes as well as absolute lymphocyte counts. There were no substantial changes in any subpopulation attributable to IFN treatment. Hence, the proportions of T cells, Fc_γ receptor-bearing cells, and complement receptor-bearing cells all remained unchanged (Tables 2 and 3). While the percent of rosetting cells did not change, the possibility of simultaneous decline and increase of specific cell subpopulations within each population exists. To examine this question, we have developed a rosetting assay to examine these specific lymphocyte subsets. We utilized commercially available mouse monoclonal antibodies (MoAbs) with specificity directed towards various lymphocyte surface markers. A universal rosetting reagent was utilized.[42] This reagent is composed of ox erythrocytes to which are reacted the IgG fraction of rabbit antiox RBC

Table 3
PROPORTION OF EA, B73.1, AND HNK-1 POSITIVE CELLS IN PBLs OF IFN-TREATED MELANOMA PATIENTS[a]

Day	No. tested	Percent EA	Percent B73.1	Percent HNK-1
0	9	20 ± 4	18 ± 12	17 ± 6
2 or 3	7	20 ± 2	19 ± 9	20 ± 12
7	9	21 ± 2	16 ± 8	22 ± 10
14	9	19 ± 3	NT[b]	NT
21 or 35	9	18 ± 2	19 ± 10	18 ± 8
42	9	18 ± 3	NT	NT

[a] Patients received partially purified human leukocyte IFN i.m. daily over 42 days. Results combined for all dosage levels (1×10^6 U/day, 3×10^6 U/day, and 9×10^6 U/day). Percentage positive rosetting cells ± S.E.M.
[b] NT = Not tested.

Table 4
PROPORTION OF T HELPER AND T SUPPRESSOR CELLS AMONG PBLs OF IFN-TREATED MELANOMA PATIENTS[a]

Day	No. tested	Percent Leu-2a	Percent Leu-3a	Ratio 3a:2a
0	6	43.3 ± 7.0	29.3 ± 11.2	0.67 ± 0.27
2 or 3	5	32.7 ± 7.4	40.2 ± 3.8	1.30 ± 0.33
7	6	32.0 ± 11.0	39.2 ± 5.3	1.47 ± 0.36
21 or 35	6	48.0 ± 7.5	29.0 ± 7.3	0.61 ± 0.19

[a] Patients received partially purified human leukocyte IFN i.m. daily over 42 days. Results combined for all dosage levels (1×10^6 U/day, 3×10^6 U/day, and 9×10^6 U/day). Percentage positive rosetting cells ± S.E.M.

antibody. Protein A is then bound to the Fc portion of the anti-RBC antibody followed by the IgG fraction of rabbit antimouse IgG binding to the protein A. By addition of this reagent to a macrophage-depleted lymphocyte population previously incubated with a specific mouse monoclonal, rosetted cells are indicative of a particular lymphocytic phenotype. This technique has allowed us to monitor the lymphocyte subsets during the course of IFN therapy.[43]

The mouse MoAb HNK-1, an antibody with specificity directed towards NK cells described by Abo and Balch,[44] was used to detect the level of NK cells. The results are depicted in Table 3. In five patients, HNK-1 positive cells increased slightly by day 7 but four other patients showed either no change or a decline in the numbers from pretreatment levels. Since NK cells express Fc receptors (FcR) on their cell surface, we also tested the MoAb B73.1, which reacts with FcRs on NK cells[43] against PBLs of IFN-treated patients. Slight increases in B73.1 positive cells were observed in only three patients while four others either remained unchanged or declined (Table 3). These results confirm the absence of change in FcR cells as determined by EA_γ-rosette formation. To determine the relative numbers of T cell, helper, and suppressor T cells among the PBLs, the MoAbs Leu-1, Leu-3a, and Leu-2a, respectively, were employed. The percent of T cells remained constant during the course of IFN treatment in all patients tested (Table 3). This corroborates evidence previously reported on the constancy of sheep erythrocyte rosette-forming cells. During the 1st week of IFN treatment, a general pattern emerged with an increase in Leu-3a (helper) positive cells and a decrease in Leu-2a (suppressor) positive cells (Table 4). Average Leu-3a values were 29 ± 12.3%

pretreatment and 42.6 ± 3.2% by day 7. Average values for Leu-2a positive cells were 43.3 ± 7.2% pretreatment and 30.8 ± 10.0% at day 7.

We then assessed the ratios of the helper subset to the suppressor subset. As seen in Table 4, all patients exhibited increased helper to suppressor cell ratios by day 7 with a gradual decline to pretreatment levels by day 21. The average pretreatment ratio was 0.67 ± 0.27% and the average peak value was 1.47 ± 0.36%. There was a correlation between the NK cytotoxic activity with the alterations in the helper to suppressor cell ratios. There is a parallel increase in both until day 7 as well as a parallel gradual decrease from day 7 to day 28, suggesting that the relative functions of T helper cells and T suppressor cells affect NK function. The mechanism for such T cell influence on NK function is unknown at present, although IL-2 production by T helper cells would be a logical candidate.

In summary, we have found that NK activity can be augmented in vivo by IFN administration and that this augmented activity subsequently declines despite continued IFN administration. The increases in NK activity are directed towards NK-sensitive targets with only modest increases seen with NK-resistant cell lines such as the M14 melanoma line. Our observations of increases in cytotoxic activity in vivo appear related to a recruitment of cells from an NK precursor population such that the total number of NK cells in the peripheral blood is increased rather than an increase in the cytotoxic activity for the preexisting mature NK cells. This increase in binding cells would appear to be in conflict with our data indicating no changes in numbers of Fc$_\gamma$+ or HNK-1+ cells during IFN treatment. One possibility is that the conversion of nonbinding cells to binding and killing cells takes place within the population of already Fc$_\gamma$+ HNK-1+ cells. Alternatively, the conversion of precursors into active NK cells may be accompanied by the exit of other inactive cells from the pool of Fc$_\gamma$+ cells. At present there is no direct evidence to differentiate among these alternatives.

Both in vivo treatment with IFN and in vitro incubation with IFN have been shown to augment NK activity, but there are several features which differ depending on the mode of IFN exposure. Einhorn et al.[46] found that in vitro incubation of lymphocytes with IFN for periods up to 48 hr caused a decrease in percentage of Fc$_\gamma$+ cells with a decrease in the percentage of E-rosetting cells and no change in EAC-rosetting cells. This suggests that the NK cells comprising a subpopulation of FcR-bearing cells may in fact be suppressed in their expression of phenotype by IFN. However, in investigations with T cell hybrids, Fridman et al.[47] found that in vitro incubation with IFN caused an increase in the percentage of Fc$_\gamma$+ cells but only on those cell lines that already expressed the Fc$_\gamma$ receptor and not on Fc$_\gamma$ cell lines. No observed changes were seen in the percentage of cells expressing the Fc$_\gamma$ receptor. Gustafsson et al.[48] reported that in vitro incubation of effector cells with IFN resulted in enhancement of the lytic mechanism and the expression of new receptors against non-IFN-inducing cell lines. This caused an increase in cytotoxic activity against previously NK-resistant cell lines. These results are in agreement with our observations of increased target recognition by effector cells after IFN treatment. Ullberg et al.[49] found that incubation of normal PBLs with IFN resulted in a dual effect — an increase in effector cell recruitment from a pre-NK precursor pool and an increase in lytic activity per cell or recycling capacity. However, these effects were not observed for all cell lines, some of whom demonstrated lack of effector cell recruitment. Thus, there does not appear to be complete agreement of the in vitro effects of IFN although there are certainly several parallel observations with some in vivo studies.

In addition, there appears to be a correlation between a predominant T helper cell effect and augmented NK activity, although the specific interactions of this relationship are unknown. The subsequent decline in NK activity after day 7 of IFN administration may be due to a relative increase in the suppressor cell population though it does not appear to be a G-10 adherent population working by a prostaglandin-mediated process. Other possible mechanisms may include IFN-induced sequestration of active NK cells from the peripheral blood to other body compartments or perhaps depression of NK cell precursors at the sites of production and maturation.

The increases in NK activity induced by IFN have been observed by several groups. We shall briefly review some of these studies in order to identify common characteristics associated with IFN modulation of NK activity. However, the timing and duration of augmented NK activity appears to vary with each study.

In a study by Kariniemi et al.,[50] six healthy volunteers were given IFN intradermally and tested for NK activity. There was a transient decline in NK activity and in the numbers of NK cells (large granular lymphocytes [LGLs]) 4 hr postinjection. The nadir of depression was observed at 20 hr and normalized at 72 hr. They detected no clear activation of NK cells for up to 120 hr. Examination of suction blister fluid at the site of IFN injection revealed no increase in NK activity or in numbers of LGLs.

Several studies have observed transient elevations in NK activity followed by a subsequent decline in NK activity following systemic administration of IFN. In a study of IFN-treated cancer patients, Huddlestone et al.[51] reported a series of five patients with non-Hodgkin's lymphoma treated with partially purified IFN i.m. for periods up to 30 days. Augmentation in NK activity was found as early as 12 hr with a gradual decline to pretreatment levels at 18 hr after a single dose of IFN. Einhorn et al.[52] examined the effects of repeated doses of IFN in a series of 43 patients with a variety of neoplasms treated with daily i.m. injections of 3×10^6 U of partially purified IFN. Using Chang liver cells as targets, they also found an increase in cytotoxic activity with a peak activity between 12 and 24 hr, with a subsequent decline. However, several patients in the report were evaluated up to 9 months following initiation of IFN therapy and were found to have persistent elevations in NK activity.

In a multi-institutional phase II trial by Borden et al.,[53] with IFN treatment of 23 patients with disseminated breast cancer, patients received 3×10^6 U/day for an initial period of 28 days. Increased levels of NK and ADCC activity were noted 48 hr after the initiation of therapy although both activities declined with the continuation of additional IFN treatment. Similar to Einhorn's observations,[52] several patients had persistently elevated levels of NK and ADCC activity despite lack of clinical response. Thus, in the patient populations of these studies, IFN treatment is associated with an elevation in NK activity in the majority of patients. However, individual responses to IFN therapy is variable, as noted by the prolonged elevations in some patients seen by Einhorn[52] and Borden.[53]

In a study designed to examine subsets of patients according to preexisting NK cytotoxic levels and subsequent response to IFN therapy, Lotzová et al.[54] studied a series of 42 cancer patients and normal volunteers treated with partially purified leukocyte or recombinant IFN over a 1-month period. In this report, subjects were classified according to pretreatment NK activity as either high, middle, or low. Those individuals exhibiting low to middle preexisting levels of NK activity had the greatest augmentation in NK activity by IFN. Patients with high pretreatment NK levels failed to show any significant augmentation by IFN. In addition, single cell analysis of PBLs was performed in three IFN-responding patients who received a single i.m. injection of 3×10^6 U of recombinant IFN-α. Assessment of binders and killers of K562 targets before and 24 hr after IFN treatment showed no significant changes in target cell binding but did show increased cytotoxic activity among binders. The lack of increase of binders by IFN-α in the latter studies is in apparent contrast to our findings.[36,37] In examining our data to determine if any correlation existed between pretreatment NK activity and subsequent NK activity, there was only a weak correlation in comparing day 0 values and day 7 values ($r = 0.35$; Pearson correlation coefficient). There was even less ($r = 0.17$) correlation between initial values and peak response. We did not attempt to classify responders before IFN treatment as did Lotzová et al.,[54] and therefore these studies are not directly comparable. The results of the single cell assays found by Lotzová agree with the findings of Ullberg[49] with in vitro incubation of PBLs with IFN. However, while these studies observed increases only in the percentage of binders mediating lysis in the single cell analysis, we found increases in both target binders and killers. The disparity of these two sets of data are probably due to differences in experimental design, as Lotzová et al.[54] studied the short-term effects of a single dose of pure recombinant IFN, while our experimental design encompassed multiple dosages of partially purified IFN at varying dosage levels. Thus, it is probable that both results reflect the variety of IFN-induced changes. In the short term, IFN may activate lytic processes while in the long-term may promote the recruitment of NK precursors.

In a study of 17 cancer patients treated with partially purified lymphoblastoid IFN, Koren et al.[55] also noted augmentation of NK activity and increased ADCC during therapy. IFN administration was performed in two separate phases in this study. The first phase examined the NK effects of IFN after a single i.m. injection. The second phase examined the levels of NK activity with chronic administration for a period up to 15 weeks. Similar to the observations of by other groups, Koren et al. found a transient depression in NK activity with a nadir at 12 hr after a single IFN dose. PBLs obtained at this time were unable to be stimulated by in vitro IFN incubation for periods up to 18 hr. In addition, studies with in vitro incubation of IFN with pretreatment PBLs paralleled the maximal responses observed in vivo and thus served as a predictive guide. Those patients who received chronic administration of IFN had maximal NK activity during the 1st week of treatment. Some patients exhibited a decline to pretreatment levels after this peak while others maintained a sustained elevation in NK activity. Paradoxically, maximal stimulation was achieved at 7 days when higher doses of IFN were administered while only patients receiving chronic low dose IFN were able to sustain this augmented NK activity. These observations regarding the effects of dosage regimen on subsequent augmentation or depression of NK response are quite similar to our experience with the dosage schedule used in melanoma patients.

The effects of different IFN preparations on modulation of NK activity were studied by Edwards et al.[56] on 15 cancer patients. The IFNs utilized were partially purified human leukocyte IFN-α and two recombinant DNA-produced IFNs (IFN-rαA and IFN-rαD). Each patient received a single i.m. injection of one type of IFN. When PBLs obtained 24 hr postinjection were assayed, 14 of 15 patients exhibited elevated NK activity compared to pretreatment values irrespective of the IFN preparation. Pretreatment PBLs incubated in vitro in the presence of the same IFN preparation also exhibited a consistent elevation of NK activity. Thus the data corroborates the observations of Koren[55] that individual response to IFN in vivo is reflected by the modulation of NK activity by in vitro incubation of pretreatment PBLs with IFN.

In a study designed to address the question of dosage and timing of administration of IFN in optimizing immune parameters, Silver et al.[57] examined the effects of high and low dose regimens of partially purified lymphoblastoid IFN on NK activity and T cell subsets in 54 cancer patients. Low dose treatment consisted of 2×10^6 U/m^2/day by i.m. injection for 28 days. Maintenance treatment was continued daily for alternate weeks if there was evidence of clinical disease stabilization. High dose treatment consisted of continuous i.v. administration over 10 days. The initial dose was 5×10^6 U/m^2/day with daily increases in dosage of 5×10^6 to 20×10^6 U/m^2/day with further increases in dose every other day. Patients in the low dose regimen exhibited a slight trend towards increases in NK activity although this did not reach statistically significance. Post-treatment NK activity showed no changes from pretreatment levels. During the period of IFN administration, the ratio of OKT4 to OKT8 in PBLs showed a significant decrease reflected by an increase in the proportion of OKT8 positive cells. Among patients in the high dose regimen, there were no changes in NK activity during the period of IFN infusion. Post-treatment NK activity did, however, exhibit long-term elevations up to 15 months. There was also a decrease in the proportion of OKT8 positive cells with a corresponding increase in the OKT4 to OKT8 ratio post-treatment. These findings differ from the results of other workers who have found inverse correlations of NK activity with IFN dosage and minimal effects of IFN on post-treatment levels of NK cytotoxicity. Similarly, Neefe et al.[58] observed that partially purified lymphoblastoid IFN at low dosages augmented NK cytotoxicity while higher doses caused either a depression of NK activity or lack of any change. Ozer et al.[59] administered recombinant DNA-produced IFN and also noted that higher doses of IFN were associated with depression of NK activity whereas lower doses augmented NK activity.

In contrast, some studies have failed to detect any augmentation of NK activity with in vivo administration of IFN. In a study of 134 cancer patients treated with recombinant leukocyte IFN-α, Maluish et al.[60] found NK activity either unchanged or decreased in the majority of patients. Dosages ranged from 1×10^5 to 135×10^6 U per injection, which were administered either twice daily or thrice weekly over a period of 28 days. In assessing NK activity irrespective of total IFN dosage, depressed levels were found in 61 to 91% of PBLs tested. They also noted a trend towards increased depression of NK activity with increasing IFN dosage. Of those patients receiving IFN dosages greater than 240×10^6 U/week, only 10 to 11% had increases in mean NK activity while 32 to 39% of those receiving less than 60×10^6 U IFN had increased activity. This is in agreement with our data and Koren's data[55] regarding the activation of NK at lower IFN dosages. The data also seemed to suggest that lower pretreatment NK activity among patient PBLs was associated with an augmentation in NK levels with IFN treatment and these results are consistent with Lotzová's previous findings.[54]

In a study of 32 cancer patients, Lotzová et al.[61] also studied the effects of recombinant leukocyte IFN-α. Depression of NK activity was observed at 4 and 8 hr after a single injection of IFN for all patients at all dosage levels. However, at 24 hr after IFN treatment, Lotzová observed augmentation of NK activity in patients who exhibited low NK activity prior to IFN treatment irrespective of dosage. In patients who exhibited moderate to high pretreatment NK activity, only 35% showed augmentation of NK activity compared to pretreatment levels. Cytotoxicity in these patients was often below pretreatment levels. The depression of NK activity in the moderate and high pretreatment NK patient groups appeared to be dose related. Of patients who received higher doses of IFN (45 to 86×10^6 U), 67% display depressed NK activity, while only 14% of patients receiving low (3.0 to 4.5×10^6 U) or intermediate (27 to 36×10^6 U) doses showed depressed NK activity.

Ernstoff et al.[62] examined the effects of dose and route of IFN administration in a study of recombinant IFN-in 29 cancer patients. Some 17 patients received i.m. dosages ranging from 3 to 100×10^6 U/day for 28 consecutive days or to tolerance; 12 patients received i.v. administration of IFN. In patients receiving IFN by the i.m. route, the NK activity increased in the 1st week of therapy from a mean pretreatment cytotoxicity of 49% to 67% after 1 week of treatment at both high and low dosages. However, patients receiving i.v. IFN exhibited either no change or depression of NK activity, particularly when dosage exceeded 30×10^6 U/day. In addition to assessment of NK activity, PBLs were assessed for their lymphocyte subpopulations using MoAb markers. In those patients who received higher IFN doses i.m. and showed augmentation of NK activity, the helper to suppressor (Leu-3a to Leu-2a) ratio was increased twofold with an increase in the proportion of Leu-3a positive (helper) cells. Patients receiving more than 30×10^6 U/day of i.v. IFN and exhibiting depression of NK activity had a decrease of the Leu-3a to Leu-2a ratio by 50% due to simultaneous rise in Leu-2a positive cells and a fall in Leu-3a positive cells. This is in agreement with our preliminary findings of augmented helper to suppressor ratios during the peak of NK activity with IFN therapy and the decrease in this ratio during the decline of NK activity later in the course of IFN treatment.

Spina et al.[63] found that the administration of lymphoblastoid IFN to 28 patients with a variety of advanced malignancies resulted in a depressed NK activity during treatment.

Patients were administered partially purified IFN-α from 1.5 to 100 × 10^6 U/day over a period of 7 days. A transient rise in NK activity was seen within 2 hr of IFN administration, particularly in those patients receiving 10 × 10^6 U/day or more. The early augmentation of NK activity with higher IFN dosages is similar to that observed by Koren et al.[55] However, after this transient rise in NK activity, the levels became significantly depressed by day 6 of therapy with NK function returning to baseline levels by days 8 to 16. Parallel studies with day 6 PBLs incubated in vitro with IFN also failed to show augmented NK activity. Preliminary cell mixing experiments with IFN patient lymphocytes and control lymphocytes failed to reveal a suppressor cell population that could account for the depressed NK activity from IFN treatment.

Thus, a wide range of NK activity has been reported with IFN administration. Some studies have clearly shown an augmentation in NK activity by IFN. However, a wide range of kinetic patterns has been observed. Peak NK activity has been seen between 18 hr and 7 days with varying levels of NK activity observed during the late phases of treatment or post-treatment periods. Others have indicated minimal changes or frank depression in NK cytotoxic activity following IFN administration. Several studies also indicated a trend towards depression of NK activity or development of a refractory state with repeated high doses of IFN administration. While selection of patient material and variations in cytotoxicity assays are a consideration, other significant factors are clearly involved. One such factor may be the purity and class of IFN. In studies where depression of NK activity has been observed, most have utilized relatively pure IFN preparations obtained by recombinant DNA technology. Others have utilized a partially purified IFN which may contain other classes of IFN or other immune modulators such as lymphokines, with varying modes and specificities of action. Another factor is the varying dosages and treatment schedules utilized in the trials. These in turn are critically dependent on accurate quantitation of the actual concentration of IFN administered.

While differences in results exist in the studies involving in vivo effects of IFN, some common features among the studies do exist. There is general agreement that the percentage of Fc positive cells remains fairly constant during treatment, although subpopulation variations have been noted. Most groups also have uniformly observed an early decline in NK cytotoxicity after initiation of IFN treatment. This phenomenon has been seen as early as 4 hr and as late as 3 days following IFN. It is interesting that despite the varying IFN preparations or the particular treatment regimen utilized, all groups have seen similarities in early NK depression. Several investigators have observed alterations in the lymphocyte subsets although their role in the modulation of NK activity remain unclear. There is also common agreement that in vivo exposure to IFN renders PBLs nonresponsive to in vitro activation by IFN. This finding, coupled with several indications that lower doses are more effective at maintaining elevated NK activity than are higher doses, suggests that with biologic agents such as IFN "more is better" is a poor starting assumption. In fact, there is evidence for depression of NK activity by larger IFN doses and the only indications of NK activation at high IFN dosage are early and transient. Perhaps some trials with low doses or frequent "rest" periods without IFN administration would provide more consistent and prolonged elevation of NK activity than the trials performed thus far.

III. STUDIES WITH BCG

Intralesional injection of BCG as immunotherapy has been intensively investigated. It has been associated with regression of tumors although its mechanisms are not completely understood.[20,21,64] The presence of macrophages and a granulomatous reaction has correlated with BCG-induced tumor regression on biopsy.[65] The presence of lymphocytic and monocytic inflammatory cells seen on histologic examination of tumor specimens indicate a cell-mediated immune response[66] and has clinically prognostic value.[67-71] Since the NK system has been proposed as a possible immune mechanism in limiting tumor growth, the NK activity at the tumor site is of express interest, as is the local influence of BCG at the tumor site.

Several studies have examined the characteristics of lymphoid infiltrates at the tumor site. Vose et al.[72] compared the NK activity of tumor-infiltrating lymphocytes (TILs) extracted from tumors of varying histologies with autochthonous lymph node lymphocytes and PBLs. In assessing the cytotoxicity against autochthonous tumor cells, they found significant cytotoxicity in only 11 of 31 cancer patients. Similar reactivity was found in the tumor-draining lymph node lymphocytes. Totterman et al.[73] observed similar results of depressed NK activity in the TILs of various tumors which were examined for their reactivity against a wide spectrum of target cells.

While there have been reports of suppression of NK activity in the lymphocytic infiltrates of solid tumors, little is known about the regulatory events governing this suppression. We undertook studies to examine the characteristics of the cellular infiltrates directly at the tumor site and how their composition and functional activity is altered in lesions locally injected with BCG. In this way, we were able to examine the specific regulation of NK activity in the tumor mass and its modulation by a known potentiator of NK activity. The procedures for intralesional injection of BCG into human pulmonary tumors have been described previously.[74]

We have shown that TILs extracted from human pulmonary tumors have decreased proportions of T cells and have a relatively high proportion of null cells.[75] These TILs have shown low responses to alloantigen-induced proliferation and poor generation of cytolytic T cells. Further characterization of the TILs also showed a high proportion (18.8%) of Fc_γ positive cells, indicating that NK activity might be expected in this population. However, by ^{51}Cr-release assay against K562 targets, TILs showed marked depression in NK cytotoxic activity compared with autochthonous PBLs. The TILs were prepared by mechanical disaggregation and separated by Ficoll-Hypaque centrifugation. Additional fractionation procedures such as nylon fiber columns, passage over a Sephadex G-10 column, or plastic adherence did not restore NK activity. Further purification to remove all residual tumor cells also failed to augment the depressed NK activity. Since macrophages from the bronchopulmonary tree have been shown to have a suppressive effect on cytotoxic activity,[76] TILs were macrophage depleted by incubation with carbonyl iron. No relief of suppression of NK activity was observed in macrophage-depleted TIL populations.

In contrast are our results with patients who had been injected intralesionally with BCG 2 weeks prior to surgical resection.[75] In this situation, the TILs exhibited higher levels of NK activity compared to uninjected tumors (20.5 ± 7.7% for 5 BCG-injected tumors compared with 7.7 ± 1.9% at 50:1 effector to target ratio for TILs from 20 uninjected tumors). Patients injected intralesionally with BCG also showed moderate increases in NK activity of regional draining lymph node lymphocytes (LNL) and PBLs compared to uninjected patients (23.3 ± 4.8% for LNLs and 36.5 ± 7.9% for PBLs in BCG-injected patients; 15.4 ± 4.8% for LNLs and 28.6 ± 4.0% for PBLs in uninjected patients). Of particular interest was our finding of low NK activity in TILs from uninjected tumors obtained from the same lung as the BCG-injected tumors. This indicates that despite local, regional, and systemic enhancement of NK activity, NK cells either cannot penetrate untreated tumors or are promptly inactivated there.

We also studied the TILs for ability to bind and lyse target cells in the single cell assay. We have found comparable proportions of cells capable of binding to K562 target cells and those mediating lysis among TILs and PBLs[77] (binding = 13.9 ± 5.0% for TILs and 12.6 ± 4.4% for PBLs; killing = 13.8 ± 8.7% for TILs and 10.1 ± 8.4% for PBLs). Thus, while there does not appear to be a lack of NK cells at the tumor site, the low NK activity as assessed by the ^{51}Cr-release assay indicates a functional impairment of these cells. Since the number of target binding cells is comparable in TILs and PBLs, the most likely defect appears to be in the kinetics of lysis or in recycling capability of NK cells among the TILs. Our unpublished observations and the findings of Moore and Vose[78] indicate that IFN cannot activate TIL NK activity. IFN has been shown to increase the recycling capacity among NK cells in vitro,[49] and might be expected to have little stimulatory effect on those cells unable to mediate multiple lytic events.

We next examined whether a suppressor cell population might account for the depressed NK activity among the TILs. Addition of TILs to autochthonous PBLs did not diminish the cytotoxic activity of PBLs. While Vose and Moore[79] reported a population of suppressor cells among TILs for proliferative responses, we found little suppressive effect of TILs on the NK activity of PBLs. To determine whether the low NK activity of TILs was due to the presence of prostaglandin-secreting cells, we incubated TILs in the presence of indomethicin for up to 18 hr. This treatment failed to restore NK activity. Thus, the microenvironment of the solid tumor has an extremely inhibitory effect on local immune function as seen by low NK activity. The low NK activity of TILs can be partially overcome with local BCG injection.

BCG has been shown to augment NK cytotoxicity in mice, healthy human volunteers, and melanoma patients.[80-82] Thatcher[81] studied the effects of i.d. BCG administration to five healthy human volunteers. An increase in NK activity was found by day 7 to 10 postadministration with a return to baseline levels by day 28. In a study with 16 patients with disseminated melanoma,[82] BCG administration was administered i.d. every 3 weeks. Elevated levels of NK cytotoxicity were detected within 1 week of BCG administration with sustained elevations seen for up to 8 weeks.

In preliminary experiments, we have seen increased NK activity against K562 targets in melanoma patients treated with BCG. Three patients who received i.v. BCG for metastatic melanoma were evaluated in addition to one patient who received intralesional injection of BCG for skin metastases. In these patients, all exhibited elevations in NK activity after BCG administration. Cytotoxicity was assessed against K562, the M14 melanoma cell line, and the L14 lymphoblastoid cell line. M14 cells express an oncofetal antigen against which many patients show a serologic reaction.[83]

In the melanoma patient injected intralesionally with BCG into skin metastases and in three patients treated with i.v. BCG, augmentation in NK activity against K562 and L14 targets was seen soon after the initiation of treatment with BCG. These levels remained high during the 1st week but subsequently declined to nearly undetectable levels 1 month post-treatment. Cytotoxic activity towards the allogeneic M14 target as assessed by 4-hr ^{51}Cr-release remained unchanged during treatment. These findings are in close agreement with the augmentation of NK activity observed with IFN administration to melanoma patients and thus suggest a similarity in the pathways of in vivo NK activation from a baseline state.

Having observed parallel results in BCG- and IFN-treated patients, we attempted to determine if BCG also increases the number of NK precursors. We tested serially obtained cryopreserved lymphocytes of two BCG-treated melanoma patients for generation of NK-like cytotoxicity in vitro after allogeneic lymphoblast stimulation. Cytotoxic activity was increased greater than twofold in PBL specimens from day 2 and 7 at all effector to target ratios compared to day 1 samples or control PBLs. These results thus suggest that BCG administration, like IFN, may be accompanied by enhancement of a pre-NK precursor pool which could increase the number of active NK cells in the peripheral blood.

Having observed augmentation of NK activity in the ^{51}Cr-release assay, we utilized the single cell assay to determine whether the increase was due to enhanced killing capability of each cell or an increase in the numbers of NK cells. Some 14 melanoma patients with advanced Stage II and III disease were treated with intralymphatic immunotherapy (ILI)

Table 5
SINGLE CELL ANALYSIS OF PBLs OF PATIENTS RECEIVING INTRALYMPHATIC IMMUNOTHERAPY[a]

	Treatment Number				
	0	**1**	**2**	**3**	**4—7**
K562					
% Binding[b]	8.3 ± 0.6	10.3 ± 0.8	13.0 ± 1.1	11.9 ± 0.9	12.6 ± 0.9
% Killing[c]	22.3 ± 3.0	21.7 ± 2.3	21.5 ± 2.8	20.4 ± 2.1	19.8 ± 1.7
% NK[d]	1.9 ± 0.3	2.2 ± 0.2	2.6 ± 0.3	2.4 ± 0.3	2.5 ± 0.3
M14					
% Binding	6.5 ± 0.9	11.3 ± 1.3	11.0 ± 1.3	12.5 ± 2.0	11.1 ± 1.6
	15.5 ± 11.6	17.9 ± 6.1	19.4 ± 9.1	21.4 ± 7.9	19.8 ± 12.1
% NK	1.0 ± 0.8	2.1 ± 0.9	1.2 ± 0.5	2.6 ± 1.3	1.8 ± 0.9
No. samples tested	14	13	13	10	12

[a] Patients received intralymphatic tumor cell vaccine (TCV) and either intradermal or intralymphatic BCG. PBL obtained 1 week following each treatment.
[b] Percent of PBL binding to targets; 200 lymphocytes scored.
[c] Percent of target binding cells mediating lysis as determined by trypan blue dye exclusion. At least 100 binders scored.
[d] Product of a × b.

consisting of i.d. BCG and intralymphatic administration of either an irradiated allogeneic tumor cell vaccine or vaccine plus BCG.[84] The tumor cell vaccine consisted of three cultured melanoma cell lines (UCLA-SO-M7, M14, and M20) which had been irradiated with 10,000 rads. ILI administration consisted of two treatments given 2 weeks apart with subsequent treatments at monthly intervals. Results are seen in Table 5. The number of cells capable of binding K562 targets increased during the initial treatment and remained elevated for the duration of ILI. However, the percent of binders that were capable of killing did not change during the course of treatment. This implies that there was an increase in the absolute number of NK cells but that the specific activity per cell remained unchanged. These results are in agreement with our results of the single cell analysis of systemically treated IFN melanoma patients. There was also an increase in the numbers of cells capable of binding M14 targets during the treatment period. However, since the M14 cell line was included as part of the trivalent tumor cell vaccine used to treat patients, the increased number of binders probably represents allospecific sensitization rather than an increase in NK cells. Since patients received both BCG and allogeneic tumor cell vaccine, the assessment of the relative roles of each in modulating NK activity was indeterminate. The route of BCG administration had only modest effects on the increase in NK activity towards K562 targets. Of the ILI patients studied, seven received intralymphatic BCG plus i.d. BCG while seven received only i.d. BCG. The intralymphatic group showed an increase from 8.9 ± 0.9% binders (pretreatment) to 14.4 ± 1.6% (after two treatments) while the i.d. BCG group showed an increase from 7.7 ± 0.6% to 10.8 ± 1.0% during the same period.

These results indicate that intralymphatic immunotherapy in conjunction with BCG is capable of augmenting systemic NK activity as reflected in the peripheral blood. The augmentation in NK activity, however, was not correlated with clinical effects.

Although we have assumed that the BCG component of the ILI is responsible for the NK effects, it is possible that the alloimmunization is the cause of elevation of NK activity. Several animal model systems have shown that alloimmunization can elevate NK activity.[85,86] Recent results also indicate that NK cells will accumulate at the site of a rejecting rat kidney allograft.[87] In humans, elevated NK activity has been correlated with graft vs. host disease in bone marrow allograft recipients.[88] There is also extensive evidence for in vitro induction of human NK activity by allostimulation in mixed lymphocyte culture. This area is reviewed extensively in Chapter 12 in Volume I. Thus, there is ample evidence to indicate that the alloimmunization, in concert with the BCG, is responsible for the changes in NK activity during ILI.

IV. CONCLUSION

The investigation of NK modulation by immunomodulatory agents in human cancer patients serves as a useful model for probing the regulation of the NK system. IFN has generated considerable controversy regarding its mode of action and its ability to alter host NK activity. While current evidence suggests that the magnitude of observed augmentation of NK activity does not correlate with the clinical efficacy, issues regarding the purity and class of IFN as well as dosage schedules need to be resolved to definitively address this question. BCG has also been associated with augmentation of NK activity both systemically and intralesionally. It is possible that BCG works as an enhancer of NK activity via induction of IFN production. Both agents may be influenced by other host produced products such as IL-2. Until the pathways involved in in vivo modulation of NK are better defined, it will remain quite difficult to predict how to consistently and effectively modulate NK activity with biologic agents.

The central issue that remains unresolved is does elevated NK activity have any therapeutic potential? Although agents such as IFN and BCG are not directed solely at the NK system, it would be inappropriate to modify dose/time schedules to maximize the NK response if elevated NK activity has no therapeutic benefit. However, the only direct evidence we are likely to get to determine the therapeutic efficacy of NK cells would be with agents such as IFN. At present, the results are not very encouraging as there has been no unequivocal correlations between NK activity and clinical response to any biological response modifier. Some evidence indicates that NK cells either do not have good access to tumor sites or are inactivated at the tumor site. In contrast, results in animal models[3,4] have indicated NK activity against circulating tumor cells capable of yielding metastatic lesions. Perhaps the ideal trial to examine the possible clinical benefits of agents capable of augmenting NK function would include an approach to maximize and maintain high NK activity in patients with minimal disease but with a high likelihood of having circulating "premetastatic" tumor cells. Postoperative adjuvant trials in diseases such as carcinoma of the breast or colon or melanoma could be better candidate situations than trials in patients with large tumor burdens. Unfortunately, efficacy in trials with extensive disease is usually the criterion for exploration of the use of an agent in an adjuvant setting.

ACKNOWLEDGMENT

This work was supported in part by U.S. National Institute of Health grant CA 12582 and CCCI.

REFERENCES

1. **Herberman, R. B. and Holden, H. T.,** Natural killer cells as anti-tumor effector cells, *J. Natl. Cancer Inst.*, 62, 441, 1979.
2. **Hanna, N. and Burton, R. C.,** Definitive evidence that natural killer (NK) cells inhibit experimental tumor metastasis in vivo, *J. Immunol.*, 127, 1754, 1981.
3. **Hanna, N.,** Inhibition of experimental tumor metastasis by selective activation of natural killer cells, *Cancer Res.*, 42, 1337, 1982.
4. **Hanna, N. and Fidler, I. J.,** Role of natural killer cells in the destruction of circulating tumor emboli, *J. Natl. Cancer Inst.*, 65, 801, 1980.
5. **Häller, O., Hansson, M., Kiessling, R., and Wigzell, H.,** Role of non-conventional killer cells in the resistance against syngeneic tumor cells in vivo, *Nature (London)*, 270, 609, 1977.
6. **Petranyi, G. G., Kiessling, R., Povey, S., Klein, G., Heizengerg, L., and Wigzell, H.,** Genetic control of natural killer cell activity and its association with an in vivo resistance against a Moloney lymphoma isograft, *Immunogenetics*, 3, 15, 1976.
7. **Riccardi, C., Santoni, A., Puccetti, P., and Herberman, R. B.,** In vivo natural reactivity of mice against tumor cells, *J. Natl. Cancer Inst.*, 63, 1041, 1979.
8. **Talmadge, J. E., Meyers, K. M., Priens, D. J., and Starkey, J. R.,** Role of NK cells in tumor growth and metastasis in beige mice, *Nature (London)*, 284, 622, 1980.
9. **Talmadge, J. E., Meyers, K. M., Priens, D. J., and Starkey, J. R.,** Role of natural killer cells in tumor growth and metastasis in C57BL/6 normal and beige mice, *J. Natl. Cancer Inst.*, 65, 929, 1980.
10. **Gorelik, E. and Herberman, R. B.,** Radioisotope assay for evaluation of in vivo natural cell mediated resistance of mice to local transplantation of tumor cells, *Int. J. Cancer*, 27, 709, 1980.
11. **O'Toole, C., Perlmann, P., Unsgaard, B., Moberger, G., and Edsmyr, F.,** Cellular immunity to human urinary bladder carcinoma. I. Correlation to clinical stage and radiotherapy, *Int. J. Cancer*, 10, 77, 1972.
12. **Pross, H. F. and Baines, M. G.,** Spontaneous human lymphocyte-mediated cytotoxicity against tumor target cells. I. Effects of malignant disease, *Int. J. Cancer*, 18, 593, 1976.
13. **Stratton, M. L., Herz, J., Loeffler, R. A., McGlurg, Reiter, A., Bernstein, P., Danley, D. L., and Benjamin, E.,** Antibody-dependent cell-mediated cytotoxicity in treated and nontreated cancer patients, *Cancer*, 40, 1045, 1977.
14. **Takasugi, M., Ramsmeyer, A., and Takasugi, J.,** Decline of natural nonselective cell-mediated cytotoxicity in patients with tumor progression, *Cancer Res.*, 37, 413, 1977.
15. **Bloom, B. R.,** Interferons and the immune system, *Nature (London)*, 284, 593, 1980.
16. **Herberman, R. B., Ortaldo, J. R., Djeu, J. Y., et al.,** Role of interferon in regulation of cytotoxicity by natural killer cells and macrophages, in *Regulatory Functions of Interferons*, Vilcek, J., Gresser, I., and Merigan, T. C., Eds., New York, Academy of Science, 350, 63, 1980.
17. **Djeu, J. Y., Heinbaugh, J. A., Holden, H. T., and Herberman, R. M.,** Augmentation of mouse natural killer cell activity by interferon and interferon inducers, *J. Immunol.*, 122, 175, 1978.
18. **Timonen, T., Ortaldo, J. R., and Herberman, R. B.,** Characteristics of human large granular lymphocytes and relationship to natural killer cells, *J. Exp. Med.*, 153, 569, 1981.
19. **Herberman, R. B., Ortaldo, J. R., and Bonnard, G. D.,** Augmentation of interferon of human natural and antibody-dependent cell-mediated cytotoxicity, *Nature (London)*, 277, 221, 1979.
20. **Hanna, M. G., Zbar, B., and Rapp, H. J.,** Histopathology of tumor regression after intralesional injection of *Mycobacterium bovis*. I. Tumor growth and metastases, *J. Natl. Cancer Inst.*, 48, 1441, 1972.
21. **Bast, R. C., Jr., Zbar, B., Borsos, T., and Rapp, H. J.,** BCG and cancer, *N. Engl. J. Med.*, 290, 1413, 1974.
22. **Golub, S. H. and Holmes, E. C.,** In vitro assay of immunocompetence in patients with lung cancer treated with levamisole, *Cancer Immunol. Immunother.*, 7, 143, 1979.
23. **Gresser, I.,** Antitumor effects of interferon, in *Cancer, A Comprehensive Treatise*, Becker, F. F., Ed., Plenum Press, New York, 1977, 521.
24. **Strander, H.,** Interferons: antineoplastic drugs?, *Blut*, 35, 279, 1977.
25. **Strander, H., Cantrell, D., Carstrom, G., and Jakobsson, P. A.,** Clinical and laboratory investigations on man: systemic administration of potent interferon to man, *J. Natl. Cancer Inst.*, 51, 733, 1973.
26. **Merigan, T. C., Sikora, K., Breeden, J. H., Levy, R., and Rosenberg, S. A.,** Preliminary observations on the effect of human leukocyte interferon in non-Hodgkin's lymphoma, *N. Engl. J. Med.*, 299, 1449, 1978.
27. **Gutterman, J. U., Blumenschein, G. R., Alexanian, R., Yap, H., Buzdar, A., Cabanillas, F., Hortobagyi, G., Hersh, E. M., Rasmussen, S., Harman, M., Kramer, M., and Pestka, S.,** Leukocyte interferon-induced tumor regression in human metastatic breast cancer, multiple myeloma, and malignant melanoma, *Ann. Intern. Med.*, 93, 399, 1980.

28. **Gutterman, J. U., Fine, S., Quesada, J., Horning, S. J., Levine, J. F., Alexanian, R., Bernhardt, L., Kramer, M., Siegal, H., Colburn, W., Trown, P., Merigan, T., and Dziewanowski, Z.,** Recombinant leukocyte-a interferon: pharmacokinetics, single dose tolerance, and biologic effects in cancer patients, *Ann. Intern. Med.*, 96, 549, 1982.
29. **Ikic, D., Brodarec, I., Padovan, I., Knezevic, M., and Soos, E.,** Application of human leucocyte interferon in patients with tumours of the head and neck, *Lancet*, 1F, 1025, 1981.
30. **Ikic, D., Maricic, X., Oresic, V., Rode, B., Nola, P., Smudj, K., Knexevic, M., Jusic, D., and Soos, E.,** Application of human leucocyte interferon in patients with urinary bladder papillomatosis, breast cancer, and melanoma, *Lancet*, 1F, 1022, 1981.
31. **Mellstedt, H., Bjorkholm, M., Johansson, B., Ahre, A., Strander, H., and Holm, G.,** Interferon therapy in myelomatosis, *Lancet*, 1F, 245, 1979.
32. **Gresser, I., Borrali, C., Levy, J. P.,** Fontaine-Bronty-Boye, D., and Thomas, M. R., Increased survival in mice inoculated with tumor cells and treated with interferon preparations, *Proc. Natl. Acad. Sci. U.S.A.*, 63, 51, 1969.
33. **Salerno, R. A., Whitmire, C. E., Garcia, I. M., and Huebner, R. J.,** Chemical carcinogenesis in mice inhibited by interferon, *Nature (New Biol.)*, 239, 31, 1972.
34. **Sarma, P. S., Shin, G., Neubauer, R. H., Bara, S., and Huebner, R. J.,** Virus-induced sarcoma of mice: inhibition by a synthetic polyribonucleotide complex, *Proc. Natl. Acad. Sci. U.S.A.*, 62, 1046, 1969.
35. **Krown, S. E., Burk, M., Kirkwood, J. M., Kerr, D., Morton, D. L., and Oettgen, H. F.,** Human leukocyte interferon in metastatic malignant melanoma: preliminary report of the American Cancer Society Clinical Trial, *Proc. Am. Assoc. Cancer Res.*, 22, 158, 1981.
36. **Golub, S. H., Dorey F., Hara, D., Morton, D. L., and Burk, M. W.,** Systemic administration of human leukocyte interferon to melanoma patients. I. Effect on NK function and cell populations, *J. Natl. Cancer Inst.*, 68, 703, 1982.
37. **Golub, S. H., D'Amore, P. J., and Rainey, M.,** Systemic administration of human leukocyte interferon to melanoma patients. II. Cellular events associated with changes in NK cytotoxicity, *J. Natl. Cancer Inst.*, 68, 711, 1982.
38. **Grimm, E. and Bonavida, B.,** Mechanisms of cell-mediated cytotoxicity at the single cell level. I. Estimation of cytotoxic T lymphocyte frequency and relative lytic efficiency, *J. Immunol.*, 35, 213, 1980.
39. **Savary, C. A. and Lotzová, E.,** Suppression of natural killer cytotoxicity by splenocytes from *Corynebacterium parvum*- injected, bone marrow tolerant, and infant mice, *J. Immunol.*, 120, 239, 1978.
40. **Cudkowicz, G. and Hochman, P. S.,** Carageenan-induced decline of natural killer activity. I. In vitro activation of adherent non-T-suppressor cells, *Cell. Immunol.*, 53, 395, 1980.
41. **Droller, J. J., Schneider, M. V., and Perlmann, P.,** A possible role of prostaglandins in the inhibition of natural and antibody-dependent cell mediated cytotoxicity against tumor cells, *Cell. Immunol.*, 39, 165, 1978.
42. **Karavodin, L. M. and Golub, S. H.,** Universal rosetting reagent for the detection of human cell surface markers, *J. Immunol. Methods*, 61, 293, 1983.
43. **Karavodin, L. M. and Golub, S. H.,** Systemic administration of human leukocyte interferon to melanoma patients. III. Increased helper: suppressor cell ratios in melanoma patients during interferon treatment, submitted.
44. **Abo, T. and Balch, C. M.,** A differentiation antigen of human NK cells and K cells identified by a monoclonal antibody (HNK-1), *J. Immunol.*, 127, 1024, 1981.
45. **Perussia, B., Stan, S., Abraham, S., Fanning, V., and Trinchieri, G.,** Human natural killer cells as analyzed by B73.1, a monoclonal antibody blocking Fc receptor function, *J. Immunol.*, 130, 2133, 1983.
46. **Einhorn, S., Blomgren, H., and Troye, M.,** Proportion of lymphocytes forming E, EA, and EAC rosettes following treatment with human interferon preparations in vitro, *Cell. Immunol.*, 56, 374, 1980.
47. **Fridman, W. H., Gresser, I., Bander, M. T., Aguet, M., and Neauport-Sautes, C.,** Interferon enhances the expression of Fc-gamma receptors, *J. Immunol.*, 5, 2436, 1980.
48. **Gustafsson, A. and Lundgren, E.,** Augmentation of natural killer cells involves both enhancement of lytic machinery and expression of new receptors, *Cell. Immunol.*, 62, 367, 1981.
49. **Ullberg, M., Merrill, J., and Jondal, M.,** Interferon-induced NK augmentation in humans. An analysis of target recognition, effector cell recruitment and effector cell recycling, *Scand. J. Immunol.*, 14, 285, 1981.
50. **Kariniemi, A. L., Timonen, T., and Kousa, M.,** Effect of leukocyte interferon on natural killer cells in healthy volunteers, *Scand. J. Immunol.*, 12, 371, 1980.
51. **Huddlestone, J. R., Merigan, T. C., and Olstone, M. B.,** Induction and kinetics on natural killer cells in humans following interferon therapy, *Nature (London)*, 282, 417, 1979.
52. **Einhorn, S., Blomgren, H., and Strander, H.,** Interferon and spontaneous cytotoxicity in man. V. Enhancement of spontaneous cytotoxicity in patients receiving human leukocyte interferon, *Int. J. Cancer*, 26, 419, 1980.

53. **Borden, E. C., Holland, J. F., Dao, T. L., Gutterman, J. U., Weiner, L., Chang, Y., and Patel, J.,** Leukocyte-derived interferon (alpha) in human breast carcinoma, *Ann. Intern. Med.*, 97, 1, 1982.
54. **Lotzová, E., Savary, C. A., Gutterman, J. U., and Hersh, E. M.,** Modulation of natural killer cell-mediated cytotoxicity by partially purified and cloned interferon, *Cancer Res.*, 42, 2480, 1982.
55. **Koren, H. S., Brandt, C. P., Tso, C. Y., and Laszlo, J.,** Modulation of natural killing activity by lymphoblastoid interferon in cancer patients, *J. Biol. Resp. Modif.*, 2, 151, 1983.
56. **Edwards, B. S., Hawkins, M. J., and Borden, E. C.,** Correlation between in vitro and systemic effects of native and recombinant interferon-α on human natural killer cell cytotoxicity, *J. Biol. Resp. Modif.*, 2, 409, 1983.
57. **Silver, H. K. B., Connors, J. M., Karim, K. A., Kong, S., Spinelli, J. J., deJong, G., McLean, D. M., and Salinas, F. A.,** Effect of lymphoblastoid interferon on lymphocyte subsets in cancer patients, *J. Biol. Resp. Modif.*, 2, 428, 1983.
58. **Neefe, J. R., Sullivan, J. E., and Silgals, R.,** Preliminary observations of immunomodulatory activity of lymphoblastoid interferon-α administered every other day or weekly, *J. Biol. Resp. Modif.*, 2, 441, 1983.
59. **Ozer, H., Gavigan, M., O'Malley, J., Thompson, D., Dadey, B., Nussbaum-Blumenson, A., Snider, C., Rudnick, S., Ferraresi, R., Norred, S., and Han, T.,** Immunomodulation by recombinant interferon-α2 in a phase I trial in patients with lymphoproliferative malignancies, *J. Biol. Resp. Modif.*, 2, 499, 1983.
60. **Maluish, A. E., Ortaldo, J. R., Conlon, J. C., Sherwin, S., Leavitt R., Strong, D. M., Fine, S., Wiernik, P., Oldham, R. K., and Herberman, R. B.,** Depression of natural killer cytotoxicity after in vivo administration of recombinant leukocyte interferon, *J. Immunol.*, 131, 503, 1983.
61. **Lotzová, E., Savary, C. A., Gutterman, J. U., Quesada, J. R., and Hersh, E. M.,** Regulation of human natural killer cell cytotoxicity by recombinant leukocyte interferon clone A, *J. Biol. Resp. Modif.*, 2, 482, 1983.
62. **Ernstoff, M. S., Fusi, S., and Kirkwood, J. M.,** Parameters of interferon action. II. Immunological effects of recombinant leukocyte interferon (IFN-α2) in phase I-II trials, *J. Biol. Resp. Modif.*, 2, 540, 1983.
63. **Spina, C., Fahey, J. L., Durkos-Smith, D., Dorey, F., and Sarna, G.,** Suppression of NK cell cytotoxicity in the peripheral blood of patients receiving interferon therapy, *J. Biol. Resp. Modif.*, in press.
64. **Morton, D. L., Eilber, F. R., Malgrem, R. A., and Wood, W. C.,** Immunological factors which influence response to immunotherapy in malignant melanoma, *Surgery*, 68, 158, 1970.
65. **Zbar, B., Bernstein, I. D., Bartlett, G. L., Hanna, M. G., and Rapp, J. J.,** Immunotherapy of cancer: regression of intradermal tumors and prevention of growth of lymph node metastases after intralesional injection of living *Mycobacterium bovis*, *J. Natl. Cancer Inst.*, 49, 119, 1972.
66. **Svennevig, J. L., Lovik, M., and Svaar, H.,** Isolation and characterization of lymphocytes and macrophages from solid, malignant tumors, *Int. J. Cancer*, 23, 626, 1979.
67. **Hamlin, I. M. E.,** Possible host resistance in carcinoma of the breast: a histological study, *Br. J. Cancer*, 22, 381, 1968.
68. **Bloom, H. J. G., Richardson, W. W., and Field, J. R.,** Host resistance and survival in carcinoma of the breast: a study of 104 cases of medullary carcinoma of breast in a series of 1411 cases of breast cancer followed for 20 years, *Br. Med. J.*, 3, 181, 1970.
69. **Elston, C. W. and Bagshawe, K. D.,** Cellular reaction in trophoblastic tumors, *Br. J. Cancer*, 28, 245, 1973.
70. **Dipaola, M., Bertolotti, A., Colizza, S., and Coli, M.,** Histology of bronchial carcinoma and regional lymph nodes as putative immune response of the host to the tumor, *J. Thorac. Cardiovasc. Surg.*, 73, 531, 1977.
71. **Lauder, I., Aherne, W., Stewart, J., and Sainsbury, R.,** Macrophage infiltration of breast tumors: a prospective study, *J. Clin. Pathol.*, 30, 563, 1977.
72. **Vose, B. M., Vanky, F., and Klein, E.,** Human tumor-lymphocyte interaction in vitro. V. Comparison of the reactivity of tumor infiltrating, blood and lymph node lymphocytes with autologous tumor cells, *Int. J. Cancer*, 20, 512, 1977.
73. **Totterman, T. H., Hayry, P., Saksela, E., Timonen, T., and Eklund, B.,** Cytological and functional analysis of inflammatory infiltrates in human malignant tumors. II. Functional investigations of the infiltrating inflammatory cells, *Eur. J. Immunol.*, 8, 872, 1978.
74. **Fon, G. T., Bein, M. E., Holmes, E. C., and Huberman, R. P.,** Intralesional BCG injection of pulmonary neoplasms: radiographic findings, *Am. J. Radiol.*, 137, 269, 1981.
75. **Niitsuma, M., Golub, S. H., Edelstein, R., and Holmes, E. C.,** Lymphoid cells infiltrating human pulmonary tumors: effect of intralesional BCG injection, *J. Natl. Cancer Inst.*, 67, 997, 1981.
76. **Bordignon, C., Villa, F., Allavena, P., et al.,** Inhibition of natural killer activity by human bronchoalveolar macrophages, *J. Immunol.*, 129, 587, 1982.

77. **Golub, S. H., Moy, P. M., Gray, J. D., Karavodin, L. M., Kawate, N., Niitsuma, M., and Burk, M. W.,** Systemic and local regulation of human NK cytotoxicity, in *Basic Mechanisms and Clinical Treatment of Cancer Metastases,* Torisu, M. and Yoshida, T., Eds., Academic Press, New York, 1982.
78. **Moore, M. and Vose, B. M.,** Extravascular natural cytotoxicity in man: anti-K562 activity of lymph node and tumor-infiltrating lymphocytes, *Int. J. Cancer,* 27, 265, 1981.
79. **Vose, B. M. and Moore, M.,** Suppressor cell activity of lymphocytes infiltrating human lung and breast tumors, *Int. J. Cancer,* 24, 579, 1979.
80. **Djeu, J. Y., Heimbaugh, J. A., Hoden, H. T., and Herberman, R. B.,** Role of macrophages in the augmentation of mouse natural killer cell activity by poly I:C and interferon, *J. Immunol.,* 122, 182, 1978.
81. **Thatcher, N. and Crowther, D.,** Changes in nonspecific lymphoid (NK, K, T cell) cytotoxicity following BCG immunization of health subjects, *Cancer Immunol. Immunother.,* 5, 105, 1978.
82. **Thatcher, N., Swindell, R., and Crowther, D.,** Effects of repeated *Corynebacterium parvum* and BCG therapy in immune paramenters: a weekly sequential study of melanoma patients. I. Changes in nonspecific (NK, K, and T cell) lymphocyte toxicity, peripheral blood counts and delayed hypersensitivity reactions, *Clin. Exp. Immunol.,* 36, 227, 1979.
83. **Irie, R. F., Giuliano, A. E., and Morton, D. L.,** Oncofetal antigen: a tumor-associated fetal antigen immunogenic in man, *J. Natl. Cancer Inst.,* 63, 367, 1979.
84. **Ahn, S. S., Irie, R. F., Weisenburger, T. H., et al.,** Humoral immune response to intralymphatic immunotherapy for disseminated melanoma: correlation with clinical response, *Surgery,* 92, 362, 1982.
85. **Betton, G. R., Gorman, N. T., and Owen, L. N.,** Cell mediated cytotoxicity in dogs following systemic or local BCG treatment alone or in combination with allogeneic tumor cell lines, *Eur. J. Cancer,* 15, 545, 1979.
86. **Clark, E. A. and Holly, R. D.,** Activation of natural killer (NK) cells in vivo with H-2 and non H-2 alloantigens, *Immunogenetics,* 12, 221, 1981.
87. **Nemlander, A., Sadsela, E., and Hayry, P.,** Are "natural killer" cells involved in allograft rejection?, *Eur. J. Immunol.,* 13, 348, 1983.
88. **Dokhaelar, M. C., Wiels, J., Lipinski, M., et al.,** Natural killer cell activity in human bone marrow recipients, *Transplantation,* 31, 61, 1981.

Chapter 5

THE IMPLICATIONS OF ABERRANT NATURAL KILLER (NK) CELL ACTIVITY IN NONMALIGNANT CHRONIC DISEASES

Jean E. Merrill

TABLE OF CONTENTS

I. INTRODUCTION

Immunologists face a thought-provoking question in considering natural killer (NK) cells and disease. Do NK cells benefit the host by eliminating virus-infected cells, or do they contribute to chronic pathological conditions, as in autoimmune diseases, by failing to control virus infection and persistence? If the latter, virally modified tissue could be the target of both specific and nonspecific cellular and humoral autoreactivity.[1,2] This simple scheme is complicated by the fact that NK cells can also be stimulated by normal cells in the absence of virus or by virus alone to lyse normal cells.

When normal cells are targets of NK cells, they usually are immature fetal cell types. Their mature counterparts have decreased NK cell sensitivity.[3-8] Not only have NK cells been described as potential regulators of lymphocyte development from bone marrow and thymus,[5] they may regulate normal development of myeloid[6] and erythroid stem cells.[4,7,8] When this regulation is excessive, diseases such as neutropenia[6] and aplastic anemia[7,8] may result. Mature normal cells[9-11] can also be targets of NK cells generated by autologous mixed lymphocyte reaction (auto-MLR)[11] or by chronic hepatitis B virus.[10] If the role of NK cells is not to lyse infected targets, what other role could they play in chronic nonmalignant disease? One possibility is that NK cells may prevent chronic infection or contribute to prevention of autoimmunity by boosting the antigen-specific immune response via production of interleukin-2 (IL-2)[12] and enhance antiviral activity by secretion of α-interferon (IFN-α).[13-17]

This chapter surveys chronic diseases of known and unknown etiology and explores two possibilities. The first is that aberrant NK cell activity is merely a response to a chronic antigenic stimulus — the result of an imbalance in the immune response due to a previously initiated autoimmune event — and thus is unrelated to the chronicity of the nonmalignant disease. The second possibility is that NK cells contribute to the pathology of autoimmune diseases, immunodeficiency, and bacterial and viral infections.

II. ARE CHANGES IN NK CELL ACTIVITY IN NONMALIGNANT DISEASE SPECIFIC FOR THE INDUCING ANTIGEN OR THE DISEASE PROCESS — OR ARE THEY TRIGGERED BY A NONSPECIFIC EVENT?

Of the events following antigenic stimulus, alterations of NK cell activity are a straightforward consequence and not likely to be specific for any antigen triggering a disease process. Macrophages are activated by antigens and T lymphokines to produce interleukin-1 (IL-1),[18,19] which stimulates IL-2 production,[18,19] which in turn induces IFN-γ.[20,21] IFN-γ induces IL-2 receptors,[20] and the immune response, including NK cell activity, is then amplified. IFN,[22,23] especially IFN-α,[23-26] boosts NK cell activity directly, as does IL-2.[27-29] NK cell recruitment, NK cell numbers, and recycling are elevated by IFN.[30] Thus, the induction of NK cell activity is IL-1 dependent,[19] IL-2 dependent,[27-29] IFN dependent,[27-30] and the natural consequence of any immune response.

So an *increase* in NK cell activity cannot be associated with chronic disease, but a *decrease* in NK activity could be due to disease: the disease-associated antigen stimulates antibody production, and the resulting immune complexes (1) directly inhibit NK cells via their $Fc_{\gamma}R$[31-33] or $Fc_{\mu}R$[33] or (2) induce prostaglandin E (PGE).[34,35] PGE can inhibit IL-2 production,[36,37] which may partly explain its suppression of NK cells,[38-40] though PGE might directly suppress NK cells.[41] Immune complexes are the hallmarks of a variety of chronic autoimmune diseases and have been claimed to be responsible for depressed NK cell activity in secondary syphilis[42,43] and in lepromatous leprosy patients undergoing an episode of erythema nodosum leprosum.[44] Immune complexes in sera of patients with systemic lupus erythematosus (SLE)[45,46] and rheumatoid arthritis[47] have also been shown to suppress NK cells.

III. DOES NK CELL ACTIVITY PLAY A ROLE IN THE PATHOLOGY OF THE DISEASE IN QUESTION?

NK cells activity probably plays no role as a mediator of antigen-associated killing or lymphokine production in such infections as malaria[48] or toxoplasmosis,[49] or in skin disorders like psoriasis[50] or pemphigus vulgaris.[51] In chronic viral infections or autoimmune diseases of viral etiology, NK cells may play a role. Virus-transformed cells can induce IFN and thereby elevate NK cell activity.[22] The result is a preferential lysis of virus-infected cells over nonvirus-infected cells by the NK cells.[52] Indeed, there is a correlation between low herpes simplex virus (HSV-1) NK activity and susceptibility to HSV infection in man.[53] HSV-1-infected targets are strong inducers of NK cell activity; virus-infected cells are preferentially lysed in relation to relative expression of HSV-1 glycoproteins.[54] Even NK-resistant cell lines can be lysed if infected with HSV-1.[55] Although no clinical data is available on the therapeutic effect of IFN administration in vivo in patients with chronic active hepatitis (hepatitis B surface antigen$^+$ [HepBsAg$^+$]), IFN stimulates NK cell activity for up to 5 weeks in vivo.[56] Acute and recovered hepatitis B virus (HBV) patients have normal NK cell activity; chronic HBV patients have elevated spontaneous NK cell activity.[57,58] This lytic activity seems to be HepBsAg directed,[59] though recognition may be for virally altered liver cell antigens,[57,58] not the viral antigen.[57]

If NK cells produce significant amounts of IFN[12-17] and if IFN regulates the pathology of the disease, NK cells are indirectly important in both virally induced infection and putative virally induced autoimmunity. Virus-like structures or transmissible agents have been isolated from endothelial cells on renal biopsy in SLE and Sjögren's syndrome (SS)[60] and from Crohn's lesions in Crohn's disease.[61] It is suggested that these autoimmune-like diseases are of a viral etiology. Treatment of Crohn's patients with IFN-β has been shown to cause improvement in two of five patients.[61] By comparison, Sjögren's syndrome is characterized by lymphoid cells infiltrating into the exocrine gland, reduced endogenous NK cell activity and IFN production, impaired IFN-induced NK cell activity, autoantibodies, and benign and malignant lymphomas.[62,63] The immune dysfunction of low IFN production could lead to reduced NK cell activity and viral persistence and result in the observed malignancies.[62] In immune-deficient patients experiencing repeated bacterial infections,[64] papova virus infections, squamous cell carcinoma, or hepatoma as in Fanconi's anemia,[65] NK cell defects may again be secondary to low IFN production, the result of which might be viral persistence and malignancy.

In multiple sclerosis (MS), where viral etiology has been suggested but no virus specific to MS patients has been isolated, there is only one piece of evidence that the NK-IFN relationship is important in the disease process. This is clouded by the lack of consensus among investigators as to IFN production by MS patients in vivo and in vitro. IFN has been reported to be undetectable in sera or CSF,[66] and yet in another article it appears to be detectably elevated compared with controls.[67] It has been said to be produced in vitro by peripheral blood mononuclear cells of MS patients at normal levels in response to a variety of viral and nonviral stimuli,[68,69] though others report abnormally low production to these same stimuli.[70-75] Most data now favor a defect in IFN production in MS. It was thus of great interest when Jacobs et al. treated MS patients with intrathecal injections of purified IFN-β. After treatment the rate of relapse of IFN recipients was less than before treatment and less than the control group, indicating a positive effect of such an antiviral and immune response-boosting therapy.[76,77]

There is some evidence of contribution by NK cells to autoimmunity, in which NK cells may be lysing normal cells. As mentioned previously, excess NK regulation of hematopoiesis may result in aplastic anemia or agranulocytosis.[6,8] Lymphocyte killing of normal human skin fibroblasts in diseases like atopic dermatitis[9] and mucocutaneous lymph node syndrome[78] has led to implication of the NK cell in autoimmunity. This is supported by the OKM1 phenotype of these effectors in atopic dermatitis.[9] It could also be argued that NK cell lysis of virally modified autologous cells might contribute to disease pathology.

IV. THE NK ABERRATION IN CHRONIC DISEASE: WHAT IS THE LEVEL OF NK CELL ACTIVITY IN VIVO AND IN VITRO? IS IT RELATED TO DISEASE PHASES?

Bacterial and parasitic infections cause an early increase in NK cell activity, but chronicity may depress it. In primary syphilis, NK cell activity is normal or elevated;[79] in secondary, latent, and lipoidal Ab-positive syphilis it is reduced. NK cell activity in syphilis thus is activated by disease but is depressed by disease progression. This parallels a concomitant generalized suppression and lymphopenia in these patients,[79] perhaps due to circulating immune complexes.[42] In contrast, mice acutely and chronically infected with *Toxoplasma gondii* had elevated endogenous NK cell activity.[49] NK cell activity is elevated in malaria-infected children, and the correlation between parasitemia and lytic activity is positive. Circulating IFN-α was elevated in sera of malaria-infected patients, and this high antiviral activity correlated positively with the degree of parasitemia and NK cell activity.[48]

In acute and chronic active HBV infection, there have been several reports that acute hepatitis patients have normal NK cell activity and antibody-dependent cellular cytotoxicity (ADCC).[57,58,80,81] There is a discrepancy as to whether the NK cell activity of chronic HBV patients is decreased,[81] normal,[80] or elevated.[57,58] As will be established later in discussing SLE patients, NK cell activity in vitro using lymphocytes washed free of serum components may be quite different from that in vivo, where such immunomodulators as IL2, IFN-γ, and PGE can have dramatic effects on NK cells. One interpretation of the differences seen in vitro is that NK cell activity may be activated by virus in vivo but suppressed both in vitro[81] and in vivo by immune complexes shown to exist in the serum of chronic active hepatitis (CAH) patients.[58] These CAH sera inhibit autologous and allogeneic NK cell activity and ADCC.[58] Nevertheless, ADCC in these patients is less sensitive to immune complex (IC) inhibition than is NK cell activity,[58] as has also been shown in normal individuals.[41] It is believed that necrosis in CAH patients is the result of cytotoxicity of hepatocytes by $T8^+$ cytotoxic cells[82,83] and K cells mediating ADCC,[81,83,84] in addition to a functional T suppressor (Ts) cell defect.[82]

In the realm of autoimmune disorders of unknown but probably infectious etiologies, investigators have examined how the disease phases of MS, SLE, rheumatoid arthritis (RA), Sjögren's syndrome (SS), Crohn's disease, and Hashimoto's thyroiditis are related to NK cell activity. MS has been the topic of many papers and reviews on NK cell activity because of the disease association with a possible virus, such as measles. One report found no defect in NK, ADCC, IFN-inducible NK, or in virus- or nonvirus-induced IFN production.[68] However, there seems to be overwhelming data that MS patients are defective in NK cell activity to a variety of tumor- and virus-infected targets.[66,69,72,73,85-94] In one study the defect was target cell-related, with lower NK cell killing to virus-infected targets.[66] There also seems to be general agreement that activity is lowest during active disease,[72,86-91] more in an acute relapse than in chronic progressive or remission stages.[87-90] Nor can NK cell activity be detected in the cerebrospinal fluid (CSF) of MS patients by a sensitive single cell assay;[86-90] however, it is detectable in the CSF of patients with acute infections of the CNS.[86,87]

Few if any reports find low NK cell activity in SLE to be independent of the disease stage;[95,96] most find it decreased in active disease.[46,62,80,97-102] Endogenous NK- and IFN-inducible NK cell activity in SS is depressed.[62,63] Impaired augmented NK (augmented by HeLa cells infected with measles) is seen only in patients with systemic manifestations of hypergammaglobulinemia and lymphoid hyperplasia.[62] In sharp contrast to other collagen diseases, RA patients have normal levels of peripheral blood NK cell activity and IFN production,[62,63,80,98,103-105] but they may have elevated NK cell activity in synovium compared with the blood.[98,103,105] Chronic NK suppression in Crohn's disease[106-108] is independent of disease duration[106] and only weakly and inversely related to disease activity.[108] There is no significant difference in NK cell activity between patients and controls in Hashimoto's thyroiditis,[109,110] where it is concluded that ADCC is a likely mechanism and related to the disease process.[110]

NK activity in skin disorders also fluctuates with disease phase. Elevated NK-like activity in mucocutaneous lymph node syndrome resolves during convalescence.[78] Reduced NK activity in atopic dermitis, to targets other than skin fibroblasts (see above[9]), is related to the severity of the disease[111,112] with mild disease showing a 50% or lower reduction in NK activity and severe disease showing a 50 to 80% reduction.[112] As discussed, chronic lepromatatous leprosy may be complicated by erythematous subcutaneous nodules; this complication is accompanied by reduction or total loss of NK cell activity.[44]

One comment should be made about the identity of populations of NK and K cells. Since NK and K cells can be distinguished functionally by different sensitivities to immunomodulating molecules,[41,113-115] it cannot be assumed that low NK cell activity in a disease automatically means concomitant low ADCC activity. This can be significant in autoimmunity where persistent viral infection and low NK cell activity contrast with an elevated ADCC contributing to the pathology of the disease. ADCC probably is important in the pathology of CAH patients[58,81] and also active in RA and Hashimoto's thyroiditis.[116-119] Interestingly, despite low NK cell activity, K cell ADCC has been observed to be normal or elevated in MS,[66,87,92] SLE,[80] Crohn's disease,[107] and some forms of immunodeficiency.[120,121]

V. WHAT CAUSES THE DEFECT IN CHRONIC NONMALIGNANT DISEASE?

Aberrant NK cell activity could be found as the result of a variety of immunodefects: (1) reduced numbers, lytic activity, or recycling of NK cells, (2) defects in producing or responding to IL-1, IL-2, or IFN by NK cells, (3) anti-DR, anti-NK, or anti-IFN antibodies, or (4) active suppressive mechanisms like PGE, immune complexes, other Mϕ or T cell suppressors, or molecules as yet unidentified. Some of these events might even be HLA-linked. In reviewing the nonmalignant diseases for explanations of their NK cell defects, one or more of the above explanations holds. There are no simple unifying causes for depressed NK cell activity in autoimmunity. NK cell activity is induced with the rest of the immune response. As many complex reasons for an aberrant NK response can be found as there are complex driving mechanisms to stimulate it.

Depressed NK cell activity in syphilis,[42] lepromatous leprosy,[44] and in chronic HBV infections[81] may be due to immune complexes.[42,58] Elevated NK cell activity in *Herpes simplex* may[121] or may not[54] be IFN-α-dependent while elevated NK is related to endogenous IFN-α production in *Plasmodium falciparum*-induced malaria.[48]

The controversy over HLA-related defects in NK cell activity and IFN production in MS patients continues. Abb and colleagues[122] have documented that low responsiveness by peripheral blood lymphocytes (PBLs) of any individual to inducers of IFN-α (flu virus, Molt 4) is associated with DR2, though they found no association of IFN-γ production and DR2. It has been shown that MS patients show a higher than normal frequency of DR2 antigen[66,72,73,85] and thus studies have been conducted to link DR2 antigen as the sole source for defective NK and IFN production in MS patients. An association of DR2 and low NK and IFN production in the general populace would make trivial the findings in MS, but such an association has not been upheld; nor has a firm association between DR and defective NK IFN circuits been established. Initial work correlating low NK cell activity and DR2 in MS patients[66,72] apparently is not statistically significant.[73,85] The finding that low NK cell activity occurs in DR2 MS patients but not in normal DR2 controls[66] or in normal (DR2$^+$) monozygotic MS twins with normal NK activity[69,94,123] makes this HLA association an unlikely explanation for defects in MS patients. That low IFN production is the cause of low NK cell activity in MS[70,75,85,91] also seems unlikely since IFN-α is not always low.[69,94,123] When it is low, it does not correlate with NK cell activity.[73,91] It would appear that NK and IFN activities are independent phenomena.

Decreased NK cell activity in MS has been demonstrated using the ^{51}Cr-release assay,[66,72,86-90,92] but the underlying defect responsible for this result may reside in the defect at the level of target cell binding or killing, or effector recycling. At the single cell level, acute relapse patients have fewer peripheral blood NK cells during an exacerbation; the defect is at both the level of binding to and lysis of the target.[86] There is an apparent defect in recycling as well.[86,87] By a similar assay, there are no binders or killers in CSF, i.e., no detectable functional NK cells.[86,87] It is misleading to quantify NK cells in a disease state by scoring cells of given phenotypes — such as OKM1$^+$,[124] large granular lymphocytes (LGLs),[125] or HNK-1$^+$[126-129] to make conclusions about activities of cell populations. This is especially true since NK cells defined by such phenotypes share markers or functions of helper T cells[125,126] or suppressor, cytotoxic T cells.[125,126,129,130] An example of this discrepancy occurs in MS patients where NK cell numbers and activity are depressed and HNK-1$^+$ cell numbers are elevated[92] or patients have normal numbers of LGLs.[87] What is also striking is that LGLs have T cell phenotypes, and T4$^+$ and T8$^+$ cells mediate NK cell activity in MS patients.[87] The best piece of evidence for immunoregulatory defects causing low NK cell activity in MS patients is suggested by the work of this laboratory in which MS patients make elevated amounts of PGE in vitro (PBLs) and in vivo (neat CSF). These elevated PGE levels are associated in MS with decreased NK cell activity and IFN production.[88,90] In addition, NK cells in MS patients are more sensitive to the effects of PGE than controls.[89,90] It has been suggested that circulating IC may activate Mϕ to produce PGE. An early observation by Rola-Pleszcynski et al. regarding the presence of blocking factors in MS sera which prevented NK killing of virus-infected targets may relate to circulating IC or PGE induction.[131] Similarly, depletion of phagocytic adherent cells in Crohn's disease,[106,107] atopic dermatitis,[111] and leprosy[44] leads to an increase in NK cell activity, suggesting a role for Mϕ-associated PGE suppression. However, there has been one report on Crohn's disease using indomethacin which concluded that PGE was not responsible for depressed NK.[108]

In SLE there may be many reasons for depressed NK cell activity. The deficiency is not related to the ability of NK cells to recognize and bind to targets,[100,102] but to the deficiency of active NK cells to kill.[100] Recycling of active NK cells probably is normal.[100] It is not clear whether an NK cell-bound inhibitor (such as IC) is relevant in SLE. One report claims overnight incubation of effectors increases NK cell activity,[132] while other reports say neither incubation[97,102] nor protease treatment[102] reverses low NK cell function. One report claims that SLE sera do not decrease normal NK activity,[100] but others show inhibitory activity[132] and assign it to anti-NK antibodies.[45,133]

IFN levels in SLE are elevated in vivo,[103,134-137] which may explain the apparent in vitro defect in IFN production and IFN-inducible NK cell activity in SLE.[46,101,134,138,139] That is, IFN production is already turned on in vivo and cannot be augmented in vitro. In addition, NK cells are depressed in activity after continuous exposure to IFN.[134] An unusual IFN system seems to be disproportionately represented in both SLE and acquired immunodeficiency syndrome (AIDS): i.e., an IFN-γ deficiency and an acid-labile IFN-α overproduction.[134,135,137,140,141] A similar pH-sensitive IFN-α is seen in other autoimmune and infectious diseases as well. AIDS patients have low NK cell activity, though the relationship of low NK cell activity to this unusual IFN-α is not clear.[142] In addition, SLE patients have selective defects in IFN production to different inducers.[46,134,138] IFN-inducible NK cell activity may be suppressed by anti-IFN produced by these patients[137] or by the insensitivity of their NK cells to IFN that results from long-term exposure in vivo.[139] Sibbitt et al.[102] have examined the suppressor effects of Mϕ in SLE and ruled out direct Mϕ suppression or PGE production as a reason for low NK cell activity. IL-2 boosts normal NK cell activity[27-29] and has been shown to boost low NK cell activity in AIDS patients.[142] IL-1 and IL-2 production[143,144] and IL-2 response[144] are decreased in SLE. The relationship of these defects to NK cell activity is worthy of further attention.

As with SLE patients, Sjögren's syndrome (SS) patients have elevated serum IFN[145] but low IFN production and low IFN-inducible NK cell activity in vitro.[62] Inhibition of NK cell activity is not associated with suppressive serum factors[62] or antilymphocytic Ab or IC.[63] The inhibitory effects on normal NK of RA sera[47] obviously have no in vitro effects on RA-peripheral NK cell activity, which is normal.[62,63,80,98] These observations do not preclude a possible in vivo inhibition of NK cell activity by IC in these patients. The evidence for activated NK cells at the site of synovial inflammation in RA is interesting.[103,105] There appear to be more LGLs present in the synovium, higher amounts of IFN in synovial fluid, and more functional NK cells.[103] Since there is no difference in peripheral blood and synovial mononuclear target binding cell numbers,[103] the differences in their activity may be related to increased lytic activity and recycling, perhaps stimulated by the elevated levels of IFN.[30] These NK cells apparently are FcR^- and not impaired by IC.[104,105] Cell-free synovial fluid, as well as supernatants from cultured synovial cells, contain a lymphotoxin-like mediator that inhibits cell growth or lyses cells.[146] An alternative explanation for increased NK cell activity by synovial fluid cells may be that they are stimulated by the increased production of IL-1 and IL-2 in the synovial fluid.[147,148]

VI. CONCLUSIONS

The role of NK cells in autoimmunity is still a mystery. To assign such cells the task of surveillance and prevention of chronic infections that may trigger an autodestructive cycle, we must identify the viruses causing these diseases, show the relationship between low NK cell activity, viral persistence, and autoimmunity, and demonstrate that therapy which induces NK cell activity prevents disease progression or has some other therapeutic benefit in these patients.

REFERENCES

1. **Lampert, P. W.,** Autoimmune and virus-induced demyelinating diseases, *Am. J. Pathol.*, 91, 176, 1978.
2. **Dal Canto, M. and Lipton, H. L.,** Ultrastructural immunohistochemical localization of virus in acute and chronic demyelinating Theiler's virus infection, *Am. J. Pathol.*, 106, 20, 1982.
3. **Timonen, T. and Saksela, E.,** Human natural cell-mediated cytotoxicity against fetal fibroblasts. I. General characteristics of cytotoxic activity, *Cell. Immunol.*, 33, 340, 1977.
4. **Hansson, M., Kiessling, R., and Beran, M.,** Natural killing of hematopoietic cells, in *NK Cells and Other Natural Effector Cells*, Herberman, R. B., Ed., Academic Press, New York, 1982, 1077.
5. **Hansson, M., Kiessling, R., and Andersson, B.,** Human fetal thymus and bone marrow contain target cells for natural killer cells, *Eur. J. Immunol.*, 11, 8, 1981.
6. **Pross, H. F., Pater, J., Dwosh, I., Giles, A., Galliner, L. A., Rubin, P., Corbett, W. E. N., Galbraith, P., and Baines, M. G.,** Studies of human natural killer cells. III. Neutropenia associated with unusual characteristics of antibody-dependent and natural killer cell mediated cytoxicity, *J. Clin. Immunol.*, 2, 126, 1982.
7. **Zoumbos, N., Gascon, P., and Young, N.,** The function of lymphocytes in normal and suppressed hematopoiesis, *Blut*, 48, 1, 1984.

8. **Mangan, K. F., Hartnett, M. E., Matis, S. A., Winkelstein, A., and Abo, T.,** Natural killer cells suppress human erythroid stem cell proliferation in vitro, *Blood,* 63, 260, 1984.
9. **Leung, D. Y. M., Parkman, R., Feller, J., Wood, N., and Geha, R. S.,** Cell mediated cytoxicity against skin fibroblasts in atopic dermatitis, *J. Immunol.,* 128, 1736, 1982.
10. **Mutchnick, M. G., Missirian, A., and Johnson, A. G.,** Lymphocyte cytotoxicity in human liver disease using rat hepatocyte monolayer cultures, *Clin. Immunol. Immunopathol.,* 16, 423, 1980.
11. **Tomonari, K.,** Cytotoxic T cells generated in the autologous mixed lymphocyte reaction. I. Primary autologous mixed lymphocyte reaction, *J. Immunol.,* 124, 1111, 1980.
12. **Herberman, R. B. and Ortaldo, J. R.,** Natural killer cells: their role in defense against disease, *Science,* 214, 24, 1981.
13. **Welsh, R. M.,** Natural killer cells in virus infections, in *Current Topics in Microbiology and Immunology,* Häller, O., Ed., Springer-Verlag, Berlin, 1980, 739.
14. **Timonen, T., Saksela, E., Virtanen, I., and Cantell, K.,** Natural killer cells are responsible for the interferon production in human lymphocytes by tumor cell contact, *Eur. J. Immunol.,* 10, 422, 1980.
15. **Peter, H. H., Dallügge, H., Zavatzky, R., Euler, S., Leibold, W., and Kirchner, H.,** Human peripheral null lymphocytes. II. Producers of type-1 interferon upon stimulation with tumor cells, *Herpes simplex* virus, and *Corynebacterium parvum, Eur. J. Immunol.,* 10, 547, 1980.
16. **Timonen, T., Ortaldo, J. R., and Herberman, R. B.,** Characteristics of human large granular lymphocytes and relationship to natural killer and K cells, *J. Exp. Med.,* 153, 569, 1981.
17. **Kato, T. and Minagawa, T.,** Enhancement of cytotoxicity of human peripheral blood lymphocytes by interferon, *Microbiol. Immunol.,* 25, 837, 1981.
18. **Smith, K.,** T cell growth factor, *Immunol. Rev.,* 51, 337, 1980.
19. **De Vries, J. E., Figdor, C. G., and Spits, H.,** Regulation of human NK activity against adherent tumor target cells by monocyte subpopulations, IL1, and IFNs, in *NK Cells and Other Natural Effector Cells,* Herberman, R. B., Ed., Academic Press, New York, 1982, 657.
20. **Kuribayashi, K., Gillis, S., Kern, D. E., and Henney, C. S.,** Murine NK cell cultures: effects of interleukin 2 and interferon on cell growth and cytotoxic reactivity, *J. Immunol.,* 126, 2321, 1981.
21. **Kern, D. E., Gillis, S., Okada, M., and Henney, C. S.,** The role of interleukin 2 (IL2) in the differentiation of cytotoxic T cells: the effect of monoclonal anti IL2 antibody and absorption with IL2 dependent T cell lines, *J. Immunol.,* 127, 1323, 1981.
22. **Trinchieri, G. and Santoli, D.,** Anti-viral activity induced by culturing lymphocytes with tumor derived or virus transformed cells, *J. Exp. Med.,* 147, 1314, 1978.
23. **Herberman, R. B., Ortaldo, J. R., and Bonnard, G. D.,** Augmentation by interferon of human natural and antibody-dependent cell mediated cytotoxicity, *Nature (London),* 277, 221, 1979.
24. **Saksela, E. and Timonen, T.,** Cellular interactions in the augmentation of human NK activity by interferon, *N.Y. Acad. Sci.,* 350, 102, 1980.
25. **Matheson, D. S., Green, B., and Tan, Y. H.,** Human interferons α and β inhibit T cell dependent and stimulate T cell independent mitogenesis and natural cell cytotoxicity: relationship to chromosome 21, *Cell Immunol.,* 165, 366, 1981.
26. **Herberman, R. B., Ortaldo, J. R., Rubinstein, M., and Pestka, S.,** Augmentation of natural and antibody-dependent cell-mediated cytotoxicity by pure human leukocyte interferon, *J. Clin. Immunol.,* 1, 149, 1981.
27. **Dempsey, R. A., Dinarello, C. A., Mier, J., W., Rosenwasser, L. J., Allegretta, M., Brown, T. E., and Parkinson, D. R.,** The differential effects of human leukocytic pyrogen/lymphocyte-activating factor, T cell growth factor, and interferon on human natural killer cell activity, *J. Immunol.,* 129, 2504, 1982.
28. **Donzig, W., Stadler, B. M., and Herberman, R. B.,** Interleukin 2 dependence of human natural killer (NK) cell activity, *J. Immunol.,* 130, 1970, 1983.
29. **Handa, K., Suzuki, R., Matsui, H., Shimizu, Y., and Kumagai, K.,** Natural killer (NK) cells as a responder to interleukin 2 (IL2). II. IL2 induced interferon-γ production, *J. Immunol.,* 130, 988, 1983.
30. **Ullberg, M., Merrill, J., and Jondal, M.,** Interferon-induced NK augmentation in humans. An analysis of target recognition, effector cell recruitment, and effector cell recycling, *Scand. J. Immunol.,* 14, 285, 1981.
31. **Saksela, E., Timonen, T., Ranki, A., and Hayry, P.,** Morphological and functional characterization of isolated effector cells responsible for human natural killer activity to fetal fibroblasts and to cultured cell line targets, *Immunol. Rev.,* 44, 71, 1979.
32. **Pape, G. R., Moretta, L., Troye, M., and Perlmann, P.,** Natural cytotoxicity of human Fcγ-receptor positive T lymphocytes after surface modulation with immune complexes, *Scand. J. Immunol.,* 9, 291, 1979.
33. **Merrill, J. E., Ullberg, M., and Jondal, M.,** Influence of IgG and IgM receptor triggering on human natural killer cell cytotoxicity measured on the level of the single effector cell, *Eur. J. Immunol.,* 11, 536, 1981.

34. **Passwell, J., Rosen, F. S., and Merler, E.,** The effect of Fc fragments of IgG on human monoclear cell responses, *Cell. Immunol.*, 52, 395, 1980.
35. **Poleshuck, L. C. and Strausser, H. R.,** Immune complex induced prostaglandin production by monocytes of normal human subjects and cancer patients, *Prostaglandin Med.*, 4, 363, 1980.
36. **Baker, P. E., Fahey, J. V., and Munck, A.,** Prostaglandin inhibition of T cell proliferation is mediated at two levels, *Cell. Immunol.*, 61, 52, 1981.
37. **Rapport, R. S. and Dodge, G. R.,** Prostaglandin E inhibits the production of human interleukin 2, *J. Exp. Med.*, 155, 943, 1982.
38. **Brunda, M. J., Herberman, R. B., and Holden, H. T.,** Inhibition of murine natural killer cell activity by prostaglandins, *J. Immunol.*, 124, 2682, 1980.
39. **Koren, H. S., Anderson, S. J., Fischer, D. G., Copeland, C. S., and Jensen, P. J.,** Regulation of human natural killing. I. The role of monocytes, interferon, and prostaglandins, *J. Immunol.*, 127, 2007, 1981.
40. **Jondal, M., Merrill, J., and Ullberg, M.,** Monocyte induced human natural killer cell suppression followed by increased cytotoxic activity during short term in vivo culture in autologous serum, *Scand. J. Immunol.*, 14, 555, 1981.
41. **Merrill, J. E.,** Natural killer (NK) and antibody dependent cellular cytotoxicity (ADCC) activities can be differentiated by their different sensitivities to interferon and prostaglandin E_1, *J. Clin. Immunol.*, 3, 42, 1983.
42. **Jensen, J. R., Jørgensen, A. S., and Thestrup-Pedersen, K.,** Depression of natural killer cell activity by syphilitic serum, *Br. J. Vener. Dis.*, 58, 298, 1982.
43. **Jensen, J. R., Thestrup-Pedersen, K., and From, E.,** Fluctuations in natural killer cell activity in early syphilis, *Br. J. Vener. Dis.*, 59, 30, 1983.
44. **Humphres, R. C., Gelber, R. H., and Krahenbuhl, J. L.,** Suppressed natural killer cell activity during episodes of erythema nodosum leprosum in lepromatous leprosy, *Clin. Exp. Immunol.*, 49, 500, 1982.
45. **Goto, M., Tanimoto, K., and Horiuchi, Y.,** Natural cell mediated cytotoxicity in systemic lupus erythematosus, *Arthritis Rheum.*, 23, 1274, 1980.
46. **Tsokos, G. C., Rook, A. H., Djeu, J. Y., and Balow, J. E.,** Natural killer cells and interferon responses in patients with systemic lupus erythematosus, *Clin. Exp. Immunol.*, 50, 239, 1982.
47. **Fink, P. C., Schedel, I., Peter, H. H., and Deicher, H.,** Inhibition of spontaneous and antibody dependent cellular cytotoxicity by sera and isolated antiglobulin preparations from rheumatoid arthritis patients, *Scand. J. Immunol.*, 173, 183, 1977.
48. **Ojo-Amaize, E. A., Salimonu, L. S., Williams, A. I. O., Kinwolere, O. A. O., Shabo, R., Alm, G. V., and Wigzell, H.,** Positive correlation between degree of parasitemia, interferon titers, and natural killer cell activity in *Plasmodium falciparum* infected children, *J. Immunol.*, 127, 2296, 1981.
49. **Hauser, W. E., Sharma, S. D., and Remington, J. S.,** Natural killer cells induced by acute and chronic *Toxoplasma* infection, *Cell. Immunol.*, 69, 330, 1982.
50. **Jansén, C. T. and Viander, M.,** Basic and interferon augmented natural killer (NK) cell activity in psoriasis, *Acta Derm. Venereol.*, 63, 384, 1983.
51. **Ahmed, A. R.,** Antibody dependent cellular cytoxicity in bullous diseases, *J. Am. Acad. Dermatol.*, 6, 481, 1982.
52. **Biron, C. A. and Welsh, R. M.,** Proliferation and role of natural killer cells during viral infection, in *NK Cells and Other Natural Effector Cells*, Herberman, R. B., Ed., Academic Press, New York, 1982, 493.
53. **Lopez, C., Kirkpatrick, D., and Fitzgerald, P.,** The role of NK (HSV-1) effector cells in resistance to herpes virus infections in man, in *NK Cells and Other Natural Effector Cells*, Herberman, R. B., Ed., Academic Press, New York, 1982, 1445.
54. **Fitzgerald, P. A., Lopez, C., and Siegal, F. P.,** Role of interferon in natural kill of Herpes virus infected fibroblasts, in *NK Cells and Other Natural Effector Cells*, Herberman, R. B., Ed., Academic Press, New York, 1982, 387.
55. **Bishop, G. A., Glorioso, J. C., and Schwartz, S. A.,** Relationship between expression of *Herpes simplex* virus glycoproteins and susceptibility of target cells to human killer activity, *J. Exp. Med.*, 157, 1544, 1983.
56. **Pape, G. R., Hadam, M. R., Eisenburg, J., and Riethmuller, G.,** Natural killer cell activity during treatment with fibroblast interferon, *Immunobiology*, 158, 450, 1981.
57. **Dienstag, J. L. and Bhan, A. K.,** Enhanced *in vitro* cell-mediated cytotoxicity in chronic hepatitis B virus infection: absence of specificity for virus-expressed antigen on target cell membranes, *J. Immunol.*, 125, 2269, 1980.
58. **Hütteroth, T. H., Poralla, T., and Meyerzum Büschenfelde, K.-H.,** Spontaneous cell-mediated (SCMC) and antibody-dependent cellular cytotoxicity (ADCC) in patients with acute and chronic active hepatitis, *Klin. Wochenschr.*, 59, 699, 1981.

59. **Chin, T. W., Hollinger, F. B., Rich, R. R., Troisi, C. L., Dreesman, G. R., and Melnick, J. L.,** Cytotoxicity by NK-like cells from hepatitis B-immune patients to a human hepatoma cell line secreting HBsAg, *J. Immunol.*, 130, 173, 1983.
60. **Shearn, M. A., Tu, W. H., Stephens, B. G., and Lee, J. C.,** Virus-like structures in Sjögren's syndrome, *Lancet*, 1, 568, 1970.
61. **Van Trappen, G., Covemans, G., Billiau, H., and De Somer, P.,** Treatment of Crohn's Disease with interferon: a preliminary clinical trial, *Acta Clin. Belg.*, 35, 238, 1980.
62. **Minato, N., Takeda, A., Kano, S., and Takaku, F.,** Studies of the functions of natural killer-interferon systems in patients with Sjögren's syndrome, *J. Clin. Invest.*, 69, 581, 1982.
63. **Goto, M., Tanimoto, K., Chihara, T., and Horiuchi, Y.,** Natural cell-mediated cytotoxicity in Sjögren's syndrome and rheumatoid arthritis, *Arth. Rheum.*, 24, 1377, 1981.
64. **Virelizier, J. L. and Griscelli, C.,** Défaut sélectif de sécrétion d'interféron associé à un déficit d'activité cytotoxique naturelle, *Arch. Fr. Pediatr.*, 38, 77, 1981.
65. **Hersey, P., Edwards, A., Lewis, R., Kemp, A., and McInnes, J.,** Deficient natural killer cell activity in a patient with Fanconi's anemia and squamous cell carcinoma. Association with a defect in interferon release, *Clin. Exp. Immunol.*, 48, 205, 1982.
66. **Hauser, S. L., Ault, K. A., Levin, M. J., Garavoy, M. R., and Weiner, H. L.,** Natural killer cell activity in multiple sclerosis, *J. Immunol.*, 127, 1114, 1981.
67. **Degré, M., Dahl, H., and Vandvik, B.,** Interferon in the serum and cerebrospinal fluid of patients with multiple sclerosis and other neurological disorders, *Acta. Neurol. Scand.*, 53, 152, 1976.
68. **Santoli, D., Hall, K., Kastrukoff, L., Lisak, R. P., Perussia, B., Trinchieri, G., and Koprowski, H.,** Cytotoxic activity and interferon production by lymphocytes from patients with multiple sclerosis, *J. Immunol.*, 126, 1274, 1981.
69. **Kaudewitz, P., Zander, H., Abb, J., Ziegler-Heitbrock, H. W., and Riethmuller, G.,** Genetic influence on natural cytotoxicity and interferon production in multiple sclerosis studies in monozygotic discordant twins, *Hum. Immunol.*, 7, 51, 1983.
70. **Neighbour, P. A. and Bloom, B. R.,** Absence of virus-induced lymphocyte suppression and interferon production in multiple sclerosis, *Proc. Natl. Acad. Sci. U.S.A.*, 76, 476, 1979.
71. **Neighbour, P. A., Miller, A. E., and Bloom, B. R.,** Interferon responses of leukocytes in multiple sclerosis, *Neurology*, 31, 561, 1981.
72. **Benczur, M., Petrányi, G. Gy., Pálffy, Gy., Varga, M., Tálas, M., Kotsy, B., Földes, I., and Hollán, S. R.,** Dysfunction of natural killer cells in multiple sclerosis: a possible pathogenic mechanism, *Clin. Exp. Immunol.*, 39, 657, 1980.
73. **Gyódi, E., Bençzur, M., Pálffy, G. Gy., Tálas, M., Petrányi, Gy., Földes, I., and Hollán, S. R.,** Association between HLA B7, DR2 and dysfunction of natural and antibody-mediated cytotoxicity without connection with the deficient interferon production in multiple sclerosis, *Hum. Immunol.*, 4, 209, 1982.
74. **Salonen, R., Ilonen, J., Reunanen, M., and Salmi, A.,** Defective production on interferon-α associated with HLA DW2 antigen in stable multiple sclerosis, *J. Neurol. Sci.*, 55, 197, 1982.
75. **Haahr, S., Møller-Larson, A., and Pedersen, E.,** Immunological parameters in multiple sclerosis patients with special reference to the herpes virus group, *Clin. Exp. Immunol.*, 51, 197, 1983.
76. **Jacobs, L., O'Malley, J., Freeman, A., and Ekes, R.,** Intrathecal interferon reduces exacerbations in multiple sclerosis, *Science*, 214, 1026, 1981.
77. **Jacobs, L., O'Malley, J., Freeman, A., Murawski, J., and Ekes, R.,** Intrathecal interferon in multiple sclerosis, *Arch. Neurol.*, 39, 609, 1982.
78. **Leung, D. Y. M., Siegel, R. L., Grady, S., Krensky, A., Meade, R., Reinherz, E. L., and Geha, R. S.,** Immunoregulatory abnormalities in mucocutaneous lymph node syndrome, *Immunopathology*, 23, 100, 1982.
79. **Jensen, J., Thestrup-Pedersen, K., and From, E.,** Natural killer cell activity in syphilis, *Arch. Derm. Res.*, 272, 163, 1982.
80. **Penschow, J. and MacKay, I. R.,** NK and K cell activity of human blood: differences according to sex, age, and disease, *Ann. Rheum. Dis.*, 39, 82, 1980.
81. **Serdengecti, S., Jones, D. B., Holdstock, G., and Wright, R.,** Natural killer activity in patients with biopsy-proven liver disease, *Clin. Exp. Immunol.*, 45, 361, 1981.
82. **Montano, L., Aranquibel, F., Boffill, M., Goodwill, H. H., Janossy, G., and Thomas, H. C.,** An analysis of the composition of the inflammatory infiltrate in autoimmune and hepatitis B virus-induced chronic liver disease, *Hepatology*, 3, 292, 1983.
83. **Eggink, H. F., Horthoff, H. J., Huitema, S., Gips, C. H., and Poppema, S.,** Cellular and humoral immune reactions in chronic active liver disease. I. Lymphocyte subsets in liver biopsies of patients with untreated idiopathic autoimmunal hepatitis, chronic active hepatitis B and primary biliary cirrhosis, *Clin. Exp. Immunol.*, 50, 17, 1982.

84. **Stefanini, G. F., Bernardi, M., Miglio, F., Mariani, E., Chiodo, F., Facchini, A., Labo, G., and Gasbarrini, G.,** Different mechanisms of *in vitro* lymphocytotoxicity against isolated rabbit hepatocytes during the course of acute viral hepatitis, *Digestion*, 22, 229, 1981.
85. **Bençzur, M., Gyódi, E., Petrányi, G., Hollán, S. R., Pálffy, G., Talás, M., Stöger, I., and Földes, I.,** Impaired natural killer cell function in multiple sclerosis and association with the HLA system, in *NK Cells and Other Natural Effector Cells*, Herberman, R. B., Ed., Academic Press, New York, 1982, 1227.
86. **Merrill, J. E., Jondal, M., Seeley, J., Ullberg, M., and Siden, A.,** Decreased NK killing in patients with multiple sclerosis: an analysis on the level of the single effector cell in peripheral blood and cerebrospinal fluid in relation to disease activity, *Clin. Exp. Immunol.*, 47, 419, 1981.
87. **Merrill, J. E., Scott, A., Myers, L., and Ellison, G.,** Cytotoxic activity of peripheral blood and cerebrospinal fluid lymphocytes from patients with multiple sclerosis and other neurological diseases, *J. Neuroimmunol.*, 3, 123, 1982.
88. **Merrill, J. E., Gerner, R. H., Myers, L. W., and Ellison, G. W.,** Regulation of natural killer cell cytotoxicity by prostaglandin E in the peripheral blood and cerebrospinal fluid of patients with multiple sclerosis and other neurological diseases. I. Association between amount of prostaglandin produced, natural killer, and endogenous interferon, *J. Neuroimmunol.*, 4, 239, 1983.
89. **Merrill, J. E., Myers, L. W., and Ellison, G. W.,** Regulation of natural killer cell cytotoxicity by prostaglandin E in the peripheral blood and cerebrospinal fluid of patients with multiple sclerosis and other neurological diseases. II. Effect of exogenous PGE_1 on spontaneous and interferon-induced natural killer, *J. Neuroimmunol.*, 4, 246, 1983.
90. **Merrill, J. E., Gerner, R. H., Myers, L. W., and Ellison, G. W.,** Regulation of NK activity and IFN production by PGE in the peripheral blood and cerebrospinal fluid of patients with multiple sclerosis and other neurological diseases, in *Intercellular Communication in Leukocyte Function*, Parker, J. W. and O'Brien, R. L., Eds., John Wiley & Sons, Chichester, 1983, 79.
91. **Neighbour, P. A., Grayzel, A. I., and Miller, A. E.,** Endogenous and interferon-augmented natural killer cell activity of human peripheral blood mononuclear cella *in vitro*. Studies of patients with multiple sclerosis, systemic lupus erythematosus, or rheumatoid arthritis, *Clin. Exp. Immunol.*, 49, 11, 1982.
92. **McGarry, R. C., Roder, J. C., and Brunet, D.,** Mechanisms of natural killer cell depression in multiple sclerosis, in *NK Cells and Other Natural Effector Cells*, Herberman, R. B., Ed., Academic Press, New York, 1982, 1219.
93. **Uchida, A., Maida, E. M., Lenzhofer, R., and Micksche, M.,** Natural killer cell activity in patients with multiple sclerosis: interferon and plasmapheresis, *Immunobiology*, 160, 392, 1982.
94. **Abb, J., Kaudewitz, P., Zander, H., Ziegler, H.-N. L., Dienhardt, F., and Riethmuller R.,** Interferon (IFN) production and natural killer (NK) cell activity in patients with multiple sclerosis: influence of genetic factors assessed by studies of monozygotic twins, in *NK Cells and Other Natural Effector Cells*, Herberman, R. B., Ed., Academic Press, New York, 1982, 1233.
95. **Oshima, K., Sumiya, M., Gonda, N., Kano, S., and Takaku, F.,** Natural killer cell activity in untreated systemic lupus erythematosus, *Ann. Rheum. Dis.*, 41, 417, 1982.
96. **Kaufman, D. B.,** Natural killer augmentation in systemic lupus erythematosus via a soluble mediator derived from human lymphocytes, *Arthritis Rheum.*, 25, 562, 1982.
97. **Hoffman, T.,** Natural killer function in systemic lupus erythematosus, *Arthritis Rheum.*, 23, 30, 1980.
98. **Neighbour, P. A., Reinitz, E., Grayzel, A. I., Miller, A. E., and Bloom, B. K.,** Studies of human NK cell functions in chronic diseases, in *NK Cells and Other Natural Effector Cells*, Herberman, R. B., Ed., Academic Press, New York, 1982, 1241.
99. **Kozlowski, S. H., Hirsue, D. J., and Jackson, E. J.,** Comparison of natural killing with antibody-dependent cell mediated cytotoxicity in patients with systemic lupus erythematosus, *J. Rheumatol.*, 9, 59, 1982.
100. **Katz, P., Zaytoun, A. M., Lee, J. H., Panush, R. S., and Longley, S.,** Abnormal natural killer cell activity in systemic lupus erythematosus: an intrinsic defect in lytic event, *J. Immunol.*, 129, 1966, 1982.
101. **Strannegard, O., Hermodsson, S., and Westberg, G.,** Interferon and natural killer cells in systemic lupus erythematosus, *Clin. Exp. Immunol.*, 50, 246, 1982.
102. **Sibbitt, W. L., Mathews, P. M., and Bankhurst, A. D.,** Natural killer cell in systemic lupus erythematosus: defects in effector lytic activity and response to interferon and interferon inducers, *J. Clin. Invest.*, 71, 1230, 1983.
103. **Reinitz, E., Neighbour, P. A., and Grayzel, A. I.,** Natural killer cell activity of mononuclear cells from rheumatoid patients measured by a conjugate-binding cytotoxicity assay, *Arthritis Rheum.*, 25, 1440, 1982.
104. **Dobloug, J. H., Førre, O., Krien, T. K., Egeland, T., and Degré, M.,** Natural killer (NK) cell activity of peripheral blood synovial fluid, and synovial tissue lymphocytes from patients with rheumatoid arthritis and juvenile rheumatoid arthritis, *Ann. Rheum. Dis.*, 41, 490, 1982.
105. **Silver, R. M., Redelman, D., Zvaifler, N. J., and Naides, S.,** Studies of rheumatoid synovial fluid lymphocytes. I. Evidence for activated natural killer (NK) like cells, *J. Immunol.*, 128, 1758, 1982.

106. **Auer, I. O., Ziemer, E., and Sommer, H.,** Immune status of Crohn's Disease, *Clin. Exp. Immunol.*, 42, 41, 1980.
107. **Auer, I. O. and Ziemer, E.,** Immune status in Crohn's Disease. An *in vitro* antibody dependent cell mediated cytotoxicity in peripheral blood, *Klin. Wochenschr.*, 58, 779, 1980.
108. **Beeken, W. L., MacPherson, B. R., Gundel, R. M., Andre-Ukena, S. St., Wood, S. G., and Sylvester, D. L.,** Depressed spontaneous cell-mediated cytotoxicity in Crohn's Disease, *Clin. Exp. Immunol.*, 51, 351, 1983.
109. **Seybold, D., Ryan, E. A., and Wall, J. R.,** Natural cytotoxicity of blood mononuclear cells from normal subjects and patients with Hashimoto's thyroiditis against normal thyroid cells, *J. Clin. Lab. Immunol.*, 6, 241, 1981.
110. **Chow, A., Baur, R. J., Schleusener, H., and Wall, J. R.,** Natural cytotoxicity of peripheral blood leukocytes from normal subjects and patients with Hashimoto's thyroiditis against human adult and fetal thyroid cells, *Life Sci.*, 32, 67, 1983.
111. **Jensen, J. R., Sand, T. T., Jørgensen, A. S., and Thestrop-Pedersen, K.,** Modulation of natural killer activity in patients with atopic dermatitis, *J. Invest. Dermatol.*, 82, 30, 1984.
112. **Kusaimi, N. and Trentin, J.,** Peripheral blood natural cell-mediated cytoxicity in patients with atopic dermatitis, in *NK Cells and Other Natural Effector Cells*, Herberman, R. B., Ed., Academic Press, New York, 1982, 1249.
113. **Santoli, D. and Koprowski, H.,** Mechanisms of activation of human natural killer cells against tumor and virus infected cells, *Immunol. Rev.*, 44, 125, 1979.
114. **Trinchieri, G., Granato, D., and Perussia, B.,** Interferon induced resistance of fibroblasts to cytolysis mediated by natural killer cells: specificity and mechanism, *J. Immunol.*, 126, 335, 1981.
115. **Nair, P. N. and Schwartz, S. A.,** Suppression of normal killer activity and antibody dependent cellular cytotoxicity by cultured human lymphocytes, *J. Immunol.*, 126, 2221, 1981.
116. **Feldman, J.-L., Becker, M. J., Moutsopoulos, H., Fye, K., Blackman, M., Epstein, W. V., and Talal, N.,** Antibody dependent cell mediated cytotoxicity in selected autoimmune diseases, *J. Clin. Invest.*, 58, 173, 1976.
117. **Michalkiewicz, J.,** Immunological characteristics of lymphocytes in synovial fluid and peripheral blood in patients with rheumatoid arthritis, *Arch. Immunol. Ther. Exp.*, 26, 801, 1978.
118. **Calder, E. A., Penhale, W. J., McLeman, D., Barnes, E. W., and Irvine, W. J.,** Lymphocyte dependent antibody-mediated cytotoxicity in Hashimoto's thyroiditis, *Clin. Exp. Immunol.*, 14, 153, 1973.
119. **Wasserman, T., von Stedingle, L.-V., Perlmann, P., and Jonsson, J.,** Antibody-induced *in vitro* lymphocyte cytotoxicity in Hashimoto's thyroiditis, *Int. Arch. Allergy*, 47, 473, 1974.
120. **Koren, H. S., Amos, D. B., and Buckley, R. H.,** Natural killing in immunodeficient patients, *J. Immunol.*, 120, 796, 1978.
121. **Lipinski, M., Virelizier, H., Tursz, T., and Giriscelli, C.,** Natural killer and killer cell activities in patients with primary immunodeficiencies or defects in immune interferon production, *Eur. J. Immunol.*, 10, 246, 1980.
122. **Abb, J., Zander, H., Abb, H., Albert, E., and Diehnardt, F.,** Associating human leukocyte low responsiveness to inducers of interferon alpha with HLA-DR2, *Immunology*, 49, 239, 1983.
123. **Zander, H., Abb, J., Kaudewitz, P., and Riethmuller, G.,** Natural killing activity and interferon production in multiple sclerosis, *Lancet*, i, 280, 1982.
124. **Breard, J., Reinherz, E. L., O'Brien, C., and Schlossman, S. F.,** Delineation of an effector population responsible for natural killing and antibody cellular cytotoxicity in man, *Clin. Immunol. Immunopathol.*, 18, 145, 1981.
125. **Rumpold, H., Kraft, D., Obexer, G., Radaszkiewicz, T., Majdic, O., Bettelheim, P., Knapp, W., and Bock, G.,** Phenotypes of human large granular lymphocytes as defined by monoclonal antibodies, *Immunobiology*, 164, 51, 1983.
126. **Abo, T., Cooper, M. D., and Balch, C. M.,** Characterization of HNK-1$^+$ (Leu 7) human lymphocytes. I. Two distinct phenotypes of human NK cells with different cytotoxic capability, *J. Immunol.*, 129, 1752, 1982.
127. **Abo, T. and Balch, C. M.,** Characterization of HNK-1$^+$ (Leu 7) human lymphocytes. II. Distinguishing phenotypic and functional properties of natural killer cells from activated NK-like cells, *J. Immunol.*, 129, 1758, 1982.
128. **Abo, T. and Balch, C. M.,** Characterization of HNK-1$^+$ (Leu 7) human lymphocytes. III. Interferon effects on spontaneous cytotoxicity and phenotypic expression of lymphocyte subpopulations delineated by the monoclonal HNK-1 antibody, *Cell. Immunol.*, 73, 376, 1982.
129. **Tilden, A. B., Abo, T., and Balch, C. M.,** Suppressor cell function of human granular lymphocytes identified by the HNK-1 (Leu 7) monoclonal antibody, *J. Immunol.*, 130, 1171, 1983.
130. **Perussia, B., Fanning, V., and Trinchieri, G.,** A human NK and K cell subset shares with cytotoxic T cells expression of the antigen recognized by antibody OKT8, *J. Immunol.*, 131, 223, 1983.

131. **Rola-Plesczynski, M., Abernathy, M., Vincent, M. M., Hansen, S. A., and Bellanti, J. A.,** Lymphocyte mediated cytotoxicity to viruses in patients with multiple sclerosis: presence of blocking factor, *Clin. Immunol. Immunopathol.*, 5, 165, 1976.
132. **Silverman, S. L. and Cathcart, E. S.,** Natural killing in systemic lupus erythematosus inhibiting effects of serum, *Clin. Immunol. Immunopathol.*, 17, 219, 1980.
133. **Rook, A. H., Tsokos, G. C., Quinnan, G. V., Balow, J. E., Ramsey, K. M., Stocks, N., Phelan, M. A., and Djeu, J. Y.,** Cytotoxic antibodies to natural killer cells in systemic lupus erythematosus, *Clin. Immunol. Immunopathol.*, 24, 179, 1982.
134. **Preble, O. T., Rothko, K., Klippel, J. H., Friedman, R. M., and Johnston, M. I.,** Interferon-induced 2′-5′ adenylate synthetase *in vivo* and interferon production *in vitro* by lymphocytes from systemic lupus erythematosus patients with and without correlating interferon, *J. Exp. Med.*, 157, 2140, 1983.
135. **Preble, O. T., Black, R. J., Friedman, R. M., Klippel, J. H., and Vilcek, J.,** Systemic lupus erythematosus: presence in human serum of an unusual acid labile leukocyte interferon, *Science*, 216, 429, 1982.
136. **Ytterberg, S. R. and Schnitzer, T. J.,** Serum interferon levels in patients with systemic lupus erythematosus, *Arthritis Rheum.*, 25, 401, 1982.
137. **Panem, S., Check, I. J., Henriksen, D., and Vilcek, J.,** Antibodies to interferon in a patient with systemic lupus erythematosus, *J. Immunol.*, 129, 1, 1982.
138. **Neighbour, P. A. and Grayzel, A. I.,** Interferon production *in vitro* by leukocytes from patients with systemic lupus erythematosus and rheumatoid arthritis, *Clin. Exp. Immunol.*, 45, 576, 1981.
139. **Fitzharris, P., Alcocer, J., Stephens, H. A. F., Knight, R. A., and Snaith, M. L.,** Insensitivity to interferon of NK cells from patients with systemic lupus erythematosus, *Clin. Exp. Immunol.*, 47, 110, 1982.
140. **Hooks, J. J., Moutsopoulos, H. M., and Geis, S. A.,** Immune interferon in the circulation of patients with autoimmune disease, *N. Engl. J. Med.*, 301, 5, 1979.
141. **Talal, N.,** A clinician and a scientist look at acquired immunodeficiency syndrome (AIDS), *Immunol. Today*, 4, 180, 1983.
142. **Rook, A. H., Masur, H., Lane, H. C., Frederick, W., Kasahara, T., Mucher, A. M., Djeu, J. Y., Manischewitz, J. F., Jackson, L., Fauci, A. S., and Quinnan, G. V.,** Interleukin-2 enhances the depressed natural killer and cytomegalovirus-specific cytotoxic activities of lymphocytes from patients with the acquired immunodeficiency syndrome, *J. Clin. Invest.*, 72, 398, 1983.
143. **Linker-Israeli, M., Bakke, A., Kitridou, R. C., Gendler, S., Gillis, S., and Horwitz, D. A.,** Defective production of interleukin 1 and interleukin 2 in patients with systemic lupus erythematosus (SLE), *J. Immunol.*, 130, 2651, 1983.
144. **Alcocer-Varela, J. and Alarcon-Segovia, D.,** Decreased production of and response to interleukin 2 by cultured lymphocytes from patients with systemic lupus erythematosus, *J. Clin. Immunol.*, 69, 1388, 1982.
145. **Hooks, J. J., Moutsopoulos, H. M., and Notkins, A. L.,** Circulating interferon in human autoimmune diseases, *Tex. Rep. Biol. Med*, 41, 164, 1982.
146. **Burmester, G. R., Beck, P., Eife, R., Peter, H. H., and Kalden, J. R.,** Induction of a lymphotoxin-like mediator in peripheral blood and synovial fluid lymphocytes by incubation with synovial fluid from patients with rheumatoid arthritis, *Rheumatol. Int.*, 1, 139, 1981.
147. **Fontana, A.,** Interleukin 1 activity in the synovial fluid of patients with rheumatoid arthritis, *Rheumatol. Int.*, 2, 49, 1982.
148. **Wilkins, J. A., Warrington, R. J., Sigurdson, S. L., and Rutherford, W. J.,** The demonstration of an interleukin 2 like activity in the synovial fluids of rheumatoid arthritis patients, *J. Rheumatol.*, 10, 109, 1983.

Chapter 6

NK CELL ROLE IN REGULATION OF THE GROWTH AND FUNCTIONS OF HEMOPOIETIC AND LYMPHOID CELLS

Eva Lotzová

TABLE OF CONTENTS

I. INTRODUCTION

Natural killer (NK) cells have been recognized primarily for their cytotoxic reactivity against malignant cells.[1,2] However, concurrently with the revelation of NK cell antitumor potential, it became evident that these cells are also involved in the regulation of the growth of semisyngeneic (parental into F_1 hybrids), allogeneic (between two different strains of the same species), and xenogeneic (between different species) bone marrow transplants.[3-5] This was initially evidenced by uninhibited growth of histoincompatible bone marrow cells after transplantation into NK cell-depleted, NK cell-deficient, or NK cell-immature mice, and conversely, by increased resistance to the same transplants in NK cell-stimulated mice.[3-6] More recently, the direct involvement of NK cells in murine bone marrow transplantation was demonstrated by abrogation of resistance to parental and allogeneic bone marrow grafts by antibody directed against NK cell-specific structure, NK 1.1 antigen,[7] and by restoration of bone marrow graft resistance in NK cell-depleted mice by transfer of cloned NK cells.[8] The role of NK cells in regulation of the growth of hemopoietic tissues was further substantiated by studies in man. The latter investigations demonstrated that NK cells displayed inhibitory activity on the in vitro colony-forming potential of myeloid and erythroid precursors.[9,10] Relatively recent data indicate that NK cells also control the proliferation and differentiation of murine and human lymphoid tissues. For instance, in vitro colony formation by T cells has been shown to be potentiated by NK cells, and on the contrary, NK cells inhibited immunoglobulin secretion and differentiation of B cells.[12-14] Furthermore, transplantation studies suggest that NK cells may be involved (in as yet not precisely determined way) in another lymphoid cell-mediated phenomenon, graft-vs.-host reaction.[15]

From these observations, it appears that the important biological function of NK cells may be the maintenance of the homeostasis of the organism. Such function would consist of defense against exogenous and endogenous invaders, as exemplified by various types of microbes and cancer cells, regulation of the growth and differentiation of hemopoietic and lymphoid cells (thus preventing hypo- or hyperplasia of these tissues and securing proper execution of their functions), and perhaps regulation of reactivity against "self", consequently restraining the manifestation of autoimmunity. That the NK cells may play this fundamental biological role is supported by their appearance early in the phylogeny and their preservation through phylogenetic development to *Homo sapiens*.

This chapter will present the most recent data on the NK cell role in bone marrow transplantation and in the control of the growth of hemopoietic and lymphoid cells. It is hoped that such information will lead not only to a better understanding of NK cell functional heterogeneity and biological importance, but will also stimulate NK cell research in these so far not fully explored areas.

II. NK CELL ROLE IN BONE MARROW TRANSPLANTATION

A. Hemopoietic Resistance: Genetic Aspects

Although the detailed genetics of murine bone marrow transplantation is beyond the scope of this chapter, it will be discussed here briefly, since its understanding is important for the comprehension of the immunobiology of bone marrow resistance. Readers who are more interested in the genetic aspect of bone marrow transplantation are referred to the original articles and reviews cited in detail in the list of references of this chapter.

The immunogenetics of murine bone marrow transplantation portrayed an enigma for transplantation immunologists for almost 2 decades. One of the most perplexing observations in this area was the failure of irradiated F_1 hybrid mice to support the growth of parental bone marrow transplants, the phenomenon designated *hybrid resistance*.[16-20] This observation clearly contrasted with the classical laws of transplantation, which state that F_1 hybrid mice between two inbred strains are universal acceptors of parental tissue grafts.

The unusual behavior of parental bone marrow transplants was further extended to transplantation of allogeneic and xenogeneic bone marrow cells, which also demonstrated growth patterns divergent from solid tissue transplants. This was exemplified by unimpaired growth of some allografts and xenografts (rat-into-mice) in spite of the major histocompatibility complex (MHC) and species-specific differences, respectively. Such "take" of histoincompatible bone marrow grafts could not be attributed to intrinsic or radiation-induced incapability of the recipients to respond to allogeneic and xenogeneic cells, since the same recipient strains of mice displayed resistance to histoincompatible bone marrow grafts from other donors. This unpredictable behavior of allogeneic and xenogeneic bone marrow grafts was designated *allogeneic* and *xenogeneic resistance*, respectively.[17,21-25] Since *hybrid, allogeneic*, and *xenogeneic resistance* phenomenon were shown to be exhibited not only to bone marrow cells, but also against other hemopoietic tissues, this phenomenon will be referred to in this article as *hemopoietic resistance*.

Studies on murine bone marrow transplantation thus indicated that the genetic determinants controlling growth of hemopoietic transplants differed from classical MHC genes in several aspects: by noncodominant inheritance (hybrid resistance phenomenon), restriction to hemopoietic tissues, and ability to initiate host antigraft reaction in total body irradiated mice. Detailed genetic and transplantation analysis, utilizing the genetic markers of murine linkage group IX, on chromosome 17, and involving multiple mouse strain combinations, disclosed that the genetic determinants of hybrid and allogeneic resistance were multiple and polymorphic,[17-20,22-24] and the majority were linked to the *H-2D* end of murine MHC.[18-23] Additionally, *H-2K*-end associated hemopoietic resistance determinants, as well as those segregating independently of murine MHC were also identified.[22,26-28] These genetic determinants of hybrid and allogeneic resistance were designated hemopoietic-histocompatibility genes (*Hh* genes),[17] to indicate their relevance for transplantation of hemopoietic tissues. The genetic control of xenogeneic resistance has not been explored so extensively; however, the limited genetic analysis indicates that multiple genes also control this phenomenon.[29,30]

Hh genes have been viewed as structural genes coding for cell surface antigens (*Hh* antigens) expressed on hemopoietic tissues and their malignant counterparts.[17,21] Expression of *Hh* antigens on the surface of hemopoietic cells is thought to be dependent on the homozygosity for the *Hh* gene. According to this postulation, *Hh* antigen would be fully expressed in inbred strains of mice which are homozygous, but not in F_1 hybrid mice which are heterozygous for *Hh* gene. Consequently, the F_1 hybrid recipients, which lack the *Hh* antigen, would recognize it as foreign on homozygous parental cells, and would mediate antiparental reactivity. Furthermore, the differences in *Hh* genetic makeup among various strains of mice, and between mice and rats (as indicated above, *Hh* genes are multiple and polymorphic) would lead to manifestation of allogeneic and xenogeneic resistance, respectively.

Even though the entire concept of murine bone marrow transplantation immunogenetics is based on the premise of *Hh* genes, there appears to be another class of genes that operates in hemopoietic resistance. Specifically, the expression of *Hh* antigen(s) is the essential, but not sufficient, condition for manifestation of hemopoietic resistance. The recognition of and the reactivity to *Hh*-incompatible bone marrow cells is regulated by immune response-like genes. When the *Hh*-incompatible recipient is a genetic "nonresponder", the transplanted bone marrow cells will proliferate without impairment. Thus, the responder status, which allows the recipient to recognize and react to the *Hh* antigens, is essential for manifestation of hemopoietic resistance. Genetic regulation of hemopoietic resistance by immune response genes has been shown to be a polygenic phenomenon, independent of murine MHC;[31] furthermore, the responsiveness to *Hh* antigens is inherited in a dominant fashion.[30,31]

It is important to accentuate that hemopoietic resistance is not a peculiarity of mouse species, since the same phenomenon has been observed in rats,[32] dogs,[33-35] and is also indicated in man.[36] Existence of hemopoietic resistance among various species, including man, indicates its biological importance and possible relevance for clinical bone marrow transplantation. However, it has to be noted that there is still an ambiguity surrounding the hemopoietic histocompatibility system, even in the species so thoroughly investigated such as mice. For instance, the *Hh* antigens are still quite hypothetical, since they were not identified directly by any of the currently available serological or immunological methods; their postulation was based solely on the bone marrow transplantation studies. Moreover, it is not clear whether *Hh* genes are indeed recessive or whether the lack of their expression on the cell surface of hemopoietic tissues of F_1 hybrid mice is mediated via some kind of interalleleic interaction (i.e., one allele may be suppressed or modified). Additionally, even though all of the *Hh* genes so far analyzed genetically displayed noncodominant inheritance patterns, it is not clear whether the *Hh* genes of all strains of mice (or other species) lack *Hh* gene product(s) when heterozygotes. Also, it has to be remembered that the mapping of *Hh* genes is still quite incomplete, since the genetic analysis of *Hh* determinants did not involve progeny testing of putative recombinant animals (the test for resistance does not permit survival of mice), and did not explore all congeneic, recombinant, and mutant strains of mice available today. Consequently, *Hh* genetics provides an open and important area for future investigations.

B. Immunobiology and the Mechanism of Hemopoietic Resistance

Interpretation of hemopoietic resistance as a host antigraft reaction led to a multitude of controversial discussions among immunologists. It was quite trying to acknowledge the existence of the cell-mediated mechanism with features deviating so sharply from classical concepts of transplantation immunology. The unusual nature of effector cells, such as the prompt reactivity (within a few hours after transplantation) without any obvious induction, their relative radioresistance, T cell-independent nature, and no MHC restriction for function, led several investigators to conclude that the phenomenon of hemopoietic resistance was not immunological. The latter interpretation was, however, incompatible with the observations that resistance to bone marrow grafts was abrogated by agents with immune suppressive properties, and could be induced in nonresponder mice by adoptive transfer of lymphocytes or their precursors from responder mice. Furthermore, immunological tolerance to incompatible bone marrow transplants could be induced in resistant mice by multiple immunization with the splenocytes of prospective bone marrow donors.[17,21,24,37] Such tolerance was highly specific for the cells used for its induction.

In an attempt to understand the mechanism of antibone marrow transplant reactivity and to dissect the cell type(s) responsible for hemopoietic resistance, an in vitro model was developed by Shearer et al.[38] Although the reactivity of F_1 hybrid mice against parental cells was detected in this model, various facets of the cytotoxic mechanism were quite discrepant from the mechanism of hemopoietic resistance. For instance, in contrast to natural occurrence of hybrid resistance, 5-day stimulation of effector cells with targets was required for manifestation of antiparental reactivity in vitro. Furthermore, whereas F_1 antiparent reactivity was demonstrated to be independent of thymus (its expression was found to be stronger in thymusless mice),[28] both phases of in vitro effector mechanism (i.e., the sensitizing, as well as the effector phase) were found to be T cell dependent.[38,39] Specifically, the athymic mice were unable to generate the hemopoietic resistance in vitro and furthermore, the cytotoxic responses were abrogated by Thy-1 antibody.[38,39] Another discordance between these two systems was demonstrated by different degree of specificity; in the in vitro model, the F_1 hybrid effector cells displayed cytotoxicity only against stimulator cells; in this regard, the F_1 hybrid reactivity in vivo is more ubiquitous. In fact, the in vitro model appears to be more compatible with conventional T cell-mediated allogeneic reaction than with hemopoietic resistance. Whether this system has any relevance to hemopoietic resistance phenomenon remains to be determined.

Table 1
COMPATIBILITY BETWEEN NK CELL CYTOTOXIC POTENTIAL AND RESISTANCE TO MURINE BONE MARROW TRANSPLANTS

Agents depressing both functions	Ref.
Cyclophosphamide	3, 4, 18, 24, 46
^{89}Sr	4, 47
Silica	3, 4, 24, 28, 55—57
Carrageenan	3, 4, 24, 28, 56, 57
Estradiol	51
Cortisone acetate	49
Glucan	6, 50
Corynebacterium parvum[a]	3, 6, 19, 45
Horse antimouse thymocyte antibody	20, 57
NK 1.1 antibody	6, 7, 53
Asialo-GM1 antibody	54, Tables 2—5
Agents potentiating both functions	
Poly I:C	6
ABPP[b]	6
Corynebacterium parvum[a]	6
Both functions are defective in	
Beige mice	8
Osteopetrotic mice	51
Infant mice	3, 4, 28
Bone marrow tolerant mice	45

[a] The effect of *Corynebacterium parvum* is time-dependent; the bacterium potentiated both functions 3 days after injection, but suppressed the same functions 6 to 12 days after injection.
[b] 2-Amino-5-bromo-6-phenyl-4-pyrimidinol.

The in vitro model for hemopoietic resistance became available with the discovery of murine NK cells.[1,2,40-44] NK cell cytotoxic activity displayed in ^{51}Cr-release assay in vitro paralleled closely the effector bone marrow cell mechanism in vivo. Both phenomena were displayed naturally (without any obvious induction) and promptly (within a few hours), both were relatively radioresistant and thymus independent (in the sense that they were manifested by congenitally athymic mice). Furthermore, both effector mechanisms were found to mature late in the ontogenetic development (reactivity is expressed within 2 to 3 weeks after birth),[3,4,24,28,44-46] appear to depend on bone marrow for their origin and differentiation,[47] display broader spectrum of reactivity (including cytotoxicity against normal hemopoietic cells) without any MHC restriction.[1-4,28-30,42-44] This almost perfect compatibility between NK cells and bone marrow effector cells indicated that the former cells could be involved in hemopoietic resistance against bone marrow transplants.

After these initial observations, we and other investigators explored the correlative studies between modulation of in vitro NK cell cytotoxicity and in vivo hemopoietic resistance. It was soon obvious that the agents that depressed NK cell in vitro cytotoxic potential were also suppressive for hemopoietic resistance.[3-7,48-51] Conversely, the agents that potentiated NK cell activity increased resistance to hemopoietic transplants.[6] Furthermore, the mice defective in NK cell cytotoxic potential exhibited also defect in bone marrow graft rejection in vivo (see for review Table 1). In the context of the comparative studies between hemopoietic resistance and NK cell resistance to tumors it is important to stress that neither of these systems is absolute with regard to its effectiveness, and both may be overridden by an excessive number of bone marrow or tumor cells. For instance, the strength of hemopoietic resistance, as measured by the number of bone marrow cells which override it, varies considerably according to the donor-recipient strain combination. Some strain combinations exhibit strong resistance (which cannot be overridden by cell inocula as large as 50 million cells),[20] whereas other strain combinations are weakly resistant (resistance can be overridden easily by 2 to 3 million bone marrow cells).[24,28] Similarly, resistance of various mouse strains against leukemias and other tumors appears to depend on their NK cell responder status. In general, strains of mice with high NK cell activity exhibit stronger resistance against malignant cells.[2,42] This is important to keep in mind when the in vivo studies on hemopoietic resistance and on NK cell involvement in resistance to tumors are conducted in order to interpret the data correctly.

In addition to classical bone marrow transplantation studies, the role of NK cells in reactivity against bone marrow cells in vivo was demonstrated in clearance experiments involving radiolabeled bone marrow cells.[52] These studies showed that mice exhibiting high NK cell cytotoxicity were more efficient in clearing radioactively labeled parental and allogeneic bone marrow cells than mice with low or depressed NK cell activity. Although all of these correlative studies were valuable in indicating the compatibility between NK cell activity and antihemopoietic reactivity effector mechanisms, they were not instrumental in directly identifying NK cell involvement in bone marrow graft rejection. This is because the majority of the agents used in these studies were not selectively depleting NK cells. Most informative experiments were those employing the antiserum directed against NK cell-associated antigen, NK 1.1. Since NK 1.1 antigen has not been shown to be expressed on any of the known effector cell populations,[84] the abrogation of hemopoietic resistance with this antibody provided direct evidence for the involvement of NK cells in in vivo reactivity against bone marrow cells.[7,28,53] This conclusion was supported by two additional observations. First, deficient bone marrow graft rejection potential could be restored by transfer of cloned NK cells;[8] second, resistance to bone marrow grafts was abrogated by another antibody directed against NK cell-associated cell surface structure, asialo-GM1.[54]

Our data, illustrated in Tables 2 and 3, indicate that pretreatment of bone marrow recipients with asialo-GM1 antibody abrogated both allogeneic and hybrid resistance to bone marrow transplants. The degree of abrogation of allogeneic resistance was dependent on the interval between administration of asialo-GM1 antibody and inoculation of bone marrow cells; specifically, growth of bone marrow transplants was most promoted when the asialo-GM1 antibody was administered 48 and 24 hr prior to transplantation and least pronounced when this antibody was injected 96 and 72 hr before transplantation (Table 2). Additionally, the effect of this antibody was more powerful on allogeneic resistance (which was completely abrogated, Table 2) than on hybrid resistance (which was only partially, but significantly abrogated, Table 3). That this antibody was destructive for NK cell cytotoxic potential of $B6D2F_1$ and B6 mice against YAC-1 target is illustrated in Tables 4 and 5. Table 5 demonstrates the effect of asialo-GM1 antibody on NK cell cytotoxic potential of irradiated mice, since irradiation is a standard procedure of bone marrow transplantation experiments. Of interest is the observation that abrogation of allogeneic resistance to bone marrow transplants and NK cell cytotoxic potential by asialo-GM1 antibody was paralleled by the decrease in the splenic large granular lymphocyte (LGL) content (Table 5). These and other currently available data demonstrate that NK cells are one of the cell components involved in hemopoietic resistance to bone marrow transplantation. Furthermore, our studies indicate that at least some of the NK cells involved in bone marrow graft rejection display LGL morphology.

We have suggested previously that macrophages may be involved in bone marrow graft rejection mechanism.[24,55-57] This suggestion was based on the abrogation of hemopoietic

Table 2
EFFECT OF ASIALO-GM1 ANTIBODY ON ALLOGENEIC RESISTANCE OF B6 MICE TO BALB/c BONE MARROW TRANSPLANTS

Recipient strain	Treatment[a]	Splenic uptake of ^{125}IUdR[b]	CFUs[c]
B6	None	0.02 ± 0.002	None
B6	−48, −24 hr	0.68 ± 0.09	Confluent
B6	−72, −48 hr	0.53 ± 0.09	Confluent
B6	−96, −72 hr	0.21 ± 0.07	15.8 ± 2.7
BALB/c	None	0.88 ± 0.05	Confluent
BALB/c	−48, −24 hr	0.68 ± 0.04	Confluent
BALB/c	−72, −48 hr	0.87 ± 0.08	Confluent

[a] Asialo-GM1 antibody was injected twice in the dose of 0.3 mℓ (1:50 dilution), i.v.

[b] Mean splenic uptake of ^{125}IUdR ± S.E. of 7 to 23 mice (11 weeks old). ^{125}IUdR technique was performed as described earlier.[24] B6 mice received 900 R, and BALB/c mice received 870 R of total body irradiation 24 hr prior to transplantation of 0.5 × 10^6 BALB/c bone marrow cells. Mean splenic uptake of ^{125}IUdR was 0.03 ± 0.006 for untreated radiation controls and 0.02 ± 0.004 for radiation controls (both BALB/c and B6 mice) treated 48 and 24 hr before transplantation with asialo-GM1 antibody.

[c] Growth of splenic colonies (CFUs) was evaluated as described previously.[49]

Table 3
EFFECT OF ASIALO-GM1 ANTIBODY ON HYBRID RESISTANCE OF B6D2F$_1$ MICE TO PARENTAL B6 BONE MARROW TRANSPLANTS

Recipient strain	Treatment[a]	Splenic uptake of ^{125}IUdR[b]	CFUs
B6	None	0.44 ± 0.007	Confluent
B6D2F$_1$	None	0.04 ± 0.02	None
B6D2F$_1$	Normal rabbit serum	0.04 ± 0.01	None
B6D2F$_1$	Asialo-GM1	0.22 ± 0.03	9.5 ± 1.0

[a] Asialo-GM1 antibody and normal rabbit serum was injected i.v. 48 and 24 hr prior to transplantation in 0.3-mℓ volume (1:50 dilution).

[b] Mean splenic uptake of ^{125}IUdR ± S.E. of 6 to 14 mice (11 weeks old). B6D2F$_1$ received 1100 R and B6 mice received 900 R of total body irradiation 24 hr prior to transplantation of 0.5 × 10^6 B6 bone marrow cells. The mean splenic uptake of ^{125}IUdR was 0.02 ± 0.003 in B6D2F$_1$ radiation controls.

resistance with, then considered macrophage specific toxins — silica and carrageenan. However, we and others demonstrated later that these agents also affected functions of NK cells.[3-4] Thus, at this time, it is unresolved whether silica and carrageen-mediated abrogation of hemopoietic resistance is related to the NK cell, macrophage, or both cell types. Consequently, the participation of macrophages in hemopoietic resistance cannot be excluded.

The mechanism by which NK cells control the growth of bone marrow transplants in vivo has not been elucidated as yet. It was suggested recently that such NK cell antibone marrow

Table 4
EFFECT OF ASIALO-GM1 ANTIBODY ON SPLENIC NK CELL ACTIVITY OF B6D2F$_1$ MICE AGAINST YAC-1

	Percent of cytotoxicity[b] (T:E cell ratio)		
Treatment[a]	1:25	1:50	1:100
None	7.8 ± 0.4	11.6 ± 1.3	17.4 ± 2.9
Normal rabbit serum	6.8 ± 0.2	10.7 ± 0.7	17.3 ± 1.9
Asialo-GM1	1.7 ± 0.2	2.3 ± 0.4	3.9 ± 0.5

[a] B6D2F$_1$ mice (11-week-old) were untreated or i.v.-injected with 0.3 mℓ of normal rabbit serum or asialo-GM1 antibody (1:50 dilution) 24 and 48 hr prior to NK cell assay.
[b] NK cell cytotoxicity was tested in a 4-hr ^{51}Cr-release assay.[49] Values represent mean ± S.E. of five mice.

Table 5
EFFECT OF ASIALO-GM1 ANTIBODY ON SPLENIC NK CELL CYTOTOXICITY AND LGL CONTENT OF B6 MICE

		Percent of LGL[c]	
Treatment[a]	Percent of cytotoxicity[b]	Unseparated	NW-filtered
None	12.4 ± 1.9	0.8 ± 0.2	2.0 ± 0.6
Irradiation	7.0 ± 0.3	3.8 ± 0.9	13.7 ± 0.8
Irradiation and normal rabbit serum	6.3 ± 0.3	2.3 ± 1.2	11.3 ± 2.1
Irradiation and asialo-GM1	1.8 ± 1.1	0.2 ± 0.2	0.3 ± 0.2

[a] B6 mice (12-week-old) (3 per each group) were either untreated or irradiated with 1100 R (12 hr prior to NK cell assay). Normal rabbit serum or asialo-GM1 antibody was i.v.-injected in 0.3 mℓ (1:50 dilution) 24 and 48 hr prior to NK cell test.
[b] Cytotoxicity of unseparated splenocytes to YAC-1 was tested in a 4-hr ^{51}Cr-release assay, at 1:50 T:E cell ratio.
[c] LGLs were evaluated by analysis of May-Grünwald- and Giemsa-stained cytocentrifuge slides.[76,77] Nylon wool (NW) filtration was performed as described previously.[76]

reactivity could be mediated by antibodies.[58] The latter study demonstrated that the growth of allogeneic bone marrow transplants in nonresponder mice could be prevented by passive transfer of serum from responder mice, and that such activity was abrogated by removal of immunoglobulin by anti-Ig affinity chromatography. Moreover, the serum from responder mice was effective in specifically arming NK cells to mediate antibody-dependent cell-mediated cytotoxicity (ADCC) against allogeneic tumor cells. In addition, sera of responder animals were cytotoxic against allogeneic splenocytes in complement-dependent cytolytic reaction.

These data, though interesting, are not conclusive as to the mechanism of NK cell-mediated antibone marrow reactivity. First, only limited numbers of strain combinations were investigated, and thus, the genetic specificity displayed by bone marrow transplants in vivo could not be precisely evaluated in those studies. Second, the transfer of resistance to nonresponder mice by serum was often quite incomplete, since significant bone marrow cell growth was observed in some of the serum-transferred mice. Furthermore, serum from responder mice also lysed some of the susceptible target cells (growing upon transplantation in vivo). Also, the interpretation of this mechanism as rejection should be used with caution, since no attempt was made to determine whether the transplanted bone marrow cells were indeed rejected or only inhibited to grow. Finally, the serum-transferred antibone marrow graft in vivo reactivity was observed only in allogeneic donor-recipient combination, but not in the hybrid resistance system. Thus, if this mechanism operates in hemopoietic resistance, it cannot represent the only mechanism responsible for this phenomenon.

In this context, it is important to indicate that our data with asialo-GM1 and also with NK 1.1 antibody suggest that some differences exist in the mechanism of allogeneic and hybrid resistance. Specifically, both antibodies have been more effective in abrogating the former than the latter phenomenon. This difference could not be explained by the strength of allogeneic vs. hybrid resistance, since the strain combinations used for transplantation studies were either equally resistant or the allogeneic resistance was even stronger. Whether these differences between allogeneic and hybrid resistance reflect involvement of different subpopulation of NK cells, and/or NK cells at different stages of differentiation, or whether different mechanisms are involved in these two types of hemopoietic resistance, remains to be elucidated.

It is important to stress that the investigations on hemopoietic resistance are important not only from the basic science angle, but also from the clinical aspect, since this phenomenon may be responsible for rejection of allogeneic bone marrow grafts in man.[59-62] The actual frequency of manifestation of hemopoietic resistance in man, however, may be obscured by overriding the resistance by inoculation of large numbers of bone marrow cells in order to ensure the "take" of the grafts. However, the larger the number of transplanted allogeneic cells, the higher is the likelihood of graft-vs.-host disease (GVHD). Thus, the understanding of the mechanism of hemopoietic resistance could lead to its abrogation and to a subsequent "take" of grafts composed of smaller bone marrow cell inocula. The final outcome of this approach could result in less severe GVHD.

C. NK Cell Role in GVHD

The role of NK cells in the physiopathology of GVHD was originally suggested by studies concerned with the NK cell cytotoxic profile of patients undergoing allogeneic bone marrow or fetal liver transplantation.[15] These investigations demonstrated that patients with normal pretransplant levels of NK cell cytotoxicity against herpes simplex virus type 1-infected fibroblasts (HSV-1) displayed GVHD, whereas patients with low pretransplant NK cell levels to the same target had no evidence of this disease.[15] The association of GVHD with host NK cell responder status was interpreted to reflect host NK cell stimulatory function for graft vs. host reaction (GVHR). Importantly, however, such a correlation between NK cell cytotoxic profile and GVHD was observed only when HSV-1 cells were used as a target, but not when K562 cells were employed,[63] suggesting that distinct populations of NK cells could have been involved in reactivity against HSV-1 vs. K562 cell lines.

In another transplantation study, GVHD was reported to be related to the post-transplant levels of NK cell activity.[64] Specifically, in patients without GVHD, peripheral blood NK cell cytotoxicity against K562 target cells was low during the 1st month after transplantation and recovered to normal levels between 30 to 50 days post-transplant. In contrast, patients with acute GVHD exhibited high NK cell cytotoxicity levels early after transplantation. These results were interpreted as a possible involvement of NK cells in the effector mechanism of GVHR. Interestingly, in the latter studies, ADCC cytotoxic pattern did not correlate with GVHR, suggesting that the effector cells mediating ADCC and the subpopulation of NK cells involved in GVHR may represent two distinct lymphocyte populations. Both of the above-described studies indicated NK cell involvement in pathogenesis of GVHD, and the possible prognostic role of NK cells in GVHR; however, neither study dissected the exact role of NK cells in this disease.

Investigations concerned with the involvement of NK cells in GVHR in experimental animals are also quite limited and noncommital with regard to the exact function of NK cells in this disease. In the murine system it has been reported that thymic, splenic, and lymph node NK cell activity increased during the early period of GVHR, but the NK cell activity of the spleen declined subsequently. The thymic NK cell cytotoxic profile after initial augmentation returned to normal levels, but displayed later another phase of increase. The authors suggested that the initial potentiation of NK cell activity could be attributed to the stimulation of NK cell cytotoxicity by interferon (IFN), which has been demonstrated to be induced during GVHR.[65] The potentiation of NK cells, however, could be mediated by interleukin-2 (IL-2), since this agent also activates NK cells, and was shown to be produced during in vitro recognition reaction in mixed lymphocyte cultures (the correlate of recognition phase of GVHR).[66,67] These studies did not dissect the function of NK cells in GVHR; however, the authors speculate that increased NK cell activity in the thymus during GVHR could have a biological significance in protecting the thymus against neoplasias, some of which have been shown to be associated with GVHD. They exemplify this postulation by the observation of a high frequency of B cell lymphomas in the spleen (the tissue with low NK cell activity) following GVHR reaction, in contrast to no incidence of tumors (thymomas or thymic leukemias) in thymus, the tissue with augmented NK cell activity, during GVHD.[65]

Enhanced NK cell cytotoxic activity of splenic, mesenteric lymph node, and intraepithelial lymphocytes was also reported during GVHR.[68] Interestingly, the high proportion of intraepithelial lymphocytes detected during GVHR displayed the morphology of LGLs.[68]

In other studies, the depression of splenic and peripheral blood NK cell activity was observed in mice after acute GVHR, whereas the chronic form of GVHD was associated with significant enhancement of NK cell cytotoxicity.[69] An increase in NK cell cytotoxic potential was also observed in the early phase of acute GVHR in rats[70] however, this initial increase was followed by depression of NK cell activity at later stages of this disease.

All of the experimental animal studies described above are only phenomenological and do not contribute to the understanding of the NK cell role in the pathogenesis of GVHR. More informative as to the role of NK cells in the GVHD phenomenon were the studies of Charley et al.,[71] who reported that the treatment of recipient mice with asialo-GM1 antibody (the treatment resulting in depletion of NK cell activity) protected mice from death from GVHD. These observations suggest, in accordance with data of Lopez et al.,[15] that NK cells may represent the host stimulatory component for initiation of GVHR by donor lymphoid cells. However, since both of these studies are only correlative, and the pathophysiology of GVHR is quite complex, other mechanisms of NK cell involvement in GVHR cannot be excluded at present. These studies, even though inconclusive, indicate that NK cells may play an important role in the prognosis or pathogenesis of GVHD. The delineation of the function of NK cells in this disease may be instrumental in developing new therapeutic and diagnostic approaches to human bone marrow transplantation.

Table 6
PERITONEAL EXUDATE NK CELL REACTIVITY OF B6D2F$_1$ MICE AGAINST PARENTAL B6 BONE MARROW CELLS

	Percent of cytotoxicity[a]	
Mouse no.	Untreated	AIPP-treated[b]
1	0	7.1
2	0	13.1
3	−7.8	11.1

[a] Cytotoxicity was tested in a 4-hr ^{51}Cr-release assay at 1:50 T:E cell ratio.
[b] AIPP was injected in the dose of 250 mg/kg, i.p., 72 hr prior to NK cell test.

III. NK CELL CYTOTOXIC AND REGULATORY ACTIVITY FOR HEMOPOIETIC AND LYMPHOID CELLS

A. NK Cell in Vitro Cytotoxic Reactivity Against Hemopoietic and Lymphoid Cells

NK cell in vivo reactivity against hemopoietic tissues is compatible with NK cells lytic activity for hemopoietic cells and some lymphocytes in cytotoxic assay in vitro. Nunn et al.[72] demonstrated that splenocytes of athymic mice displayed modest, but significant, NK cell cytotoxicity against syngeneic and allogeneic bone marrow cells and thymocytes. NK cell antithymocyte-directed cytotoxicity was later confirmed by other groups of investigators.[73,74] In the latter studies, the age of the thymocytes was found to be an important factor for killing by mouse NK cells.[74] Specifically, the thymocytes of fetal or young mice were preferentially sensitive to NK cell killing. Furthermore, the susceptible target in the thymus was defined as a cortical, relatively large and immature cell. Similarly, the stage of maturation of bone marrow cells was found to be important for sensitivity to NK cell attack. Using competitive inhibition assay, it was demonstrated that less mature hemopoietic cells were more competitive with NK cell-sensitive target, YAC-1, in a ^{51}Cr-release assay.[75] We have also found that peritoneal exudate cells of B6D2F$_1$ mice stimulated with IFN inducer 2-amino-5-iodo-6-phenyl-4 pyrimidinone (AIPP)[76,77] mediated cytotoxicity against parental B6 bone marrow (Table 6). In addition to thymocytes and bone marrow cells, normal peritoneal macrophages were found to be sensitive to lysis by splenocytes of athymic mice.[72]

Peripheral blood NK cell reactivity against hemopoietic cells was also observed in humans.[74] Also in this system, target cell sensitivity to NK cell killing was age-dependent; bone marrow cells of fetal origin displayed twofold sensitivity to NK cell lysis than did adult bone marrow tissues.[74] Similar observations were made with thymus. A population of fetal human thymocytes was found to represent a highly susceptible target for NK cells, whereas adult human thymus was found to be relatively resistant to NK cell killing.[78] In compatibility with NK cell reactivity against malignant targets, reactivity against normal bone marrow cells was independent of MHC and species-specific differences, since the lysis was manifested by autologous, allogeneic, and xenogeneic NK cells.[74] Xenogeneic reactivity was exemplified by lytic activity of human PBLs against mouse spleen cells.[79]

B. NK Cell Role in Regulation of Hemopoiesis In Vitro

The observation that NK cell in vitro cytotoxicity has been displayed primarily against more primitive hemopoietic and lymphoid cells, together with the demonstration of inhibition of spleen colony-formation (the function performed by hemopoietic stem cells) after transplantation of murine hemopoietic cells in vivo[7,24,49] indicated that NK cells may control the growth of clonogenic stem cells. This notion was indeed confirmed by experiments involving human clonogenic in vitro assay for granulocyte-macrophage colony-forming cells (GM-CFC).[9] In these investigations, preincubation of bone marrow cells with PBLs prior to initiation of clonogenic assay resulted in substantial inhibition of the colony-forming potential of granulocytes and macrophages. Such inhibition was observed independently whether the inhibitory cells were of autologous or allogeneic origin. The involvement of NK cells in this phenomenon was demonstrated by studies involving NK cell-enriched and NK cell-depleted fractions obtained after Percoll density gradient separation. Specifically, the low-density fractions composed of a high proportion of LGLs displayed high GM-CFC inhibitory activity, whereas the high-density fractions (containing <2% LGLs) displayed inferior inhibitory activity.[9] The mechanism of NK cell regulation of GM-CFC potential was not determined by these studies; however, it has been shown that inhibition was contact-dependent since preincubation of bone marrow and NK cells was necessary for manifestation of the inhibitory effect. These data provided an evidence that NK cells play a role in the control of the proliferation and differentiation of autologous and allogeneic myeloid cell series in vitro. Similar inhibition of human granulopoiesis was reported earlier by Morris et al.[80] In the latter studies, the type of the regulatory cells was not analyzed, but their characteristics, such as non-T and non-B lymphocyte profile and independence of regulatory activity of MHC, indicated their NK cell nature.

The effect of NK cell-enriched populations was also tested on the in vitro proliferative activity of erythroid stem cells at different stages of maturation, i.e., on bone marrow and blood erythroid burst-forming units (BFU-E) and on bone marrow erythroid colony-forming units (CFU-E).[10] NK cells were obtained from peripheral blood and enriched by two methods: by Percoll density gradient centrifugation and by fluorescence-activated cell sorting, using HNK-1 monoclonal antibody.[10] These experiments demonstrated that Percoll density gradient-separated NK cells significantly suppressed bone marrow CFU-E formation (approximately by 60%). These cells were characterized as OKM-1 and HNK-1-positive and OKT-3-negative lymphocytes, of low density, LGL morphology, with high NK cell cytotoxic potential against K562. NK cell-mediated CFU-E-directed inhibitory effect was potentiated by IFN and abolished by treatment with HNK-1 antibody and complement.

Contrasted to the inhibitory effect on CFU-E, the Percoll-enriched NK cell population did not display any inhibitory effect on bone marrow or blood BFU-E. In fact, NK cell-enriched suspensions exhibited a slight stimulatory effect on blood BFU-E. The latter observation is in accordance with that of Pistoia et al.[11] reported earlier. Interestingly, HNK-1-positive cells, obtained by fluorescence cell sorting, displayed an inhibitory effect on both bone marrow CFU-E and BFU-E, whereas the HNK-1-negative population had no effect on any of these populations of erythropoietic cells. The discrepancy between effect of Percoll-separated vs. fluorescence cell sorter-separated NK cells on bone marrow BFU-E may be explained by various possibilities. For instance, the Percoll-separated NK cell fraction may have contained other cell populations promoting BFU-E formation and thus, masking the NK cell inhibitory effect. Alternatively, it has been recognized that not all LGLs are HNK-1 positive, and consequently, a higher concentration of the HNK-1-positive NK cell subpopulation may be required for manifestation of an inhibitory effect on BFU-E.

The mechanism of NK cell regulation of proliferation on CFU-E and BFU-E has not been dissected as yet. However, it was shown that the NK cells did not require preincubation with bone marrow cells for manifestation of CFU-E inhibitory effect and that both autologous and allogeneic NK cells were effective inhibitors. One of the possible mechanisms operating in inhibition of erythropoiesis may be the production of endogenous IFN by NK cells, which may exhibit a suppressive effect on erythroid stem cell proliferation. In fact, suppression of erythroid stem cells by IFN was previously observed.[81]

Regulation of the growth of hemopoietic cells by NK cells was also observed in the murine system. It has been shown quite recently that Percoll-enriched F_1 hybrid NK cells inhibited proliferation of parental BFU-E and GM-CFC in vitro. The cell contact in this system was a prerequisite for expression of inhibitory activity.[82] The latter observation is in agreement with our unpublished data, indicating that F_1 hybrid splenocytes suppressed proliferation of GM-CFC in vitro.[85]

C. NK Cell Regulation of Lymphocyte Growth and Functions

NK cells were implicated also in promotion of the colony-forming potential of T cells. The report of Pistoia et al.[11] indicates that the LGL population obtained from Percoll density gradient centrifugation substantially increased the clonogenic capacity of T cells. In this system, a direct contact between NK cells and T cells was not required, since LGL-produced factors were efficient in promoting T cell proliferative activity. It was suggested by the authors, but not experimentally proven, that mediators related to IL-2 may have been involved. Indeed, this postulation is compatible with the NK cell ability to produce IL-2, and with the ability of T cells to proliferate in response to this substance.

Recent reports indicate that NK cells control differentiation and antibody production by human and murine B cells. In human studies, NK cell-enriched low-density fractions obtained after separation of PBLs on Percoll gradient were effective in suppressing IgM and IgG production by autologous B cells.[13] Such inhibition was observed after coculture of NK cells with B cells and T cells in the presence of pokeweed mitogen. The suppressive effect was abolished by treatment of NK cells with HNK-1 antibody and complement. The suppression of IgM and IgG production by NK cells was manifested only in the presence of helper T cells, but not when these cells were replaced by soluble helper T cell factor. This suggests that the NK effect was exerted on helper T cells and not directly on B cells. The mechanism of NK cell inhibitory effect on antibody production has not been explored in these studies. However, the authors reported that the light-density Percoll fractions when stimulated with pokeweed mitogen produced acid-labile IFN, and that such production was inhibited by treatment with HNK-1 antibody. Since IFN has been shown to suppress antibody production,[83] it is possible that this substance could be involved in NK cell-mediated suppression of antibody production in this study.

Suppression of antibody production by NK cells was also demonstrated in mice by two groups of investigators.[12,14] In one of these investigations, in vitro-cloned NK cells were effective in inhibiting immunoglobulin secretion by splenocytes both in vitro and in vivo as measured in plaque-forming assay involving trinitrophenyl-coupled sheep erythrocytes.[12] NK cell-mediated suppression of immunoglobulin production in this system was nonspecific, since inhibition was manifested to sheep as well as to chicken erythrocytes. In contrast to human studies, the mechanism of inhibition of immunoglobulin secretion in these studies appeared to be mediated through the direct effect on B cells, as suggested by manifestation of inhibitory activity in the presence of T cell helper factor. This suggestion was also substantiated by the observation that cloned NK cells exhibited lytic activity against lipopolysaccharide-activated B cells.[12] The cell contact was required for manifestation of suppression of immunoglobulin production, since the supernatants from NK cell clones did not exert inhibitory activity. In the other investigation, inhibition of murine antibody response to sheep erythrocytes was exhibited by a poly I:C-activated NK cell-enriched population.[14] In the latter studies the adherent, antigen-processing cells were considered as the targets of NK cell regulatory activity.

IV. CONCLUSIONS

From this short review, it is evident that NK cells, in addition to their role in defense against malignancies, are involved in the regulation of various components of hemopoietic and lymphoid compartments. These function include (1) regulation of the growth of hemopoietic cells upon transplantation in vivo; (2) regulation of clonogeneic capacity of granulocytic, macrophage, erythroid, and T cell series in vitro; (3) immunoregulation of the antibody production circuit; (4) possible role in the mechanism or prognosis of GVHR.

The understanding of the mechanism of NK cell role in these functions may contribute to new therapeutic or prognostic approaches in the areas of human bone marrow transplantation, immune-deficiency diseases, and malignant and benign hemo- and lymphopathies.

ACKNOWLEDGMENT

The author wishes to express her thanks to Dr. C. A. Savary, Mr. A. Khan, and Mr. M. Lowlachi for the contribution to the studies from this laboratory, and to Mrs. A. Childers for her excellent secretarial assistance in preparation of this manuscript. The support of this research by Grant CA 31394 from the National Cancer Institute is greatly appreciated.

REFERENCES

1. **Kiessling, R., Klein, E., and Wigzell, H.,** Natural killer cells in the mouse. I. Cytotoxic cells with specificity for mouse Moloney leukemia cells. Specificity and distribution according to genotype, *Eur. J. Immunol.*, 5, 112, 1975.
2. **Herberman, R. B., Djeu, J. Y., Kay, H. D., Ortaldo, J. R., Riccardi, C., Bonnard, G. D., Holden, H. T., Fagnani, R., Santoni, A. S., and Puccetti, P.,** Natural killer cells: characteristics and regulation of activity, *Immunol. Rev.*, 44, 43, 1979.
3. **Lotzová, E. and Savary, C. A.,** Possible involvement of natural killer cells in bone marrow graft rejection, *Biomedicine*, 27, 341, 1977.
4. **Kiessling, R., Hochman, P. S., Häller, O., Shearer, G. M., Wigzell, H., and Cudkowicz, G.,** Evidence for a similar or common mechanism for natural killer cell activity and resistance to hemopoietic grafts, *Eur. J. Immunol.*, 7, 655, 1977.
5. **Lotzová, E.,** Natural bone marrow graft rejection phenomenon in mice, *Surv. Immunol. Res.*, 1, 155, 1982.
6. **Lotzová, E. and Savary, C. A.,** Natural resistance to foreign hemopoietic transplants: a possible model of leukemia surveillance, *Int. Cancer Congress, 13th, Part C, Biology of Cancer*, Mirand, E. A., Hutchinson, W. B., and Mihich, E., Eds., Alan R. Liss, New York, 983, 125.
7. **Lotzová, E., Savary, C. A., and Pollack, S. B.,** Prevention of rejection of allogeneic bone marrow transplants by NK 1.1 antiserum, *Transplantation*, 35, 490, 1983.
8. **Warner, J. F. and Dennert, G.,** Effects of cloned cell line with NK activity on bone marrow transplants, tumor development and metastasis in vivo, *Nature (London)*, 300, 31, 1982.
9. **Hansson, M., Beran, M., Andersson, B., and Kiessling, R.,** Inhibition of in vitro granulopoiesis by autologous allogeneic human NK cells, *J. Immunol.*, 129, 126, 1982.
10. **Mangan, K. F., Hartnett, M. E., Matis, S. A., Winkelstein, A., and Abo, T.,** Natural killer cells suppress human erythroid stem cell proliferation in vitro, *Blood*, 63, 260, 1984.
11. **Pistoia, U., Nocera, A., Ghio, R., Leprini, A., Perata, A., Pistone, M., and Ferrarini, M.,** PHA-induced human T cell colony formation: enhancing effect of large granular lymphocytes, *Exp. Hematol.*, 11, 249, 1983.
12. **Nabel, G., Allard, W. J., and Cantor, H.,** A cloned cell line mediating natural killer cell function, *J. Exp. Med.*, 156, 658, 1982.
13. **Arai, S., Yamamoto, H., Itoh, K., and Kumagai, K.,** Suppressive effect of human natural killer cells on pokeweed mitogen-induced B cell differentiation, *J. Immunol.*, 131, 651, 1983.
14. **Abruzzo, L. B. and Rowley, D. A.,** Homeostasis of the antibody response: immunoregulation by NK cells, *Science*, 222, 581, 1983.
15. **Lopez, C., Kirkpatrick, D., Sorell, M., and O'Reilly, R. J.,** Association between pre-transplant natural kill and graft-versus-host disease after stem cell transplantation, *Lancet*, 24, 1103, 1979.
16. **Cudkowicz, G. and Stimpfling, J. H.,** Deficient growth of C57BL marrow cells transplanted in F_1 hybrid mice. Association with the histocompatibility-2 locus, *Immunology*, 7, 291, 1964.

17. **Cudkowicz, G.,** Hybrid resistance to parental grafts of hemopoietic and lymphoma cells, in *The Proliferation and Spread of Neoplastic Cells. XXI. Annual M. D. Anderson Symposium on Fundamental Cancer Research*, Williams & Wilkins, Baltimore, 1968, 661.
18. **Lotzová, E. and Cudkowicz, G.,** Hybrid resistance to parental NZW bone marrow grafts. Association with the D-end of H-2, *Transplantation*, 12, 130, 1971.
19. **Lotzová, E. and Cudkowicz, G.,** Hybrid resistance to parental WB/Re bone marrow grafts. Association with genetic markers of linkage group IX, *Transplantation*, 13, 256, 1972.
20. **Lotzová, E. and Cudkowicz, G.,** Resistance of irradiated F_1 hybrid and allogeneic mice to bone marrow grafts of NZB donors, *J. Immunol.*, 110, 791, 1973.
21. **Cudkowicz, G.,** Genetic regulation of bone marrow transplantation, in *Cellular Interactions in the Immune Response*, 2nd Int. Convoc. Immunology, Buffalo, N.Y., S. Karger, New York, 1970, 93.
22. **Cudkowicz, G. and Lotzová, E.,** Hemopoietic cell-defined components of the major histocompatibility complex of mice: identification of responsive and unresponsive recipients for bone marrow transplants, *Transplant. Proc.*, 4, 1399, 1973.
23. **Lotzová, E.,** Involvement of MHC-linked hemopoietic histocompatibility genes in allogeneic bone marrow transplantation in mice, *Tissue Antigens*, 9, 148, 1977.
24. **Lotzová, E.,** Resistance to parental, allogeneic and xenogeneic hemopoietic grafts in irradiated mice, *Exp. Hematol.*, 5, 215, 1977.
25. **Rauchwerger, J. M., Gallagher, M. T., and Trentin, J. J.,** "Xenogeneic resistance" to rat bone marrow transplantation. II. Relationship of hemopoietic regeneration and survival, *Biomedicine*, 18, 109, 1973.
26. **Cudkowicz, G. and Warner, J. F.,** Natural resistance of irradiated 129-strain mice to bone marrow allografts: Genetic control by the H-2K region, *Immunogenetics*, 8, 13, 1979.
27. **Cudkowicz, G. and Rossi, G. B.,** Hybrid resistance to parental DBA/2 grafts: independence from H-2 locus. I. Studies with normal hemopoietic cells, *J. Natl. Cancer Inst.*, 48, 131, 1972.
28. **Lotzová, E.,** Hemopoietic histocompatibility: genetic and immunological aspects, in *Compendium of Immunology*, Vol. 3, 2nd ed., Schwartz, L. M., Ed., Van Nostrand Reinhold, New York, 1983, 468.
29. **Lotzová, E., Gallagher, M. T., and Trentin, J. J.,** Genetic control of resistance to rat bone marrow grafts in mice, *Biomedicine*, 23, 335, 1973.
30. **Lotzová, E., Dicke, K. A., Trentin, J. J., and Gallagher, M. T.,** Genetic control of bone marrow transplantation in irradiated mice: classification of mouse strains according to their responsiveness to bone marrow allografts and xenografts, *Transplant. Proc.*, IX, 289, 1977.
31. **Cudkowicz, G.,** Genetic control of bone marrow graft rejection. I. Determinant specific difference of reactivity in two pairs of inbred mouse strains, *J. Exp. Med.*, 134, 281, 1971.
32. **Rodday, P., Bennett, M., and Williams, M.,** Homozygosity at the major histocompatibility complex is required for optimal immunogenicity of bone marrow cell allografts in irradiated rats, *Tissue Antigens*, 17, 486, 1981.
33. **Rapaport, F. T., Ozaki, A., and Cannon, F. D.,** Parameters of allogeneic unresponsiveness in canine radiation chimeras, with particular reference to the possible existence of three closely linked genetic systems relevant to bone marrow transplantation, *Transplant. Proc.*, V, 845, 1973.
34. **Weiden, P. L., Storb, R., Graham, C. T., Sale, G., and Thomas, E. D.,** Resistance to DLA nonidentical marrow grafts in lethally irradiated dogs, *Exp. Hematol.*, 4 (Suppl.), 27, 1976.
35. **Vriesendorp, H. M., Löwenberg, G., Visser, T. P., Knaan, S., and van Bekkum, D. W.,** Influence of genetic resistance and silica particles on survival after bone marrow transplantation, in *Immunobiology of Bone Marrow Transplantation*, Dupont, B. and Good, R. A., Eds., Grune & Stratton, New York, 1976, 157.
36. **van Bekkum, D. W.,** Current developments in bone-marrow transplantation, *Transplant. Proc.*, VIII, 805, 1975.
37. **Lotzová, E.,** Induction of unresponsiveness to bone marrow grafts, *J. Immunol.*, 119, 543, 1977.
38. **Shearer, G. M., Waksal, H., and Cudkowicz, G.,** An in vitro model of hybrid resistance to bone marrow grafts, in *Immunobiology of Bone Marrow Transplantation*, Dupont, B. and Good, R. A., Eds., Grune & Stratton, New York, 1976, 143.
39. **Shearer, G. M.,** In vitro models of Hh mediated resistance and MHC incompatibility, in *Natural Resistance Systems Against Foreign Cells, Tumors, and Microbes*, Cudkowicz, G., Landy, M., and Shearer, G. M., Eds., Academic Press, New York, 1978, 121.
40. **Herberman, R. B., Nunn, M. E., and Lavrin, D. H.,** Natural cytotoxic reactivity of mouse lymphoid cells against syngeneic and allogeneic tumors. I. Distribution of reactivity and specificity, *Int. J. Cancer*, 16, 216, 1975.
41. **Kiessling, R., Klein, E., and Wigzell, H.,** Natural killer cells in the mouse. I. Cytotoxic cells with specificity for mouse Moloney leukemia cells. Specificity and distribution according to genotype, *Eur. J. Immunol.*, 5, 112, 1975.
42. **Lotzová, E. and McCredie, K. B.,** Natural killer cells in mice and man and their possible biological significance, *Cancer Immunol. Immunother.*, 4, 215, 1978.

43. **Roder, J. C., Kärre, K., and Kiessling, R.,** Natural killer cells, *Prog. Allergy*, 28, 66, 1981.
44. **Lotzová, E.,** Function of natural killer cells in various biological phenomena, *Surv. Synth. Pathol. Res.*, 2, 41, 1983.
45. **Savary, C. A. and Lotzová, E.,** Suppression of natural killer cell cytotoxicity by splenocytes from *Corynebacterium parvum* -injected, bone marrow-tolerant and infant mice, *J. Immunol.*, 120, 239, 1978.
46. **Cudkowicz, G. and Bennett, M.,** Peculiar immunobiology of bone marrow allografts. II. Rejection of parental grafts by resistant F_1 mice, *J. Exp. Med.*, 134, 1513, 1971.
47. **Bennett, M.,** Prevention of marrow allograft rejection with radioactive strontium: evidence for marrow dependent effector cells, *J. Immunol.*, 110, 510, 1973.
48. **Lotzová, E.,** Analogy between rejection of hemopoietic transplants and natural killing, in *Natural Cell-Mediated Immunity Against Tumors*, Herberman, R. B., Ed., Academic Press, New York, 1980, 117.
49. **Lotzová, E. and Savary, C. A.,** Parallelism between the effect of cortisone acetate on hybrid resistance and natural killing, *Exp. Hematol.*, 9, 766, 1981.
50. **Lotzová, E. and Gutterman, J.,** Effect of glucan on natural killer (NK) cells. Further comparison between NK cells and bone marrow effector cell activities, *J. Immunol.*, 123, 607, 1979.
51. **Seaman, W. E., Gindhart, T. D. Greenspan, J. S., Blackman, M. A., and Talal, N.,** Natural killer cells, bone, and the bone marrow: studies in estrogen-treated mice and in congenitally osteopetrotic (mi/mi) mice, *J. Immunol.*, 122, 2541, 1979.
52. **Riccardi, C., Santoni, A., Barlozzari, T., and Herberman, R. B.,** In vivo reactivity of mouse natural killer (NK) cells against normal bone marrow cells, *Cell. Immunol.*, 60, 136, 1981.
53. **Lotzová, E., Pollack, S. B., and Savary, C. A.,** Direct evidence for the involvement of natural killer cells in bone marrow transplantation, in *NK Cells and Other Natural Effector Cells*, Herberman, R. B., Ed., Academic Press, New York, 1982, 1535.
54. **Okumura, K., Habu, S., and Shimamura, K.,** The role of asialo $GM1^+$ ($GA1^+$) cells in the resistance to transplants of bone marrow or other tissues, in *NK Cells and Other Natural Effector Cells*, Herberman, R. B., Ed., Academic Press, New York, 1587, 1982.
55. **Lotzová, E. and Cudkowicz, G.,** Abrogation or resistance to bone marrow grafts by silica particles. Prevention of silica effect by the macrophage stabilizer poly-2-vinylpyridine *N*-oxide, *J. Immunol.*, 113, 198, 1974.
56. **Lotzová, E., Gallagher, M. T., and Trentin, J. J.,** Involvement of macrophages in genetic resistance to bone marrow grafts. Studies with two specific antimacrophage agents, carrageenan and silica, *Biomedicine*, 22, 387, 1974.
57. **Lotzová, E., Gallagher, M. T., and Trentin, J. J.,** Macrophage involvement in genetic resistance to bone marrow transplantation, in *Immunology of Bone Marrow Transplantation*, Dupont, B. and Good, R. A., Eds., Grune & Stratton, New York, 1976, 151.
58. **Warner, J. F. and Dennert, G.,** Bone marrow graft rejection as a function of antibody-directed natural killer cells, *J. Exp. Med.*, in press.
59. **Parkman, R., Rosen, F. S., Rappeport, J., Camitta, B., Levey, R. L., and Nathan, D. G.,** Detection of genetically determined histocompatibility antigen differences between HL-A identical and MLC nonreactive siblings, *Transplantation*, 21, 110, 1976.
60. **Storb, R.,** for the Seattle Marrow Transplant Team, Decrease in the graft rejection rate and improvement in survival after marrow transplantation for severe aplastic anema, *Transplant. Proc.*, 11, 196, 1979.
61. **Elfenbein, G. J., Anderson, P. N., Klein, D. L., Schachter, B. Z., and Santos, G. W.,** Difficulties in predicting bone-marrow graft rejection in patients with aplastic anemia, *Transplant. Proc.*, 10, 441, 1978.
62. **Gluckman, E., Devergie, A., Marty, M., Bussel, A., Rottenbourg, J., Dousset, J., and Bernard, J.,** Allogeneic bone marrow transplantation in aplastic anemia — report of 25 cases, *Transplant. Proc.*, 10, 441, 1978.
63. **Lopez, C., Kirkpatrick, D., Livnat, S., and Storb, R.,** Natural killer cells in bone marrow transplantation, *Lancet*, 8, 1025, 1980.
64. **Dokhelar, M. C., Wiels, J., Lipinski, M., Tetaud, C., Devergie, A., Gluckman, E., and Tursz, T.,** Natural killer cell activity in human bone marrow recipients, *Transplantation*, 31, 61, 1981.
65. **Roy, C., Ghayor, T., Kongshaun, P. A. L., and Lapp, W. S.,** Natural killer activity by spleen, lymph node, and thymus cells during the graft-versus-host reaction, *Transplantation*, 34, 144, 1982.
66. **Zawatsky, R., Lapp, W. S., Shirrmacher, V., and Kirchner, H.,** Interferon production in the murine mixed lymphocyte culture (MLC) and graft-versus-host reaction, *Can. Fed. Biol. Sci.*, 22, 415, 1979.
67. **Okada, M. and Henney, C. S.,** The differentiation of cytotoxic T cells in vitro. II. Amplifying factor(s) produced in primary mixed lymphocyte cultures against K/D stimuli require the presence of Lyt 2^+ cells but not Lyt 1^+ cells, *J. Immunol.*, 125, 300, 1980.
68. **Borland, A., Mowatt, A., and Parrott, D. M. V.,** Augmentation of intestinal and peripheral natural killer cell activity during the graft-versus-host reaction in mice, *Transplantation*, 36, 513, 1983.

69. **Pattengale, P. K., Ramstedt, U., Gidlund, M., Örn, A., Axberg, I., and Wigzell, H.,** Natural killer activity in (C57BL/6 × DBA/2)F_1 hybrids undergoing acute and chronic graft-vs.-host reaction, *Eur. J. Immunol.*, 13, 912, 1983.
70. **Clancy, J., Jr., Mauser, L., and Chapman, A. L.,** Level and temporal pattern of naturally cytolytic cells during acute graft-versus-host disease (GVHD) in the rat, *Cell. Immunol.*, 79, 1, 1983.
71. **Charley, M. R., Mikhael, A., Bennett, M., Gilliam, J. N., and Sontheimer, R. D.,** Prevention of lethal, minor-determinate, graft-*vs*-host disease in mice by the *in vivo* administration of anti-asialo GM, *J. Immunol.*, 131, 2101, 1983.
72. **Nunn, M. E., Herberman, R. B., and Holden, H. T.,** Natural cell-mediated cytotoxicity in mice against nonlymphoid tumor cells and some normal cells, *Int. J. Cancer*, 20, 381, 1977.
73. **Hansson, M., Kiessling, R., Andersson, B., Kärre, K., and Roder, J.,** NK cell-sensitive T-cell subpopulation in thymus: inverse correlation to host NK activity, *Nature (London)*, 278, 174, 1979.
74. **Kiessling, R. and Wigzell, H.,** Surveillance of primitive cells by natural killer cells, in *Natural Resistance to Tumors and Viruses*, Häller, O., Ed., Springer-Verlag, New York, 1981, 107.
75. **O'Brien, T., Kendra, J., Stephens, H., Knight, R., and Barrett, A. J.,** Recognition and regulation of progenitor marrow elements by NK cells in the mouse, *Immunology*, 49, 717, 1983.
76. **Lotzová, E., Savary, C. A., and Stringfellow, D. A.,** 5-Halo-6-phenyl pyrimidinones: new molecules with cancer therapeutic potential and interferon-inducing capacity are strong inducers of murine natural killer cells, *J. Immunol.*, 130, 965, 1983.
77. **Lotzová, E., Savary, C. A., Khan, A., and Stringfellow, D. A.,** Stimulation of natural killer cells in two random-bred strains of athymic rats by interferon-inducing pyrimidinone, *J. Immunol.*, 132, 2566, 1984.
78. **Ohno, A., Amos, D. B., and Koren, H. S.,** Selective cellular natural killing against human leukemic T cells and thymus, *Nature (London)*, 266, 547, 1977.
79. **Yamamoto, K., Blalock, J. E., and Johnson, J. M.,** Human natural killer-like activity against mouse spleen cells, *Eur. J. Immunol.*, 12, 222, 1982.
80. **Morris, T. C., Vincent, P. C., Sutherland, R., and Hersey, P.,** Inhibition of normal human granulopoiesis in vitro by non-T lymphocytes, *Br. J. Haematol.*, 45, 451, 1980.
81. **Ortega, J. A., Ma, A., Shore, N. A., Dukes, P. P., and Merigan, T. C.,** Suppressive effect of interferon on erythroid cell proliferation, *Exp. Hematol.*, 7, 145, 1979.
82. **Nakamura, I., Bordignon, C., and Daley, J. P.,** Role of NK cells in hybrid resistance to bone marrow grafts, in *Mechanism for Cytotoxicity by NK Cells*, Academic Press, in press.
83. **Johnson, J. M., Smith, B., and Baron, S.,** Inhibition of primary in vitro antibody response by interferon preparation, *J. Immunol.*, 114, 403, 1979.
84. **Pollack, S.,** personal communication.
85. **Lotzová, E.,** unpublished observation.

Chapter 7

NATURAL KILLER CELLS ACTIVE AGAINST VIRAL, BACTERIAL, PROTOZOAN, AND FUNGAL INFECTIONS

Patricia A. Fitzgerald and Carlos Lopez

TABLE OF CONTENTS

I. INTRODUCTION

Natural killer (NK) cells were originally described in 1975 as effector cells capable of in vitro lysis of certain tumor targets.[1,2] Uniquely different than elements of adaptive immunity, i.e., T and B cell functions, NK cells were found in nonsensitized hosts and were postulated to have a role as the first line of defense against arising neoplasia. Although most NK cell studies have been carried out using tumor cell lines, it has become clear in the last several years that these effectors can recognize and lyse a wide variety of other target cells. For example, NK cells have been shown to lyse a number of relatively primitive normal cells including thymocytes[3-5] and bone marrow cells[4,6] as well as to inhibit in vitro granulopoiesis.[6] Furthermore, NK cells have been identified as responsible, at least in part, for mediating marrow allograft rejection.[7,8] Of great interest is the growing body of data which indicates that NK cells have an important role in early resistance to a variety of infectious pathogens. The NK activities against virus-infected cells are the best studied of these infectious systems with considerable evidence being developed to suggest that these effector cells contribute to resistance against many viral pathogens in vivo. More recently, data has also been developed to suggest that NK cells are also capable of recognizing and destroying certain bacterial, fungal, and protozoan parasites. Thus, NK cells may play an important protective role against a variety of infectious diseases, perhaps serving to limit the extent of dissemination during the earliest phases of infection before the more specific immune responses become operative.

NK responses to tumor cells and virus-infected targets is often accompanied by the production of interferon (IFN).[9,10] This factor is made in response to virus-infected targets by effector cells similar to, but slightly different than, NK cytolytic effectors.[11-15] Although IFN can augment NK cell activity, this cytokine is not necessary for normal NK lytic function in vitro.[16-19] There is, however, evidence which suggests that IFN may play an important role in vivo by recruiting active NK effector cells to the site of infection or by enhancing preexisting NK activity.[17,20-23]

It is the purpose of this chapter to summarize the data which indicate that NK cells recognize and destroy virus-infected target cells and to present the evidence suggesting that these effector cells play important roles conferring resistance to infectious agents in vivo. Because of the paucity of information on NK activity against bacteria, fungi, and protozoan parasites, this review will emphasize the considerably larger data base which has been developed on the role of NK cells in virus infections. Specifically, the types of virus-infected targets known to be lysed by NK cells, the properties of the NK effector cells, the role of IFN in lysis of infected targets, and the possible nature of the interaction between effectors and targets leading to recognition and lysis of virus-infected cells will be discussed. In addition, studies which provide evidence suggesting that NK cells operate in vivo to confer resistance to certain virus infections will be considered. Finally, we will discuss the evidence indicating that NK cells can also recognize some bacteria, fungi, and protozoan parasites and perhaps play a role in early resistance to these microorganisms.

II. NK CELLS IN VIRAL INFECTIONS

The interaction of an invading virus with the defense systems of the host is complex and elements of both natural resistance and adaptive immunity are required to provide protection from the pathogen. Elements of natural resistance, including NK cells, macrophages, and IFN-α probably act as relatively nonspecific, early defense mechanisms whereas the antigen-specific immune mechanisms, i.e., specific antibody, cytotoxic T cells, and delayed-type hypersensitivity, develop later in the course of infection.

The earliest clues that NK cells (or "nonspecific" cytolytic effectors) might be active against virus-infected targets came from investigations of virus-specific T cell cytotoxicity. Nonspecific lytic activity, peaking before specific cytotoxic T cell activity, was reported in lymphocytic choriomeningitis (LCMV),[24] ectromelia,[25] and Semliki forest[26] virus infections. This nonspecific cytotoxicity was originally attributed to either T cells or macrophages, but in retrospect, was probably the augmented NK cell activity typically found in mice 2 to 4 days after virus infection. In concurrent studies, NK effector cells, first described as troublesome background lysis in studies of "specific" tumor immunity, were being recognized as a distinct class of cytolytic effectors.[1,2] Early in the study of these new effectors, investigators reported that the activity of these cells, given the name NK cells by Kiessling et al.,[12] was greatly augmented by virus infections of mice. Inoculation of mice with any of a wide variety of either DNA or RNA viruses was found to augment in vitro NK activity (reviewed by Welsh[27]).

Evidence that NK cells from uninfected human donors could preferentially lyse virus-infected cells in culture came from studies using infected and uninfected fibroblasts as targets. In 1977 Diamond[28] reported that effector cells from the peripheral blood of nonimmune donors could preferentially lyse cytomegalovirus (CMV)-infected human fibroblasts as compared to uninfected cells. The activity was found to be independent of T cells, specific antibody or macrophages and was found to be low in cord bloods. This study was followed by reports of lysis of herpes simplex virus type 1 (HSV-1), influenza, paramyxo, and measles virus-infected fibroblasts by Santoli et al.[29] and HSV-1 infected fibroblasts by Ching and Lopez.[30] Since these early studies, many reports have been published describing lysis of a variety of virus-infected targets by effector cells from uninfected murine and human donors.

A. Characteristics of NK Cells which Lyse Virus-Infected Targets

NK cells have been shown to be capable of lysing a number of virus-infected target cells in vitro and, in general, virus-infected cells are lysed more efficiently than the uninfected targets. Most of these studies have attributed the lytic activity against virus-infected targets to NK cells using a rather broad set of criteria. These include a lack of the requirement for presensitization of the effector cells and the absence of cell surface markers uniquely expressed on mature T cells, B cells, or macrophages. Using these criteria, nonsensitized NK cells have been found to lyse targets infected with herpes simplex,[10,29-34] cytomegalo,[28,35-39] Epstein-Barr,[40-42] varicella,[43,44] vaccinia,[29,31] vesicular stomatitis,[10,45] Sendai,[10,46,47] measles,[29,45,48] mumps,[29,45,49] Sindbis,[10] influenza,[29] and paramyxo[29] viruses. In recent years, considerable attention has been focused on the cell surface markers of NK cells and on the cell lineage to which they belong. Evidence has been put forth to indicate that NK cells might belong to the macrophage, T cell, or even an independent cell lineage. The issues of NK cell lineage and phenotype are complicated by a number of recent studies which have shown that murine and human NK cells are heterogeneous populations.

1. Heterogeneity of NK Cells

Considerable evidence has been developed demonstrating that murine NK cells are heterogeneous and can be differentiated on the basis of sensitivity to ^{89}Sr, cell surface markers, ontogeny, and sensitivity to lymphokines.[50-53] Studies of cold target inhibition, adsorption to target monolayers, and cell surface markers have suggested that, as in the murine system, human NK cells are also heterogeneous.[54-57]

The cold competition assay has been used to compare the target specificity of virus-infected targets and tumor targets. In this assay, nonradioactive targets are evaluated for their ability to act as cold competitors for lysis of ^{51}Cr-labeled target cells. The results of such studies have varied widely depending both upon the infecting virus and on the target cell which is infected. For example, Blazar et al.[40] studied the effect on NK cell activity of EBV superinfection of Raji and Daudi cells, transformed cell lines which carry the EBV genome. Superinfection or treatment with *n*-butyrate caused the cells to go into cell cycle, express more viral antigen, and become good NK targets. The superinfected targets were good cold competitors for the lysis of Molt-4 tumor cells whereas uninfected Raji and Daudi cells were ineffective. Uninfected Raji were found, however, to partially compete for the lysis of superinfected Raji cells. Similarly, Yasukawa and Zarling[34] found that HSV-1-infected EBV positive lymphoblastoid cell lines and K562 cells are good cold competitors for each other. In contrast to the results of Blazar et al.,[40] Yasukawa and Zarling[34] failed to demonstrate any cold competition between the HSV-infected and -uninfected lymphoblastoid cell lines.

We have compared the lysis of HSV-1-infected and HSV-1-uninfected human fibroblasts (FS) to that of K562 erythroleukemia cells and found that uninfected FS are excellent competitors for the lysis of HSV-infected FS whereas both infected and uninfected FS are relatively poor competitors of K562 lysis.[56] Similarly, K562 cells were poor competitors for the lysis of HSV-infected FS targets but were good autologous cold competitors. We have used these observations as part of the evidence indicating that some of the NK activity against HSV-1-infected fibroblasts is mediated by effector cells different from those lysing K562 targets. Further evidence which supports this contention will be discussed below.

In a murine system, Minato et al.[45] showed that spleen cells were capable of killing tumor targets persistently infected with three different RNA viruses: measles, mumps, or vesicular stomititis virus (VSV). This NK activity correlated with the ability of nude mice to reject the persistently infected, but not the uninfected, parental tumor cell lines. When evaluated by the cold competition assay, lysis of one of the persistently infected targets, e.g., HeLa-measles, could be blocked only by unlabeled HeLA-measles and not by uninfected HeLa or HeLa infected with either of the other two viruses. These results suggest rather specific recognition of the virus-infected cells by the NK effectors. Weston et al.,[54] adding cellular immunoadsorption techniques to the analysis of target selectivity, found that monolayers of persistently infected SV-Hep2 cells were able to adsorb out NK activity against SV-Hep2, Molt-4, K562, and HSB cells. When K562 targets were used as the adsorbant monolayer, there was a partial but incomplete depletion of SV-Hep2 lysis. In parallel experiments, these two targets also acted as partial cold competitors for each other. Of interest was the observation that although uninfected Hep2 were good cold competitors for infected Hep2 targets, they did not act as good absorbants for NK activity.

Taken together, the results of the cold competition studies are somewhat difficult to interpret. Evidence for both limited viral specificity of NK effector cells, as well as for common or shared specificities between virus-infected and tumor targets has been presented. The different results with HSV-1-infected fibroblasts vs. lymphoblastoid cell lines[34,36] suggest that the target cell, as well as the infecting agent, may determine effector cell specificity. Since recent studies have shown that binding and lysis are separable steps in NK cell activity and that binding by itself is not sufficient to induce lysis, cold target inhibition might reflect a block at either of these steps. For example, Newman et al.[58] showed that monoclonal antibody (MoAb) 13.3, which recognizes a T200 determinant on human cells, is able to inhibit lysis of K562 cells without inhibiting binding of this target. Likewise, this antibody is able to inhibit the cold competition of K562 for Jurkat cells without being able to inhibit binding of the cold target. Similarly, target sites utilized by NK(HSV-FS) and NK(K562) may be different since antibody 13.3 blocked the latter but not the former.[164] These results suggest that until we understand more about the relationship between binding and lysis of NK cells, the interpretation of cold competition experiments will remain somewhat ambiguous.

The target cell for virus infection, rather than just the infecting virus itself, might determine which effector cell is responsible for lysing a particular virus-infected target. For example, Yasukawa and Zarling,[34] in their study of NK directed against HSV-1-infected lymphoblastoid cell lines (LCLs), were unable to distinguish between the effectors which lysed HSV-

LCLs and and those which lysed K562 targets. In contrast, our studies have indicated that K562 and HSV-FS targets are lysed by partially nonoverlapping subpopulations.[56] Other studies in our laboratory have also provided preliminary evidence suggesting that the target cell infected with HSV-1 is an important determinant of which effector cell subpopulation lyses that target cell.[165] In these studies, the cell surface phenotype of murine effector cells which lyse YAC-1, HSV-infected and HSV-uninfected PU51R (a monocytic tumor line), infected and uninfected WEH1-164 (a classic natural cytotoxic (NC) target[50]), and infected and uninfected M50L3 (a 3T6-derived fibroblast line) have been compared. The infected PU51R target as well as YAC-1 cells appeared to be killed by "classical" Ly-5$^+$, Qa 5$^+$, NK-1$^+$, NK effector cells whereas HSV-1-infected WEH1-164 cells were lysed exclusively by an NC-like effector lacking these cell surface markers. HSV-infected M50L3 cells were lysed by a combination of the two effector types. Thus, although the HSV infection converts all three of these poorly lysed cells into good NK targets, the virus infection by itself did not confer effector cell specificity.

Recently studies in our laboratory using the single cell assay have indicated that there are more effector cells capable of binding K562 than HSV-FS targets and, among the target binding cells, lytic conjugates are more frequently observed among the K562 than the HSV-FS target binding cells.[166] Similarly, the effectors for NK(K562) were found to have a higher V_{max} than those for NK(HSV-FS) when analyzed according to the kinetic method of Ullberg and Jondal.[21,166] These observations have been used to further distinguish the effectors which lyse these two target cells.

MoAb studies also support the concept of heterogeneity of NK effector cells. Studies from our laboratory have compared the effectors which lyse HSV-FS vs. those lysing K562 targets and found that they were phenotypically different.[56] Approximately half of the NK(HSV-FS) activity was depleted by treatment with anti-Ia plus complement while NK(K562) effectors were insensitive to similar treatment. In contrast, NK(K562) activity was markedly reduced by treatment with OKT11A or anti-Lyt-3 (E-rosette receptor) plus complement while NK(HSV-Fs) activity was relatively insensitive to this treatment. Although these data indicate that the two subpopulations can be distinguished by these antisera, studies with other MoAbs indicate that they also share other cell surface markers: both NK(HSV-Fs) and NK(K562) express Leu-11 which reacts with Fc receptors (FcR) on NK cells, as well as OKM1, and Leu-7 (HNK-1).

Patient studies have provided some of the strongest evidence that, not only are NK cells heterogeneous with respect to NK(HSV-FS) and NK(K562) activity, but also that these activities are under independent regulation in vivo. Certain individuals were found to have consistently low levels of NK(K562) activity while having normal NK(HSV-FS) activity whereas other individuals were found to have normal levels of NK(K562) but low levels of NK(HSV-FS) activity.[56] Since deficiencies of each of these activities have been found to be independent of the other, a trivial reason for selective lysis is much less likely. In sum, these data demonstrate heterogeneity of NK cells in man and suggest that these populations can be, and are in some cases, regulated independently of each other in vivo.

2. NK Cells Activated by In Vivo Virus Infection

As has been previously discussed,[27] experimental infection of animals with a wide variety of viruses is known to lead to activation of NK cells. This enhanced activity of NK cells is probably due to activation and/or recruitment of NK cells by IFN, although viral glycoproteins may also be involved in a direct, IFN-independent activation of these effectors.[18] The infection-activated NK cells not only show augmented lysis of classic NK targets, but are also able to lyse a variety of targets not usually lysed by resident NK effectors.[59]

Recent studies from Welsh's laboratory[60] have shown that in vivo infection of mice with LCMV caused blastogenesis of NK effectors, i.e., NK cells from infected mice incorporated

^{3}H-thymidine, and were larger than unstimulated spleen cells. These effector cells were fully capable of binding and lysing NK targets. Blastogenesis of NK cells presumably occurs through an IFN-dependent mechanism since IFN administration by itself has been subsequently shown to induce the same phenomenon.[61] Studies by Minato et al.[17,53] showed that IFN is able to activate a pre-NK subpopulation, phenotypically distinct from mature NK cells to become mature NK effectors. Thus, virus infection of the host has positive self-regulatory effects on NK cell activity in several different ways. First, virus-infected cells become directly susceptible to NK cell lysis in an IFN-independent manner; second, induction of IFN by the virus infection may act to recruit and stimulate the differentiation of NK precursors, and increase the lytic efficiency and recycling ability of preexisting NK effectors.

3. Role of IFN in Lysis of Virus-Infected Targets

We and others have shown that normal cells infected with certain viruses are better targets for human and murine NK cells than are uninfected cells. One possible explanation for the preferential lysis of the virus-infected cells was that effector cells generate IFN in response to the virus-infected target and that this IFN would lead to nonspecifically augmented kill against the infected targets.[9-11,27,59,62] Although such positive self-regulation of NK cell activity by IFN does undoubtedly occur, several studies have clearly shown that the preferential lysis of HSV-infected human cells and persistently infected targets is not dependent on the IFN generated during the NK assay.

Working with human effector cells, Trinchieri et al.[9,63] and Santoli et al.[11] noted that many NK targets were able to induce IFN production during routine NK assays. The IFN was produced by cells sharing many properties with NK cells themselves. These authors suggested that the induction of IFN during the NK cell assays led to the nonspecific augmentation of NK cell activity, i.e., that NK cell preference for lysing infected targets could be explained by the nonspecific augmentation of the NK cell activity by the IFN produced during the course of the assay. These conclusions were based on a number of observations. First, these investigators observed no preferential lysis of virus-infected over uninfected targets in the first hours of the NK assay and found that virus-infected cells were preferentialy lysed only after IFN became detectable in the supernatants. Second, when effector cells were pretreated with IFN, both infected and uninfected cells were lysed equally well. Third, when effector cells were incubated overnight at 37°C, there was a concomitant loss of the ability to lyse virus-infected target cells and to produce IFN. In contrast to these studies, Minato et al.,[17] using murine effector cells and persistently infected xenogeneic targets, demonstrated that the preferential lysis of virus-infected over uninfected cells was not diminished by the addition of anti-IFN antibodies during the first 9 to 12 hr of culture. Addition of anti-IFN antibodies did reduce, somewhat, the levels of NK cell activity observed at 18 to 24 hr of culture. Thus, although augmentation of NK by IFN generated during the assay could eventually account for a portion of the increased lysis of the infected targets, it was not solely responsible. Similarly, in a nonviral system, lysis of K562 cells was also shown to be independent of the IFN generated in vitro.[19]

We have studied the IFN produced by human cells during NK cell assays using HSV-1 infected fibroblasts (NK[HSV-FS]) as targets to determine what role this IFN has in the preferential lysis of virus-infected targets.[16] Several of our findings demonstrate that IFN production during this NK assay cannot account for the preferential lysis of the virus-infected cells. IFN was produced during 14-hr NK(HSV-Fs) assays by effector cells from both HSV-1 seropositive and seronegative individuals and was found to have the properties of IFN-α. The IFN could be induced by either fibroblasts infected with live HSV-1 or by band-purified, UV-inactivated virus antigen. No correlation was found between the levels of cytotoxicity developed against the virus-infected targets and the amount of IFN generated during the NK(HSV-FS) assay. If NK(HSV-FS) were dependent on the generation of IFN, one would expect similar levels of lysis of infected and uninfected target cells when effector cells were optimally pretreated with IFN in vitro. Instead, however, we found that after pretreatment of effector cells of 17 control individuals with IFN-α, there remained a preferential lysis of the virus-infected targets.[16] These results have recently been confirmed by Bishop et al.,[64] also using HSV-1-infected targets. The suggestion that the preferential lysis of the virus-infected cells is independent of IFN production is further supported by experiments in which we added anti-IFN-α antibody to the NK cell assays.[16] If IFN produced during the assay were responsible for the increased kill of infected over uninfected targets, then one would expect that the presence of anti-IFN should lower NK(HSV-Fs) activity to the level of lysis found with uninfected targets. In fact, although all the IFN produced during the assay was neutralized by the anti-IFN, cytotoxicity against the virus-infected targets was not reduced. Similar results have recently been obtained by Bishop et al.,[64] who also reported that inhibition of IFN-α production by actinomycin-D failed to eliminate the preferential lysis of HSV-1-infected targets. Our patient studies have also demonstrated that NK(HSV-FS) activity and IFN production can be regulated independently of each other in vivo. We found many patients with acquired immunodeficiency syndrome (AIDS) with opportunistic infections who had normal levels of NK(HSV-FS) activity despite their inability to produce IFN during the cytotoxicity assay.[65] In addition, we have studied other patients with Wiscott-Aldrich syndrome who had abnormally low levels of NK(HSV-FS) activity but who had normal in vitro capacity to generate IFN.[167]

Taken together, these results indicate that IFN generated during NK assays is not required for lysis of virus-infected targets. However, it is likely that IFN, made in response to a virus infection in vivo, would lead to the recruitment and activation of NK cells. Such a positive self-regulation would allow for increased NK activity at the place and time of greatest need.

4. Mechanisms which Might Account for Selective Lysis of Virus-Infected Targets

Since IFN generation cannot account for the selective lysis of virus-infected over uninfected targets, other mechanisms must be considered. One possible explanation for the increased susceptibility of virus-infected targets to NK cell lysis is that the virus, by destabilizing the host cell membrane and impairing the ability of the cell to repair itself, is leaving the infected target inherently more susceptible to lysis than the intact uninfected target. With respect to HSV-1-infected fibroblasts, our studies indicate that this does not appear to be the case. In 14-hr NK assays, the HSV-infected fibroblasts do not spontaneously release more ^{51}Cr than the uninfected fibroblasts,[168] suggesting that the infected targets are not inherently more "leaky" than their uninfected counterparts. Brooks et al.[66] have suggested that relative susceptibility of rat tumor cells to NK cell lysis can be correlated with the relative resistance of the cell lines to osmotic disruption. We have subjected ^{51}Cr-labeled HSV-FS and uninfected FS cells to hypotonic conditions ranging from 0 to 67% distilled water for 14 hr and have observed no differences between the osmotic stability of the two cells,[168] again suggesting that infected targets are not inherently less stable. A third observation arguing against inherent instability of the HSV-infected targets was that infected and uninfected FS were equally susceptible to lysis by cytotoxic T cells directed against major histocompatibility determinants.[169]

Other possible explanations to account for the preferential lysis of virus-infected targets are that: (1) specific virus components are being recognized by the effector cells or (2) the virus infection leads to alterations or rearrangements of the normal cell membrane components, causing the cell to be recognized as "foreign" by the NK effector. These two hypotheses are not necessarily mutually exclusive and, in addition, different mechanisms may be found to be operative in lysis of different virus-infected targets. Strong evidence has been put forward which clearly indicates that binding and lysis of NK targets occurs through a multistep process, and that binding of the effector cell to the target is not sufficient to lead to lysis. With some infected targets, such as HSV-1-infected fibroblasts, there is good cross-competition between the infected and uninfected targets[56] and both the infected and uninfected targets are bound in the single cell assay whereas only the virus-infected target is efficiently lysed.[166] In contrast, uninfected LCLs were poor competitors of lysis of HSV-infected LCLs and, unlike infected LCLs, failed to bind NK effectors.[34,170] Thus, for these two HSV-infected targets, somewhat different initial recognition mechanisms may be operative and, in fact, the targets may be recognized by distinct effector cell subpopulations (see Section II.A.1). Direct comparisons of these two effector/target cell systems will be required in order to more fully understand these differences.

Evidence for a role of HSV-1 specific glycoproteins in conferring susceptibility of the infected target to lysis comes from the recent studies of Bishop et al.[64,67,68] These investigators found that target cells infected with HSV mutants which poorly expressed gB and gC, viral glycoproteins usually expressed on the infected cell surface, were lysed to a somewhat lesser extent than cells infected with wild-type virus. In addition, these authors claimed that F(ab)2 fragments of antibody against either gB or gC could partially block NK lysis of the targets whereas complete antibody, as would be expected, boosted lysis through an antibody-dependent mechanism. These results suggest that viral glycoproteins may be important recognition or trigger sites for NK effector cells. A similar role for VSV proteins has been indicated by the studies of Rager-Zisman et al.[69] These investigators studied the lysis of B16 tumor cells infected with temperature-sensitive mutants of VSV: one mutant being defective in the production of viral glycoprotein and the other in the matrix protein, a viral product found inside the infected cell. Neither mutant-infected cell was killed at the non-permissive temperature but both were lysed at the permissive temperature whereas a poly-merase mutant-infected cell was killed at both temperatures. Since defects in either the glycoprotein or the matrix protein are sufficient for failure of these targets to be lysed, there are two possible explanations for these results: first, the properly inserted G and M proteins may lead to alterations in the normal cellular components allowing the effector cell to recognize the infected cell as foreign, or second, properly configured G and M are required for the recognition of the viral glycoprotein by the effector cell.

As is clear from the preceding discussion, the mechanism of recognition and lysis of virus-infected targets is still very poorly understood. Confusing this issue are the problems of NK cell heterogeneity as well as differences inherent to the various viruses and even to the target cells used. A number of recent technological advances should help provide the tools necessary to define the determinants involved. For example, the availability of cloned viral DNA segments (coding for a specific glycoprotein) which can be inserted and expressed in normal cells, might more clearly define the role of that specific viral product. This is especially important with large, complex viruses such as herpesviruses, which induce many changes in infected cells and cause the expression of a large number of antigens on the surface of the infected cells. This approach also circumvents the use of viral mutants which are often "leaky" and may fail to give clear-cut answers to these questions. Studies with cloned NK effectors should also diminish the complexity of the study of virus-effector interactions by eliminating the contribution of NK cell heterogeneity to the confusion. Finally, the increasing availability of MoAbs directed against specific viral products should provide valuable probes for the roles of viral products in binding and lysis of infected targets.

B. IFN and NK Cells

1. Augmentation of NK by IFN

An interest in the role of IFN in the augmentation of NK cell activity was prompted by the observation that NK cell activity was greatly augmented during virus infections in mice.[70-72] This NK-augmenting effect of virus infections has now been found in rat, mouse, and hamster systems with a variety of RNA and DNA viruses (for a listing of these studies, see the excellent review by Welsh[27]). Increased NK activity following virus infection was similar to that found following administration of IFN or IFN inducers in vivo.[73] Since virus infection was known to induce IFN, it seemed likely that the boosting of NK was probably due to the induction of IFN by the virus infection.[74] Confirming evidence for this hypothesis came from a study by Gidlund et al.,[73] who found that treatment of mice with anti-IFN antibodies prior to challenge with Newcastle disease virus abrogated the augmentation of NK activity.

Welsh et al.[59,75] studied the target cell specificity of NK cells from mice infected with LCMV and found that a variety of continuous and early passage cell lines, many of which are not normally lysed by effector cells from uninfected mice, were lysed by cells taken 3 days after infection. LCMV-infected and uninfected L cell targets were lysed equally well by the activated NK cells whereas effector cells from uninfected animals failed to lyse either the infected or uninfected cells.

IFN induced in vivo by virus infections probably leads to the recruitment and activation of NK cells and is therefore an important component of the response to a virus infection. Such a positive self-regulation would allow for increased NK cell activity at the time of greatest need. For example, a positive interaction of NK cells and IFN was noted in the murine cytomegalovirus (MCMV) studies of Grundy et al.[76] These authors found that the ability of mice to mount an early IFN response to MCMV correlated with genetic resistance to this viral pathogen. IFN by itself, however, did not appear to mediate resistance since bg/bg mice were less resistant to MCMV infection than their heterozygous littermates despite high levels of early IFN production. It therefore appears that the early IFN induction leading to NK cell augmentation was critical for conferring resistance to this virus.

2. Protection of Uninfected Cells by IFN

IFN has also been shown to protect uninfected but not virus-infected targets from NK-mediated lysis. Preincubation of target cells with IFN resulted in lower cytolysis of uninfected targets but had no effect on lysis of virus-infected cells.[77-80] These observations have led to the theory that induction of IFN in vivo by a virus infection has two antagonistic effects on target cell lysis by NK cells, i.e., IFN could augment NK lysis of virus-infected cells while serving to protect normal cells from the deleterious effects of the NK cell lysis. A possible mechanism for the protective effect of IFN has recently been suggested by the studies of Wright et al.[81] These investigators have shown that IFN pretreatment of YAC-1 cells render them poor inducers of NK cytotoxic factors (NKCF). It is possible, therefore, that IFN pretreatment of uninfected cells renders them unable to induce or be insensitive to the activity of NKCF while infected targets induce this factor and remain sensitive to its toxic action.

3. Properties of the IFN-Generating Cells

A number of investigators have studied the effector cells which produce IFN-α subsequent to incubation with tumor cells or virus-infected targets. Large granular lyphocytes (LGLs) have been identified as the cells which produce most of the IFN-α in response to tumor targets and to infectious HSV-1 virus or HSV-1-infected fibroblasts,[12-15] although B cells[82] and macrophages[83] have also been implicated as producers of IFN-α. Results from a study by Peter et al.[84] have indicated that IFN-α can be produced by a human "null" cell distinct from most NK cells in that it is an FcR negative cell.

We have studied the cells which produce IFN-α during NK(HSV-FS) assays and have found them to be similar to, but distinct from, NK effectors. Like NK cells, the IFN-α-producing cells were found in Percoll gradient fractions enriched for LGLs, but were slightly less dense than the majority of NK effector cells.[15,171] The IFN-α-producing cells can be further distinguished from NK effector cells on the basis of cell surface phenotype as well as by "experiments of nature". The cells which make IFN-α were found to lack Lyt-3,

OKM1, Leu-7, and Leu-11, markers found on all or most cytolytic NK cells. Conversely, the IFN-α-generating cells express Ia on their cell surface, a marker also expressed on some NK(HSV-FS) but not on a significant proportion of NK(K562) effectors.[85,86] Furthermore, patient studies indicate that NK and IFN-α generation are independently regulated functions. We have found patients with normal NK(HSV-FS) lytic activity but with marked deficiency of IFN-α-generating capacity and vice versa. For example, many patients with AIDS were found to have normal levels of NK(HSV-FS) activity but failed to generate IFN-α during the same assay.[65] In contrast, a number of individuals with other immunodeficiencies have been found to have normal IFN-α production but low NK activity.[167,172] These studies indicate that the IFN-α-generating cells are probably a subpopulation of LGLs which are different than NK lytic effectors and are under independent regulation.

C. Role of NK in Host Defense Against Virus Infections

1. Role of NK in Resistance to Murine Virus Infections

A number of investigations have provided indirect evidence that murine NK cells are required for conferring resistance to certain viral infections.

a. HSV-1 Infection

Much of the data suggesting a possible role for NK effector cells in resistance to herpesvirus infection has come from the study of a mouse model of genetic resistance to HSV-1.[87] Inbred strains of mice were evaluated for resistance or susceptibility to i.p. infection with HSV-1. Resistant C57BL/6 mice were found to survive 10^6 plaque-forming units (PFUs) of HSV-1 while susceptible A/J strain mice died after challenge with as little as 10^2 PFUs. Studies of backcross mice indicated that two independently segregating genes were involved in determining resistance and that neither was linked to H-2 genes.[88] Several observations indicated that resistance was a function of the hematopoietic defense system of the host. C57BL/6 mice were found to be highly resistant to 10^6 PFUs of HSV-1 given i.p. but were susceptible to as little as 10^1 PFUs of the virus inoculated into the brain, indicating that resistance in these mice depended upon their ability to inhibit virus from reaching the central nervous system (CNS), which is the target organ for this virus. Fibroblasts from resistant and susceptible strains were found to replicate HSV-1 equally well, arguing against an inherent resistance of all cells of resistant mice to virus replication.[87] Transplantation of bone marrow stem cells from resistant mice into lethally irradiated susceptible mice resulted in chimeras with greatly enhanced resistance,[89] demonstrating that the cells responsible for resistance are derived from bone marrow stem cells. Marrow dependence of resistance, i.e., the requirement of an intact bone marrow, was evaluated by challenge of ^{89}Sr-treated C57BL/6 mice with HSV-1. In addition to losing their ability to reject bone marrow grafts and mediate in vitro NK activity against YAC-1 targets, ^{89}Sr mice were found to have lost their resistance to HSV-1.[90-92] The lack of NK cells, which have been shown to mediate resistance to bone marrow cell grafts,[7,8,92] was postulated to also be responsible for the inability of these mice to resist HSV-1 infection. In other studies, mice treated with estradiol or mice carrying the bg/bg phenotype (both of which are associated with low NK cell activity[93,94]), were found to be slightly more susceptible to HSV-1 infection than were their normal littermates, again suggesting a role for NK cells in resistance.[173] In contrast, a deficiency of T cell function and cell-mediated immunity was not associated with increased susceptibility to i.p. challenge with HSV-1.[89,95,96] Because of these observations, we have studied NK activity of resistant and susceptible strains of mice.[172] Genetically resistant mice were found to have good NK responses whereas most susceptible strains lacked significant lysis of HSV-1 infected cells. Of interest was the observation that, although CBA mice had high NK activity, they were moderately susceptible to HSV-1 infection. Since CBA mice lack only one of the two resistance genes, NK may be necessary but not sufficient for resistance and some other function must also be operative.

Studies by Kohl et al.[97-99] have also suggested a role for NK cells and ADCC in conferring resistance to HSV-1 infection in mice. These investigators were able to transfer resistance to susceptible newborn mice by transfer of peripheral blood mononuclear cells from adult but not newborn humans. Even greater protection was conferred by including HSV-specific human antibody with the mononuclear cells but antibody by itself was not protective suggesting that an ADCC mechanism was also operative.

The studies of Kirchner and colleagues[100-105] have led to the suggestion that the early production of IFN by resistant but not susceptible mice rather than NK is necessary for resistance to HSV-1 infection in mice. These investigators cite SJL mice as relatively resistant mice which have low NK activity but relatively high production of early IFN, results which they conclude indicate that early IFN might be more important than NK in conferring resistance to HSV-1. Strong evidence that IFN plays a role in resistance to HSV-1 derives from the studies of Gresser et al.,[106] which have been confirmed in our laboratory:[165] resistance to HSV-1 was dramatically lowered in mice which had been treated with heterologous anti-mouse IFN.

The data generated by Kirchner's group appears to contradict our results supporting a role for NK cell function in resistance to HSV-1. In fact, both groups are probably right and a combination of the early production of IFN and NK cell response are required for maximum resistance to HSV-1 in the mouse. Therefore, reduction of either function could result in decreased resistance and the appearance that it alone is responsible for genetic resistance. In sum, NK cell function and its amplification by IFN probably constitute an important aspect of genetic resistance to HSV-1.

b. Cytomegalovirus Infection

A role for NK cells in early resistance to MCMV infection has been suggested by a number of studies. Bancroft et al.[107] found that NK responses were augmented in mice as early as 10 hr after infection with murine CMV (MCMV). A correlation between degree of augmentation of NK and resistance of the mouse strain to MCMV infection was observed in 10 of 11 mouse strains tested. Bg/bg mice, which were susceptible to infection,[108] showed low levels of NK augmentation. In a later study by this group,[76] they suggested that the early production of IFN in resistant but not susceptible mice led to the augmentation of NK in these mice. That both IFN induction and NK response to the IFN were important in resistance was indicated by the finding that bg/bg mice showed a poor NK boost but high levels of early IFN production even though they were highly susceptible to MCMV infection in terms of greater susceptibility to lethal infection and in allowing greater replication of MCMV in their organs. Thus, the protective mechanism of the early IFN is probably not a direct antiviral effect but rather is medicated through its ability to boost NK activity.

Other studies suggesting a role for NK cells in resistance to MCMV include a study by Quinnan et al.,[109] who demonstrated that hydrocortisone administration to MCMV-infected C3H/HeN mice did not affect late serum IFN production, T cell function, or antibody production, but did lower the boost of NK activity which is typically found 3 to 6 days postinfection. The hydrocortisone-treated mice demonstrated increased susceptibility to lethal infection as well as increased spleen and pulmonary virus replication. Bukowski et al.[110] have recently provided additional evidence suggesting a role for NK cells in limiting MCMV infection using antiasialo-GM1, an agent more NK specific than hydrocortisone. Mice were treated with the antisera 4 to 6 hr before challenge with MCMV and virus titers were measured in organs 3 days later. Mice treated with antiasialo-GM1 had higher titers of MCMV in their livers and spleens than their untreated controls and also showed higher levels of serum IFN and more extensive hepatitis. These authors did not measure the effect of antiasialo-GM1 on *early* IFN production.

Somewhat contradictory evidence regarding the role of NK cells in MCMV infection comes from a study by Masuda and Bennett.[111] These authors found that, as in the case of HSV-1 infection, treatment of C3H mice with ^{89}Sr lowered resistance to MCMV infection. These mice, however, developed very high levels of NK(YAC) activity 3 to 4 days after infection with MCMV. Thus, it appears that NK by itself, or at least the NK measured in this study, is not sufficient to explain resistance of C3H mice to MCMV.

c. Other Viral Infections

Minato and colleagues[45] have examined the effect of persistent viral infection upon resistance of nude mice to tumor cell inocula. Both HeLa and BHK21 cells, which are highly tumorigenic in nude mice, were found to be nontumorigenic when persistently infected with measles, mumps, influenza, VSV, or rabies viruses. These persistently infected targets, but not their uninfected parent lines, were found to be good in vitro NK targets for spleen cells from nude mice. The cells responsible for lysis were found to have the properties of NK cells and their activity was augmented in the spleens of mice inoculated with the persistently infected tumor cells. These studies support the hypothesis that NK cells may play a role in resistance to persistent viral infection.

Several groups have considered the role of NK cells in resistance to different strains of murine hepatitis virus (MHV). Tardieu et al.,[112] studying MHV3 infections, found that they could confer resistance to susceptible newborn mice by the transfer of a combination of adherent spleen cells, T cells, and "M" or marrow cells, similar in their properties to NK cells. Spleen cells from ^{89}Sr-treated A/J mice lacked the "M" or NK cells necessary for transfer of resistance. In other studies, Bukowski et al.[110] found that depleting asialo-GM1 positive cells in vivo resulted in depletion of NK cell activity and higher levels of MHV replication in livers and spleens of treated mice as compared to mice with intact NK systems. These higher levels of virus replication and more extensive hepatitis existed despite the finding of more IFN in the serum of antiasialo-GM1-treated mice than in nontreated mice at 3 days postinoculation. Similarly increased titers of virus were found in organs of antiasialo-GM1-treated mice inoculated with MCMV and vaccinia virus while depletion of NK cells in this manner had no effect on LCMV infection (to be discussed below).

Kirchner's group came to different conclusions regarding the role of NK cells in MHV3 infections in mice.[113] These authors found that NK activity and IFN production were high in the peritoneum of susceptible C57BL/6 mice 20 to 50 hr after infection and that high peritoneal virus titers could be detected at 48 hr. In contrast, resistant A/J mice had lower levels of NK and IFN and also lower viral titers than the susceptible mice at 48 hr postinoculation. Thus, there appeared to be an inverse relationship between NK and resistance to replication of virus in the period immediately after infection. It is of interest that these authors did not observe an early peak of IFN production in the peritoneum of the MHV3-infected mice since such IFN is what this group has correlated with resistance to HSV-1 infection in mice.

d. Viral Infections in which NK does not Appear to Contribute to Resistance

Some of the earliest studies showing that in vivo viral infection could boost NK were carried out by Welsh et al.[59,74,75,114,115] with LCMV. Following acute infection of mice with LCMV, an antibody response was detected as early as 4 days postinfection (PI) and specific cytotoxic T cells were found at 5 to 6 days PI. From 1 to 4 days following infection with LCMV, mice were found to develop augmented levels of NK activity capable of lysing classical NK targets such as YAC-1 as well as certain primary cells and nearly all tested continuous cell lines that were normally resistant to lysis by endogenous NK cells. In addition, these investigators found equivalent lysis of both LCMV-infected and uninfected L cells.[10] The enhanced NK activity was found to correlate with the LCMV-induced IFN levels. Although NK activity is augmented in mice inoculated with LCMV, Welsh and colleagues[114] have found no evidence to support a role for these effectors in protection of mice against acute LCMV infection. For example, bg/bg mice infected with LCMV were found to replicate similar levels of virus in their organs and had similar levels of IFN as their heterozygous littermates despite the poor augmentation of NK found in these mice. Further evidence against a role for NK cells in LCMV infection derives from the study by Bukowski et al.[110] which showed that treatment with antiasialo-GM1 failed to increase the viral titers of LCMV in spleens and livers of mice while, as noted above, replication of MCMV, MHV, and vaccinia viruses were found to be augmented in mice so depleted of NK cells.

In a study of resistance to Sindbis virus infection, Hirsch et al.[117] could not demonstrate any protective effect of NK cells despite strong augmentation of NK activity by Sindbis virus infection. Studies by Gee et al.[118] showed that Pichinde virus infection was associated with increased numbers of cytolytic NK cells but also, more of these cells were apparently infected with this virus in susceptible than in resistant hamsters. Thus, although NK cells can be augmented by a wide variety of viruses, such NK activity is not always important in conferring resistance to the viral infection.

In many virus infections, the immune response of the host to a virus can cause as much or more damage than the virus itself.[119] One consideration, not often discussed, is the possibility that NK cell cytotoxicity might contribute to this immunopathology. It is of some interest that NK cell function is greatly enhanced in LCMV infections of the mouse since this is an excellent model system for demonstrating the immunopathology associated with virus infections.

2. In Vitro Suppression of HSV-1 Replication by NK Cells

In order for NK cells to be a viable defense against herpesvirus infections in vivo, the NK cell must not only be able to lyse virus-infected targets but must do so before the infected cell produces infectious viral progeny. To determine whether NK cells limit HSV-1 replication during the in vitro assay, we have measured HSV-1 titers in supernatants of cultures of effector cells and HSV-1-infected targets at the termination of NK assays and compared these to HSV-1 produced by infected fibroblasts in the absence of effector cells.[174] Human mononuclear cells from HSV-1 seropositive and seronegative individuals inhibited virus replication in a dose-dependent manner with the greatest inhibition being observed with the highest concentration of effectors tested, effector to target cell ratio of 800:1. To determine which population of effector cells was responsible for the reduction of virus titer, effector cells were fractionated on Percoll density gradients. Virus titers were significantly lower when fractions enriched for NK cells were used as compared to the other fractions. Since IFN-α is produced during NK(HSV-FS) assays,[16] it was important to determine whether the newly generated IFN was responsible for the reduction of HSV-1 production by the effector cells. To evaluate this, antibodies to IFN-α were added to the effector cells prior to and throughout culture with the infected targets. Although all of the IFN was neutralized, there was no difference in virus production in groups containing the anti-IFN or control antibodies. Further, the majority of the IFN-producing cells can be separated from peak NK activity on Percoll gradients and reduction of virus titer was associated with cytotoxic NK cell activity rather than IFN production. Thus, the NK cytolytic effectors themselves appear to directly inhibit virus replication, most likely by lysing the infected target cells prior to the production of infectious viral progeny. Phenotypically, the effector cells responsible for the inhibition of viral replication were confirmed to be NK cells: they lacked Leu-4, a pan-T cell antigen and were positive for the NK-specific antigen Leu-11b. These in vitro results complement our observations of low NK(HSV-FS) activity in patients susceptible to severe herpesvirus infections[118] and suggest that NK cells may significantly reduce the virus load with which the infected host must deal.

3. Role of NK Cells in Resistance to Human Virus Infections

In order to determine whether NK effectors might play a role in resistance to virus infections in man, we have studied NK responses in groups of patients known to be highly susceptible to severe herpesvirus infections.[120] Cells from cord bloods and newborns were studied because of the newborn's known susceptibility to disseminated herpesvirus infections, primarily HSV-2. When effector cells were evaluated against HSV-1-infected fibroblasts, only 30% had responses within two standard deviations of the normal, adult mean. Peripheral blood cells from nine premature infants were also tested and they all had responses greater than 3 SD below the normal mean.[120,169] Kohl et al.[33] have also found cord bloods to be deficient in their lysis of HSV-1-infected targets. In addition, we have studied NK cell activity in patients with Wiscott-Aldrich syndrome (WAS), an X-linked, primary immunodeficiency disorder characterized by exzema, thrombocytopenia, and recurrent infections.[120] Only one of eight individuals studied had normal NK(HSV-FS) activity and in each case low NK(HSV-FS) correlated with a history of persistent or recurrent virus infections. Of interest was the observation that when NK activity of two of these patients was evaluated with both K562 and HSV-FS targets, they had very low NK(HSV-Fs) but normal NK(K562) activity. This finding of normal K562 activity is consistent with the observations of Lipinski et al.[121] and suggests that the heterogeneity of NK cells may reflect different biological roles for the subpopulations of effectors. Newborns and patients with WAS have been shown to have deficiencies of other aspects of their defense systems which might also contribute to their susceptibility to infection.[122,123] We have, therefore, evaluated NK responses in a number of individuals with no known underlying primary cellular immunodeficiency but who were suffering from unusually severe virus infections at the time of study.[120] The mean response of this group of individuals was below the normal range (which was within two standard deviations of the normal mean) for NK(HSV-FS) responses. Two of these individuals were also evaluated between bouts of infection and each demonstrated equally depressed responses, suggesting that low NK(HSV-FS) activity might predispose such patients to unusually severe disease caused by herpesviruses. In contrast, individuals with normal, self-limiting viral infections were not found to have abnormal NK(HSV-FS) responses. Several of the individuals with severe herpesvirus infections who had low NK(HSV-FS) responses were simultaneously evaluated for NK(K562) activity. Although many individuals had low NK against both targets, three had normal levels of NK(K562) activity. As discussed in Section II.A.1, we have demonstrated that the effector cells for NK(HSV-FS) and NK(K562) can be phenotypically separated and are regulated independently of one another in vivo. The studies of patients with WAS and patients with unusually severe herpesvirus infections suggest that the activity against the HSV-1-infected targets may be more relevant to evaluating susceptibility to virus infections than NK(K562) activity.

Other investigators have observed correlations between low NK activity and susceptibility to virus infections as well as other diseases.[38,124-130] Sullivan et al.[124] demonstrated low NK(K562) activity in patients with X-linked lymphoproliferative syndrome, a disorder associated with susceptibility to Epstein-Barr virus infections. More recent studies, however, suggest that deficient NK(K562) in these patients is a response to infection rather than predisposing patients to it.[125] In other studies, Virelizier and colleagues[126-128] have demonstrated low NK(K562) activity in a group of patients unusually susceptible to a variety of infectious agents. Quinnan et al.[38] have found that bone marrow transplant recipients suffering from severe cytomegalovirus (CMV) infections have abnormally low levels of NK activity against CMV-uninfected fibroblasts, a finding which is in agreement with our findings of low NK(HSV-FS) activity in similar patients.[129] NK has also been studied in patients with chronic diseases of putative viral origin.[131-137] Neighbour et al.[137] found that 30% of individuals with multiple sclerosis (MS) and 40% of individuals with systemic lupus erythematosus (SLE) had NK(K562) activity greater than two standard deviations below the normal mean. Hauser et al.[30] found low NK against measles virus-infected HeLa cells but not against K562 targets in MS patients. Studies from several laboratories suggest that the defect in NK in MS patients may be related to deficiencies in numbers of NK cells as well as deficiencies in the production of and response to IFN.[132-136]

We have studied NK activity against HSV-1-infected fibroblasts and K562 targets as well as production of IFN in response to the HSV-FS targets in patients with AIDS. In our initial study of five AIDS patients with ulcerative herpesvirus infections, all of the individuals were found to have very low levels of NK activity.[138] In subsequent studies of over 200 individuals with either Kaposi's sarcoma, opportunistic infections with and without Kaposi's sarcoma, lymphadenopathy, "AIDS-related complex", generalized lymphadenopathy, and homosexual controls, we have failed to demonstrate a clear-cut relationship between low NK activity against either K562 or HSV-Fs targets and susceptibility to AIDS.[65,172] Although many AIDS patients with KS and/or opportunistic infections had low NK activity against one or the other targets and *mean* NK responses of these groups of individuals were below the mean responses of normal controls, many individuals were found to have NK responses well within the normal range. Further, individual NK values could not be used to distinguish those susceptible to infection or malignancy. When AIDS patients were studied serially, NK responses tended to deteriorate with progression of the disease, therefore suggesting that the diminished NK activity may be a response to, as opposed to a cause of, the syndrome. It is possible that these deteriorating NK levels along with deterioration of other parameters of cellular immunity might contribute to the profound susceptibility of AIDS patients to severe, recurrent infections. A more likely candidate for an early event leading to susceptibility to opportunistic infections in AIDS patients is the deficiency in IFN-α production we have consistently found in these patients.[65]

III. NK IN RESISTANCE TO BACTERIAL INFECTIONS

Compared to the studies with viral systems, there have been few studies to suggest that NK cells play a role in resistance to bacterial infections. Recent evidence, however, suggests that NK cells may be responsible for destruction of some bacteria, both by direct lysis or through ADCC mechanisms.

Early studies by Bennett et al.[139] demonstrated that mice treated with ^{89}Sr were deficient in an early defense mechanism against *Listeria monocytogenes*. ^{89}Sr treatment of mice leads to osteopetrosis with ablation of the marrow cavity. So-called "marrow dependent" (or "M") cell functions, which include hybrid resistance and NK cell activities, are deficient in these animals while T and B cell functions remain normal. One possible explanation for the impaired early immunity to *L. monocytogenes* in ^{89}Sr-treated mice was that NK cells were important for dealing with this obligate intracellular organism. More direct evidence for a role of NK cells, however, has not been developed. In contrast, studies by Skamene et al.[140] and Cheers et al.[141] suggest that early resistance to listeria is a macrophage function, with resistance being governed by a single, dominant gene. Bg/bg mice, despite having low NK activity, were not found to be more susceptible to listeria infection than their heterozygous littermates, suggesting that NK cells are not important in this system.

Direct evidence that NK cells can destroy bacteria was shown in the recent studies of Nencioni, Tagliabue et al.[142-144] These investigators found that in vitro coculture of mouse splenic or intestinal cells with *Salmonella typhimurium* bacteria resulted in a dramatically reduced plating efficiency of the bacteria. The cells from the gut responsible for killing the bacteria were histologically large granular lymphocytes (LGLs) and were asialo-GM1 and Thy-1 positive; the splenic effector cells were found to be asialo-GM1 positive and Thy-1 negative. Antibody increased the efficiency of lysis by these effector cells, presumably through an antibody-dependent mechanism. The authors suggest that these gut NK cells may be available to provide a defense against bacterial pathogens at the initial site of bacterial invasion. A recent abstract by Kleinman and Hunt[145] suggests that NK cells may also be active against *Escherichia coli* and acinetobacter. Although the evidence is still highly preliminary, taken together these studies suggest that NK cells may have a broader role in resisting infection than previously anticipated.

IV. NK IN RESISTANCE TO PROTOZOAN PARASITES

A number of recent publications have raised the possibility that NK cells may contribute to resistance against protozoan parasites. Eugui and Allison[146,147] found both an increase in spleen cell number and NK activity against YAC-1 targets in mice inoculated with babesia or malaria parasites. The augmentation of NK and spleen cell numbers was not observed in highly susceptible A/He mice. When nu/nu mice were challenged with the malarial agent *Plasmodium chabaudi,* the characteristic increase in NK and spleen cell numbers were also not observed. Since intact T cell functions are known to be important in resistance to these parasites, the authors suggest that the augmentation in NK activity is dependent upon the recruitment and activation of NK cells by T cell-dependent soluble mediators. Studies of Ruebush and Burgess[148] have shown that when mice are inoculated with *Babesia microti,* a naturally occurring parasite of wild rodents, there is an initial boost of NK activity followed several days later with a suppression of NK activity. Similar results were obtained by Hunter et al.[149] Furthermore, when bg/bg mice were injected with *B. microti,* Ruebush and Burgess[148] observed that not only did these animals fail to mount a strong NK response, they developed a much higher level of early parasitemia than did their heterozygous littermates. Both bg/bg and bg/+ mice made comparable levels of IFN, suggesting that failure to induce IFN was not responsible for the NK deficiency or increased paristemia. Thus, it is possible that NK cells may play a role in the early resistance against these parasites, serving to limit the degree of parasitemia before the development of the necessary T cell immunity.[150]

Hatcher and Kuhn[151-155] have provided direct evidence that NK cells can destroy *Trypanosoma cruzi* in vitro. Spleen cells from mice treated with pI:pC or infected with *T. cruzi* were able to destroy both the epimastigotes and blood form trypomastigotes. The cells mediating the in vitro resistance were found to have the characteristics of NK cells; they were NK 1.2+, Thy 1.2 +/−, and S Ig−. The in vivo relevance of these findings, however, remains to be determined since both highly susceptible C3H and resistant C57BL/6 mice showed similar levels of stimulated NK activity.

Studies by Albright et al.[161] of another parasite, *Trypanosoma musculi,* have suggested that although there is an early rise of NK activity in mice 2 to 4 days following infection with this parasite, there was a subsequent rapid decline to subnormal levels that persisted for more than 3 weeks and included the phase of rapid parasite elimination. Peritoneal cell NK activity was depressed to a lesser degree than that of splenic NK. The cause of the decline in NK activity was not determined, but is consistent with the findings of other investigators using different parasitic infection models. The authors suggest that although the *T. musculi* parasites induce early NK and may be, as in the case of *T. cruzi,* susceptible to lysis or inactivation by these cells,[151-155] NK cells may not be available when such lysis or inactivation would be beneficial to the host. The authors further suggest that although their results tend to rule out a role for NK in resistance to *T. musculi,* which is a free-living parasite, they cannot be assumed to apply to *T. cruzi,* which is an intracellular parasite. With *T. cruzi,* the epimastigote forms were found to be highly susceptible to NK lysis,[151-155] which might suggest that NK cells could have a significant in vivo role in resistance to this parasite. Evidence from in vivo studies will be necessary to determine whether they play a defensive role.

V. NK IN RESISTANCE TO FUNGI

Strong evidence for a role of NK cells in resistance to *Cryptococcus neoformans,* a yeast-like organism, comes from the work of Murphy and colleagues.[157-159] These authors have evaluated the clearing of *C. neoformans* in vivo and the mechanisms responsible and have developed an in vitro assay for the inhibition of growth of the organism. In an early study, Cauley and Murphy[159] noted that 7 days after infecting BALB/c nude and euthymic heterozygote mice with *C. neoformans,* nude mice had lower numbers of cryptococci in tissues than their nu/+ littermates. This early resistance in animals lacking T cell immune responses suggested that natural resistance mechanisms might be contributing to defense against this microorganism. In a more recent study, bg/bg mice were found to clear *C. neoformans* from their lungs less well than their heterozygous littermates, again suggesting a role for NK cells.[157,158] In an in vitro model, Murphy and McDaniel[157,158] developed an assay to measure the ability of murine and rat effector cells to inhibit the growth of cryptococci. In this assay, effector cells were incubated with cryptococci for 18 hr prior to enumerating the viable cryptococci by a plating technique. The effector cell activity which inhibited the cryptococci growth was found to be nylon wool nonadherent, higher in 7-week-old than 20-week-old CBA/N mice, and was augmented by pI:pC or *C. parvum.* In addition, these murine effector cells were found to be resistant to treatment with anti-Thy-1 + C′ but were sensitive to antiasialo-GM1 + C′. Finally, rat effector cells which inhibited the cryptococci growth were found in Percoll gradient fractions enriched for LGLs. Taken together, these data strongly support a role for NK cells in resistance to *C. neoformans.*

Other studies, while not directly addressing the issue of a role for NK cells in resistance to fungi, are consistent with the hypothesis that NK cells can be active against fungal cells in vivo. As was seen with *C. neoformans,* nu/nu mice infected with *Candida albicans* had longer survival and lower levels of culturable fungi than their heterozygous littermates.[159] Mice treated with cyclophosphamide were susceptible to early deaths from *C. neoformans,*[160] and had greater numbers of *Histoplasma capsulatum* in their tissues 5 days after infection,[161] results suggesting that the cyclophosphomide had depleted an early defense mechanism, most likely NK cells. Tewari and colleagues[162] were able to isolate effector cells from human peripheral blood that were cytotoxic to *H. capsulatum* in vitro. Like NK cells, these effectors were mononuclear nonadherent cells which did not require presensitization. Again, these studies provide strong suggestive evidence that NK cells may be an important first line of defense against fungal infections.

VI. CONCLUSIONS

Defense of the host against viral, bacterial, parasitic, and fungal pathogens requires the participation of several subpopulations of leukocytes and many different humoral factors interacting to resist and finally clear the infection.[163] Depending on the specific microorganism involved and the pathogenesis of infection, some aspects of host defense will be more important than others. For certain of these pathogens, a rapidly growing literature suggests that NK cells are probably a necessary component of host defense. NK cells are immediately ready to respond to invading microorganisms and are quickly activated by IFN in response to infection. These cells probably constitute one of the first barriers of host defense and probably act to sequester the infection and inhibit dissemination before the more specific components of adaptive immunity come into play.

Although by far the majority of the data suggesting a role of natural resistance mechanisms in infection have been developed in studies of viral pathogens, a number of very recent studies have now suggested that these mechanisms might also play a major role in resistance to bacterial, protozoan, and fungal infections. The observations that NK and other natural effector cells can be found in the intestinal and respiratory tracts as well as in peripheral blood, peritoneum, and various lymphoid organs suggest that NK cells probably function both at the portal of entry of many infections (i.e., the lungs and the gut) as well as systemically. The wide spread tissue distribution of natural effector mechanisms potentially allow them to be active when and where they are needed most.

The growing evidence for heterogeneity of NK and other naturally cytotoxic effector cells in both humans and mice complicated the studies of the biological roles of these effector mechanisms in vivo. In humans, for example, our studies have demonstrated that although the effector cells which lyse HSV-Fs targets, K562 targets, and the cells which produce IFN during NK assays are all found in Percoll gradient fractions enriched for LGLs, these effectors were found to be not only phenotypically distinct but were also shown to be independently regulated in vivo. This was most evident with our studies of patients susceptible to herpesvirus infections. If these studies had been carried out with the commonly used K562 targets only, then deficiencies of NK would not have been found in about one third of the patients with severe herpesvirus infections. Definition of heterogeneity of NK cells and the interaction between the subpopulations of effector cells will be important to our evaluation of the biological roles of these effector cells.

Heterogeneity also confuses studies of the basic biology of NK effector cells since results with one target (and thus perhaps with one effector subpopulation) may not characterize the other subpopulations. This is further complicated by the possibility that the target cells or the virus infecting those cells may determine the subpopulation of lytic cells which are operative.

Specific deficiencies of NK cell functions have been associated with unusual susceptibility to infections. An understanding of the basic biology of these effector cells and the interactions needed for a normal response is the necessary first step toward developing new modalities of treatment which augment these defense mechanisms to the benefit of the host.

ACKNOWLEDGMENTS

This work was supported in part by NIH Grants CA 42093, CA 34989, and CA 23766 and American Cancer Society Faculty Research Award 193 to CL.

REFERENCES

1. **Herberman, R. B., Nunn, M. E., and Lavrin, D. H.,** Natural cytotoxic reactivity of mouse lymphoid cells against syngeneic and allogeneic tumors. I. Distribution of reactivity and specificity, *Int. J. Cancer,* 16, 216, 1975.
2. **Kiessling, R., Klein, E., and Wigzell, H.,** "Natural" killer cells in the mouse. I. Cytotoxic cells with specificity for mouse Moloney leukemia cells. Specificity and distribution according to genotype, *Eur. J. Immunol.,* 5, 112, 1975.
3. **Hansson, M., Kiessling, R., Andersson, E., Kärre, K., and Roder, J.,** Natural killer (NK) cell sensitive T-cell subpopulation in the thymus: inverse correlation to NK activity of the host, *Nature (London),* 278, 174, 1979.
4. **Hansson, M., Kiessling, R., and Anderson, B.,** Human fetal thymus and bone marrow contain target cells for natural killer cells, *Eur. J. Immunol.,* 11, 8, 1981.
5. **Hansson, M., Kärre, K., Kiessling, R., Roder, J. C., Andersson, B., and Hayry, P.,** Natural NK cell targets in the mouse thymus: characteristics of the sensitive cell population, *J. Immunol.,* 123, 765, 1979.
6. **Hansson, M., Miroslav, B., Andersson, B., and Kiessling, R.,** Inhibition of in vitro granulopoiesis by autologous allogeneic human NK cells, *J. Immunol.,* 129, 126, 1982.
7. **Lotzová, E., Savary, C. A., and Pollack, S. B.,** Prevention of rejection of allogeneic bone marrow transplants by NK 1.1 antiserum, *Transplantation,* 35, 490, 1983.

8. **Warner, J. F. and Dennert, G.,** Effects of a cloned cell line with NK activity on bone marrow transplants, tumor development and metastasis in vivo, *Nature (London),* 300, 31, 1982.
9. **Trinchieri, G., Santoli, D., Dee, R. R., and Knowles, B. B.,** Anti-viral activity induced by culturing lymphocytes with tumor-derived or virus-transformed cells. Identification of the anti-viral activity as interferon and characterization of the human effector lymphocyte subpopulation, *J. Exp. Med.,* 147, 1299, 1978.
10. **Welsh, R. M. and Hallenbeck, L. A.,** Effect of virus infection on target cell susceptibility to natural killer cell mediated lysis, *J. Immunol.,* 124, 2491, 1980.
11. **Santoli, D., Trinchieri, G., and Koprowski, H.,** Cell-mediated cytotoxicity against virus-infected target cells in humans. II. Interferon induction and activation of natural killer cells, *J. Immunol.,* 121, 532, 1978.
12. **Djeu, J. Y., Stocks, N., Zoon, K., Stanton, G. J., Timonen, T., and Herberman, R. B.,** Positive self regulation of cytotoxicity in human natural killer cells by production of interferon upon exposure to influenza and herpes viruses, *J. Exp. Med.,* 156, 1222, 1982.
13. **Blalock, J. E., Langford, M. P., Georgiades, J., and Stanton, G. J.,** Nonsensitized lymphocytes produce leukocyte interferon when cultured with foreign cells, *Cell. Immunol.,* 43, 197, 1979.
14. **Timonen, T., Saksela, E., Virtanen, I., and Cantell, K.,** Natural killer cells are responsible for the interferon production induced in human lymphocytes by tumor cell contact, *Eur. J. Immunol.,* 10, 422, 1980.
15. **Fitzgerald, P. A., Kirkpatrick, D., Schindler, T., and Lopez, C.,** NK(HSV-1), NK(K562) and interferon production are independent functions of large granular lymphocytes, *Fed. Proc., Fed. Am. Soc. Exp. Biol.,* 42, 6131, 1983.
16. **Fitzgerald, P. A., von Wussow, P., and Lopez, C.,** Role of interferon in natural kill of HSV-1 infected fibroblasts, *J. Immunol.,* 129, 819, 1982.
17. **Minato, N., Reid, L., Cantor, H., Lengyel, P., and Bloom, B. R.,** Mode of regulation of natural killer cell activity by interferon, *J. Exp. Med.,* 152, 124, 1980.
18. **Casali, P., Sissons, J. G., Buchmeier, M. G., and Oldstone, M. B. A.,** In vitro generation of human cytotoxic lymphocytes by virus. Viral glycoproteins induce nonspecific cell-mediated cytotoxicity without release of interferon, *J. Exp. Med.,* 154, 840, 1981.
19. **Copeland, C. S., Koren, H. S., and Jensen, P. J.,** Natural killing can be independent of interferon generated in vivo, *Cell. Immunol.,* 62, 220, 1981.
20. **Saksela, E., Timonen, T., and Cantell, K.,** Human natural killer cell activity is augmented by interferon via recruitment of 'pre-NK' cells, *Scand. J. Immunol.,* 10, 257, 1978.
21. **Ullberg, M. and Jondal, M.,** Recycling and target-binding capacity of human natural killer cells, *J. Exp. Med.,* 153, 615, 1981.
22. **Roder, J. and Kiessling, R.,** Target-effector interaction in the natural killer cell system. I. Covariance and genetic control of cytolytic and target-cell binding subpopulations in the mouse, *Scand. J. Immunol.,* 8, 135, 1978.
23. **Targan, S. and Dorey, F.,** Interferon activation of "pre-spontaneous killer" (pre-SK) cells and alteration in kinetics of lysis of both pre-SK and active SK cells, *J. Immunol.,* 124, 2157, 1980.
24. **Pfizenmaier, K., Trostmann, H., Rollinghoff, M., and Wagner, H.,** Temporary presence of self-reactive cytotoxic T lymphocytes during murine lymphocyte choriomeningitis, *Nature (London),* 258, 238, 1975.
25. **Blanden, R. V. and Gardner, J.,** The cell-mediated immune response to ectromelia virus infection. I. Kinetics and characteristics of the primary effector T cell response in vivo, *Cell. Immunol.,* 22, 271, 1976.
26. **Rodda, S. J. and White, D. O.,** Cytotoxic macrophages: a rapid, non-specific response to viral infection, *J. Immunol.,* 117, 2067, 1976.
27. **Welsh, R. M.,** Natural cell-mediated immunity during viral infections, in *Natural Resistance to Tumors and Viruses,* Haller, O., Ed., Springer-Verlag, Berlin, 1981, 83.
28. **Diamond, R. D., Keller, R., Lee, G., and Finkel, D.,** Lysis of cytomegalovirus-infected human fibroblasts and transformed human cells by peripheral blood lymphoid cells from normal human donors (39650), *Proc. Soc. Exp. Biol. Med.,* 154, 259, 1977.
29. **Santoli, D., Trinchieri, G., and Lief, F. S.,** Cell-mediated cytotoxicity against virus infected target cells in humans. I. Characterization of the effector lymphocyte, *J. Immunol.,* 121, 526, 1978.
30. **Ching, C. and Lopez, C.,** Natural killing of herpes simplex virus type-1 infected target cells: normal human responses and influence of antiviral antibody, *Infect. Immun.,* 26, 49, 1979.
31. **Piontek, G. E., Weltzin, R., and Tompkins, W. A. F.,** Enhanced cytotoxicity of mouse natural killer cells for vaccinia and herpes virus-infected targets, *J. Reticuloendothel. Soc.,* 127, 175, 1980.
32. **Bishop, G. A., Glorioso, J. C., and Schwartz, S. A.,** Relationship between expression of Herpes simplex virus glycoproteins and susceptibility of target cells to human natural killer activity, *J. Exp. Med.,* 157, 1544, 1983.
33. **Kohl, S., Frazier, J. J., Greenberg, S. B., Pickering, L. K., and Loo, L.-S.,** Interferon induction of natural killer cytotoxicity in human neonates, *J. Pediatr.,* 98, 379, 1981.

34. **Yasukawa, M. and Zarling, J. M.,** Autologous herpes simplex virus-infected cells are lysed by human natural killer cells, *J. Immunol.*, 131, 2011, 1983.
35. **Lee, G. D. and Keller, R.,** Natural cytotoxicity to murine cytomegalovirus-infected cells mediated by mouse lymphoid cells: role of interferon in the endogenous natural cytotoxicity reaction, *Infect. Immun.*, 35, 5, 1982.
36. **Quinnan, G. V. and Manischewitz, J. F.,** The role of natural killer cells and antibody-dependent cell-mediated cytotoxicity during murine cytomegalovirus infection, *J. Exp. Med.*, 150, 1549, 1979.
37. **Kirmani, N., Ginn, R. K., Mittal, K. K., Manischewitz, J. F., and Quinnan, G. V., Jr.,** Cytomegalovirus-specific mediated by non-T lymphocytes from peripheral blood of normal volunteers, *Infect. Immun.*, 34, 441, 1981.
38. **Quinnan, G. V., Kirmani, N., Rook, A. H., Manischewitz, J. F., Jackson, L., Moreschi, G., Santos, G. W., Sarai, R.,and Burns, W. H.,** Cytotoxic T cells in cytomegalovirus infection. HLA-restricted T-lymphocyte and non-T-lymphocyte cytotoxic responses correlate with recovery from cytomegalovirus infection in bone-marrow-transplant recipients, *N. Engl. J. Med.*, 307, 6, 1982.
39. **Starr, S. E. and Garrabrant, T.,** Natural killing of cytomegalovirus-infected fibroblasts by human mononuclear leucocytes, *Clin. Exp. Immunol.*, 46, 484, 1981.
40. **Blazar, B., Patarroyo, M., Klein, E., and Klein, G.,** Increased sensitivity of human lymphoid lines to natural killer cells after induction of the Epstein-Barr viral cycle by superinfection or sodium butyrate, *J. Exp. Med.*, 151, 614, 1980.
41. **Patel, P. C. and Menezes, J.,** Epstein-Barr virus (EBV)-lymphoid cell interactions. II. The influence of the EBV replication cycle on natural killing and antibody-dependent cellular cytotoxicity against EBV-infected cells, *Clin. Exp. Immunol.*, 48, 589, 1982.
42. **Shope, T. C. and Kaplan, J.,** Inhibition of the *in vitro* outgrowth of Epstein-Barr virus-infected lymphocytes by Tg lymphocytes, *J. Immunol.*, 123, 2150, 1979.
43. **Patel, P. A., Yoonessi, S., O'Malley, J., Freeman, A., Gershon, A., and Ogra, P. L.,** Cell-mediated immunity to varicella-zoster virus infection in subjects with lymphoma or leukemia, *J. Pediatr.*, 94, 223, 1979.
44. **Ihara, T., Starr, S. E., Arbeter, A. M., and Plotkin, S. A.,** Effects of interferon on natural killing and antibody-dependent cellular cytotoxicity against Varicella-Zoster virus infected and uninfected target cells, *J. Interferon Res.*, 3, 263, 1983.
45. **Minato, N., Bloom, B. R., Jones, C., Holland, J., and Reid, L. M.,** Mechanism of rejection of virus persistently infected tumor cells by athymic nude mice, *J. Exp. Med.*, 149, 1117, 1979.
46. **Anderson, M. J.,** Innate cytotoxicity of CBA mouse spleen cells to Sendai virus-infected L cells, *Infect. Immun.*, 20, 608, 1978.
47. **Weston, P. A., Jensen, P. J., Levy, N. L., and Koren, H. S.,** Spontaneous cytotoxicity against virus-infected cells: relationship to NK against uninfected cell lines and to ADCC, *J. Immunol.*, 126, 1220, 1981.
48. **Ault, K. A. and Weiner, H. L.,** Natural killing of measles-infected cells by human lymphocytes, *J. Immunol.*, 122, 2611, 1979.
49. **Harfast, B., Andersson, T., and Perlmann, P.,** Immunoglobulin-independent natural cytotoxicity of Fc receptor-bearing human blood lymphocytes to mumps virus-infected target cells, *J. Immunol.*, 121, 755, 1978.
50. **Lust, J. A., Kumar, V., Burton, R. C., Bartlett, S. P., and Bennett, M.,** Heterogeneity of natural killer cells in the mouse, *J. Exp. Med.*, 154, 306, 1981.
51. **Stutman, O., Paige, C. J., and Figarella, E.,** Natural cytotoxic cells against solid tumors in mice. I. Strain and age distribution and target cell susceptibility, *J. Immunol.*, 121, 1819, 1978.
52. **Lattime, E. C., Pecoraro, G. A., and Stutman, O.,** The activity of natural cytotoxic cells is augmented by interleukin 2 and interleukin 3, *J. Exp. Med.*, 157, 1070, 1983.
53. **Minato, N., Reid, L., and Bloom, B.,** On the heterogeneity of murine natural killer cells, *J. Exp. Med.*, 154, 750, 1981.
54. **Weston, P. A., Levy, N. I., and Koren, H. S.,** Spontaneous cytotoxicity against virus-infected cells: cellular immunoadsorption on infected cell monolayers, *J. Immunol.*, 125, 1387, 1980.
55. **Zarling, J. M., Clouse, K. A., Biddison, W. E., and Kung, P. C.,** Phenotype of human natural killer cell populations detected with monoclonal antibodies, *J. Immunol.*, 127, 2575, 1981.
56. **Fitzgerald, P. A., Evans, R., Kirkpatrick, D., and Lopez, C.,** Heterogeneity of human NK cells: comparison of effectors that lyse HSV-1 infected fibroblasts and K562 erythroleukemia targets, *J. Immunol.*, 130, 1663, 1983.
57. **Lopez, C., Kirkpatrick, D., Fitzgerald, P. A., Ching, C. Y., Pahwa, R. N., Good, R. A., and Smithwick, E. M.,** Studies of the cell lineage of the effector cells that spontaneously lyse HSV-1 infected fibroblasts [NK(HSV-1)], *J. Immunol.*, 129, 824, 1982.
58. **Newman, W., Fast, L. D., and Ross, L. M.,** Blockade of NK cell lysis is a property of monoclonal antibodies that bind to distinct regions of T-200, *J. Immunol.*, 131, 1742, 1983.

59. **Welsh, R. M., Jr., Zinkernagel, R. M., and Hallenbeck, L. A.,** Cytotoxic cells induced during lymphocytic choriomeningitis virus infection of mice. II. ''Specificities'' of the natural killer cells, *J. Immunol.*, 122, 475, 1979.
60. **Biron, C. A., Lurgiss, L. R., and Welsh, R. M.,** Increase in NK cell number and turnover rate during acute viral infection, *J. Immunol.*, 131, 1539, 1983.
61. **Biron, C. A., Sonenfeld, G., and Welsh, R. M.,** Interferon induces natural killer cell blastogenesis *in vivo*, *J. Leuko. Biol.*, 35, 31, 1984.
62. **Trinchieri, G., Santoli, D., Granato, D., and Perussia, B.,** Antagonistic effects of interferon on the cytotoxicity mediated by natural killer cells, *Fed. Proc., Fed. Am. Soc. Exp. Biol.*, 40, 2705, 1981.
63. **Trinchieri, G., Santoli, D., and Koprowski, H.,** Spontaneous cell-mediated cytotoxicity in humans: role of interferon and immunoglobulins, *J. Immunol.*, 120, 1819, 1978.
64. **Bishop, G. A., Glorioso, J. C., and Schwartz, S. A.,** Role of interferon in human natural killer activity against target cells infected with HSV-1, *J. Immunol.*, 131, 1849, 1983.
65. **Lopez, C., Fitzgerald, P. A., and Siegal, F. P.,** Severe acquired immune deficiency syndrome in male homosexuals: diminished capacity to make interferon-alpha in vitro is associated with servere opportunistic infections, *J. Infect. Dis.*, 148, 962, 1983.
66. **Brooks, C. G., Wayner, E. A., Webb, P. J., Gray, J. D., Kenwick, S., and Baldwin, R. W.,** The specificity of rat natural killer cells and cytotoxic macrophages on solid tumor derived target cells and selected variants, *J. Immunol.*, 126, 2477, 1981.
67. **Bishop, G. A., Glorioso, J. C., and Schwartz, S. A.,** Association of herpes-specific glycoproteins with susceptibility to natural killer cells, *Fed. Proc., Fed. Am. Soc. Exp. Biol.*, 42, 851, 1983.
68. **Bishop, G. A., Glorioso, J. C., and Schwartz, C. A.,** Relationship between expression of herpes simplex virus glycoproteins and susceptibility of target cells to human natural killer activity, *J. Exp. Med.*, 157, 1544, 1983.
69. **Rager-Zisman, B., Ouan, P.-C., Schatter, A., Panish, D., and Bloom, B. R.,** NK cell lysis of targets infected with ts mutants of VSV, *Fed. Proc., Fed. Am. Soc. Exp. Biol.*, 42, 1338, 1983.
70. **Herberman, R. B., Nun, M. E., Holden, H. T., Staal, S., and Djeu, J. Y.,** Augmentation of natural cytotoxic reactivity of mouse lymphoid cells against syngeneic and allogeneic target cells, *Int. J. Cancer*, 19, 555, 1977.
71. **Macfarlan, R. I., Burns, W. H., and White, D. O.,** Two cytotoxic cells in peritoneal cavity of virus-infected mice: antibody-dependent macrophages and nonspecific killer cells, *J. Immunol.*, 119, 1569, 1977.
72. **Welsh, R. M. and Zinkernagel, R. M.,** Hetero-specific cytotoxic cell activity induced during the first three days of acute lymphocytic choriomeningitis virus infection in mice, *Nature (London)*, 268, 646, 1977.
73. **Gidlund, M., Örn, A., Wigzell, H., Senik, A., and Gesser, I.,** Enhanced NK activity in mice infected with interferon and interferon inducers, *Nature (London)*, 273, 759, 1978.
74. **Welsh, R. M., Jr.,** Cytotoxic cells induced during lymphocytic choriomeningitis virus infection of mice. I. Characterization of natural killer cell induction, *J. Exp. Med.*, 148, 163, 1978.
75. **Welsh, R. M.,** Mouse natural killer cells: induction, specificity and function, *J. Immunol.*, 121, 1631, 1978.
76. **(Chalmer) Grundy, J. E., Trapman, J., Allan, J. E., Shellam, G. R., and Melief, C. J. M.,** Evidence for a protective role of interferon in resistance to murine cytomegalovirus and its control by non-H-2-linked genes, *Infect. Immun.*, 37, 143, 1982.
77. **Trinchieri, G. and Santoli, D.,** Anti-viral activity induced by culturing lymphocytes with tumor-derived or virus-transformed cells. Enhancement of natural killer cell activity by interferon and antagonistic inhibition of susceptibility of target cells to lysis, *J. Exp. Med.*, 147, 1314, 1978.
78. **Trinchieri, G., Santoli, D., Granato, D., and Perussia, B.,** Antagonistic effects of interferons on the cytotoxicity mediated by natural killer cells, *Fed. Proc., Fed. Am. Soc. Exp. Biol.*, 40, 2705, 1981.
79. **Welsh, R. M., Kärre, K., Hansson, M., Kunkel, L. A., and Kiessling, R.,** Interferon-mediated protection of normal and tumor target cells against lysis by mouse natural killer cells, *J. Immunol.*, 126, 219, 1981.
80. **Moore, M., White, W. J., and Potter, M. R.,** Modulation of target cell susceptibility to human natural killer cells by interferon, *Int. J. Cancer*, 25, 565, 1980.
81. **Wright, S. C. and Bonavida, B.,** Studies on the mechanism of natural killer cell-mediated cytotoxicity. IV. Interferon-induced inhibition of NK target cell susceptibility to lysis is due to a defect in their ability to stimulate release of natural killer cytotoxic factors (NKCF), *J. Immunol.*, 130, 2965, 1983.
82. **Weigent, D. A., Langford, M. P., Smith, E. M., Blalock, J. E., and Stanton, G. J.,** Human B lymphocytes produce leukocyte interferon after interaction with foreign cells, *Infect. Immun.*, 32, 508, 1981.
83. **Stanwick, T. L., Campbell, D. E., and Nahmias, A. J.,** Cytotoxic properties of human monocyte macrophages for human fibroblasts infected with herpes simplex virus: interferon production and augmentation, *Cell. Immunol.*, 70, 132, 1982.
84. **Peter, H. H., Dallugge, H., Zawatzky, R., Euler, S., Liebold, W., and Kirchner, H.,** Human peripheral null lymphocytes. II. Producers of type-1 interferon upon stimulation with tumor cells, herpes simplex virus and *Corynebacterium parvum*, *Eur. J. Immunol.*, 10, 547, 1980.

85. **Ortaldo, J. R., Sharrow, S. O., Timonen, T., and Herberman, R. B.,** Determination of surface antigens on highly purified human NK cells by flow cytometry with monoclonal antibodies, *J. Immunol.*, 127, 2401, 1981.
86. **Ng, A.-K., Indiveri, F., Pellegrino, M. A., Molinaro, G. A., Quaranta, V., and Ferrone, S.,** Natural cytotoxicity and antibody-dependent cellular cytotoxicity of human lymphocytes depleted of HLA-DR bearing cells with monoclonal HLA-DR antibodies, *J. Immunol.*, 124, 2336, 1980.
87. **Lopez, C.,** Genetics of natural resistance to herpes virus infections in mice, *Nature (London)*, 258, 152, 1975.
88. **Lopez, C.,** Resistance to HSV-1 in the mouse is governed by two major, independently segregating non-H-2 loci, *Immunogenetics*, 11, 87, 1980.
89. **Lopez, C.,** Immunological nature of genetic resistance of mice to herpes simplex virus-type 1 infection, in *Oncogenesis and Herpes Viruses*, Vol. 3, de The, G., Henle, W., and Rapp., F., Eds., World Health Organization, Lyon, France, 1978, 775.
90. **Cudkowicz, G. and Bennett, M.,** Peculiar immunobiology of bone marrow allografts. II. Rejection of parental grafts by resistant F_1 hybrid mice, *J. Exp. Med.*, 134, 153, 1971.
91. **Lopez, C., Ryshke, R., and Bennett, M.,** Marrow dependent cells depleted by ^{89}Sr mediate genetic resistance to herpes simplex virus 1 infection, *Infect. Immun.*, 28, 1028, 1980.
92. **Kiessling, R., Hochman, P. S., Häller, O., Shearer, G. M., Wigzell, H., and Cudkowicz, G.,** Evidence for a similar or common mechanism for natural killer activity and resistance to hemopoietic grafts, *Eur. J. Immunol.*, 7, 655, 1977.
93. **Seaman, W. E., Gindhart, T. D., Greenspan, J. C., Blackman, M. A., and Talal, N.,** Natural killer cells, bone and bone marrow: studies in estrogen treated mice and congenitally osteoporotic mice, *J. Immunol.*, 122, 2541, 1979.
94. **Roder, J. and Duur, A.,** The beige mutation in the mouse selectively impairs natural killer cell function, *Nature (London)*, 278, 45, 1979.
95. **Schlabach, A. J., Martinez, D., Field, A. K., and Tytell, A. A.,** Resistance of C57 mice to primary systemic herpes simplex virus infection, macrophage dependence and T-cell independence, *Infect. Immun.*, 26, 615, 1979.
96. **Zawatsky, R., Hilfenhaus, J., and Kirchner, H.,** Resistance of nude mice to herpes simplex virus and correlation with (in vitro) production of interferon, *Cell. Immunol.*, 47, 424, 1979.
97. **Kohl, S., Lawman, M. J. P., Rouse, B. T., and Cahall, D. L.,** Effect of herpes simplex virus infection on murine antibody-dependent cellular cytotoxicity and natural killer cytotoxicity, *Infect. Immun.*, 31, 704, 1981.
98. **Kohl, S. and Loo, L. S.,** Protection of neonatal mice against herpes simplex virus infection. Probable *in vivo* antibody-dependent cellular cytotoxicity, *J. Immunol.*, 129, 370, 1982.
99. **Kohl, S., Loo, L. S., and Greenberg, S. B.,** Protection of newborn mice from herpes simplex virus by human interferon, antibody and leukocytes, *J. Immunol.*, 128, 1107, 1982.
100. **Kirchner, H., Engler, H., Schroder, C. H., Zawatzky, R., and Storch, E.,** Herpes simplex virus type-1 induced interferon production and activation of natural killer cells in mice, *J. Gen. Virol.*, 64, 437, 1983.
101. **Zawatzky, R., Kirchner, H., DeMayer-Guignard, J., and DeMaeyer, E.,** An X-linked locus influences the amount of circulating interferon induced in the mouse by herpes simplex virus type 1, *J. Gen. Virol.*, 63, 325, 1982.
102. **Zawatzky, R., Hilfenhaus, J., Marcucci, F., and Kirchner, H.,** Experimental infection of inbred mice with herpes simplex virus type 1. I. Investigation of humoral and cellular immunity and of interferon induction, *J. Gen. Virol.*, 53, 31, 1981.
103. **Engler, H., Zawatzky, R., Goldbach, A., Schroder, C. H., Weyand, C., Hammerling, G. J., and Kirchner, H.,** Experimental infection of inbred mice with herpes simplex virus. II. Interferon production and activation of natural killer cells in the peritoneal exudate, *J. Gen. Virol.*, 55, 25, 1981.
104. **Engler, H., Zawatzky, R., Kirchner, H., and Amerding, D.,** Experimental infection of inbred mice with herpes simplex virus. IV. Comparison of interferon production and natural killer cell activity in susceptible and resistant adult mice, *Arch. Virol.*, 74, 239, 1982.
105. **Zawatzky, R., Gresser, I., DeMaeyer, E., and Kirchner, H.,** The role of interferon in the resistance of C57BL/6 mice to various doses of herpes simplex virus type 1, *J. Infect. Dis.*, 146, 405, 1982.
106. **Gresser, I., Tovey, M. G., Maury, C., and Bandu, M.-T.,** Role of interferon in the pathogenesis of virus diseases in mice as demonstrated by the use of anti-interferon serum. II. Studies with herpes simplex, Maloney sarcoma vesicular stomatitis, Newcastle disease, and influenza viruses, *J. Exp. Med.*, 144, 1316, 1976.
107. **Bancroft, G. J., Shellam, G. R., and Chalmer, J. E.,** Genetic influences on the augmentation of natural killer (NK) cells during murine cytomegalovirus infection: correlation with patterns of resistance, *J. Immunol.*, 126, 988, 1981.
108. **Shellam, G. R., Allan, J. E., Papdimitriou, J. M., and Bancroft, G. J.,** Increased susceptibility to cytomegalovirus infection in beige mutant mice, *Proc. Natl. Acad. Sci. U.S.A.*, 78, 5104, 1981.

109. **Quinnan, G. V., Jr., Manischewitz, J. F., and Kirmani, N.,** Involvement of natural killer cells in the pathogenesis of murine cytomegalovirus interstitial pneumonitis and the immune response to infection, *J. Gen. Virol.*, 58, 173, 1982.
110. **Bukowski, J. F., Woda, B. A., Habu, S., Okumura, K., and Welsh, R. M.,** Natural killer cell depletion enhances virus synthesis and virus-induced hepatitis *in vivo*, *J. Immunol.*, 131, 1531, 1983.
111. **Masuda, A. and Bennett, M.,** Murine cytomegalovirus stimulates natural killer cell function but kills genetically resistant mice treated with radioactive strontium, *Infect. Immun.*, 34, 970, 1981.
112. **Tardieu, M., Hery, C., and Dupuy, J. M.,** Neonatal susceptibility to MHV_3 infection in: II. Role of natural effector marrow cells in transfer of resistance, *J. Immunol.*, 124, 418, 1980.
113. **Schindler, I., Engler, H., and Kirchner, H.,** Activation of natural killer cells and induction of interferon after injection of mouse hepatitis virus type 3 in mice, *Infect. Immun.*, 35, 869, 1982.
114. **Welsh, R. M., Biron, C. A., Parker, D., Bukowski, J. F., Habu, S., Okumura, K., Haspel, M. V., and Holmes, K. V.,** Regulation and role of natural cell-mediated immunity during virus infections, in *Human Immunity to Viruses*, Ennis, F., Ed., Academic Press, New York, 1983, 21.
115. **Welsh, R. M.,** Do natural killer cells play a role in virus infections?, *Antiviral Res.*, 1, 5, 1981.
116. **Welsh, R. M., Jr. and Kiessling, R. W.,** Natural killer cell response to lymphocytic choriomeningitis virus in beige mice, *Scand. J. Immunol.*, 11, 363, 1980.
117. **Hirsch, R. L.,** Natural killer cells appear to play no role in the recovery of mice from Sindbis virus infection, *Immunology*, 49, 81, 1980.
118. **Gee, S. R., Clark, D. A., and Rawls, W. E.,** Differences between Syrian hamster strains in natural killer cell activity induced by infection with Pichinde virus, *J. Immunol.*, 123, 2618, 1979.
119. **Metcalf, J. F., Hamilton, D. S., and Reichert, R. W.,** Herpetic keratitis in athymic (nude) mice, *Infect. Immun.*, 26, 1164, 1979.
120. **Lopez, C., Kirkpatrick, D., Read, S. E., Fitzgerald, P. A., Pitt, J., Pahwa, S., Ching, C. Y., and Smithwick, E. M.,** Correlation between low natural killing of fibroblasts infected with herpes simplex virus type 1 and susceptibility to herpesvirus infections, *J. Infect. Dis.*, 147, 1030, 1983.
121. **Lipinski, M., Virelizier, J.-L., Turz, T., and Griscelli, C.,** Natural killer and killer cell activities in patients with primary immunodeficiencies or defects in immune interferon production, *Eur. J. Immunol.*, 10, 246, 1980.
122. **Stiehm, R. E.,** The human neonate as an immunocompromised host, in *Pathogenesis, Prevention and Therapy*, Verhoef, J., Peterson, P. K., and Quie, P. E., Eds., Elsevier/North-Holland, Amsterdam, 1980, 77.
123. **Blaese, M., Strober, W., and Waldman, T. A.,** Immunodeficiency in the Wiscott-Aldrich Syndrome, In *Immunodeficiency in Man and Animals*, Bergsma, D., Good, R. A., and Finstad, J., Eds., Sinauer Assoc., Sunderland, Md., 1975, 250.
124. **Sullivan, J. L., Byron, K. S., Brewster, F. E., and Purtillo, D. T.,** Deficient natural killer cell activity in X-linked lymphoproliferative syndrome, *Science*, 210, 543, 1980.
125. **Sullivan, J. L., Byron, K. S., Brewster, F. E., Baker, S. M., and Ochs, H. D.,** X-linked lymphoproliferative syndrome, *J. Clin. Invest.*, 71, 1765, 1983.
126. **Virelizier, J. L.,** Viral infections in patients with selective disorders of the interferon system, 5th Int. Congr. Virology, Strasbourg, France, 1981, 152.
127. **Virelizier, J. L., Lenoir, G., and Griscelli, C.,** Persistent Epstein-Barr virus infection in a child with hypergammaglobulinemia and immunoblastic proliferation associated with a selective defect in immune interferon secretion, *Lancet*, 1, 231, 1978.
128. **Virelizier, J. L., Lipinski, M., Tursz, T., and Griscelli, C.,** Defects of immune interferon secretion and natural killer activity in patients with immunological disorders, *Lancet*, 1, 696, 1979.
129. **Quinnan, G. V., Kirmani, N., Rook, A. H., Manishewitz, J. H., Jackson, L., Moreschi, G., Santos, G. W., Saral, R., and Burns, W. H.,** HLA-restricted T-lymphocyte and non T-lymphocyte cytotoxic responses correlate with recovery from cytomegalovirus infection in bone-marrow transplantation, *N. Engl. J. Med.*, 307, 7, 1982.
130. **Starr, S. E., Tolpin, M. D., Friedman, H. M., Paucker, K., and Plotkin, S. A.,** Impaired cellular immunity to cytomegalovirus in congenitally infected children and their mothers, *J. Infect. Dis.*, 140, 500, 1979.
131. **Benczur, M., Petranyi, G. G., Palffy, G., Varger, M., Tala, M., Kotsy, B., Foldes, I., and Hollan, S. R.,** Dysfunction of natural killer cells in multiple sclerosis: a possible pathogenetic factor, *Clin. Exp. Immunol.*, 39, 657, 1980.
132. **Hauser, S. L., Aulk, K. A., Levin, M. J., Garovoy, M. R., and Weiner, H. L.,** Natural killer cell activity in multiple sclerosis, *J. Immunol.*, 127, 114, 1981.
133. **Santoli, D., Hall, W., Kastrukoff, L., Lisak, R. P., Perussia, B., Trinchieri, G., and Koprowski, H.,** Cytotoxic activity and interferon production by lymphocytes from patients with multiple sclerosis, *J. Immunol.*, 126, 1274, 1981.

134. **Merrill, J., Jondal, M., Seeley, J., Ullberg, M., and Siden, A.,** Decreased NK killing in patients with multiple sclerosis: an analysis on the level of the single effector cell in peripheral blood and cerebrospinal fluid in relation to the activity of the disease, *Clin. Exp. Immunol.,* 47, 419, 1982.
135. **Lucas, C. J. and McFarland, H. F.,** Induction of measles virus-specific cytotoxic T cells, natural killer cells and interferon in cultures of human peripheral blood lymphocytes from normal volunteers and patients with multiple sclerosis, in *Human Immunity to Viruses,* Ennis, F., Ed., Academic Press, New York, 1983, 293.
136. **Merrill, J. E., Gerner, R. H., Myers, L. W., and Ellison, G. W.,** Regulation of NK and IFN production by PGE in the peripheral blood and cerebrospinal fluid of patients with multiple sclerosis and other neurological disorders, in *Intercellular Communication in Leucocyte Function,* Parker, J. and O'Brien, R., Eds., John Wiley & Sons, Chichester, 1983, 79.
137. **Neighbor, P. A., Reinite, E., Grayzel, A. I., Miller, A. E., and Bloom, B. R.,** Studies of human NK cell function in chronic diseases, in *NK Cells and Other Natural Effector Cells,* Herberman, R., Ed., Academic Press, New York, 1982, 1241.
138. **Siegal, F. P., Lopez, C., Hammer, G. S., Brown, A. E., Kornfeld, S. J., Gold, J., Hassett, J., Hirschman, S. Z., Cunningham-Rundles, C., Adelsberg, B. R., Parham, D. M., Siegal, M., Cunningham-Rundles, S., and Armstrong, D.,** Severe acquired immunodeficiency in male homosexuals, manifested by chronic perianal ulcerative herpes simplex lesions, *N. Engl. J. Med.,* 305, 1439, 1981.
139. **Bennett, M., Baker, E. E., Eastcott, J. W., Kumar, V., and Yonkosky, D.,** Selective elimination of marrow precursors with the bone seeking isotope ^{89}Sr: implication for hemopoiesis, lymphopoiesis, viral leukemogenesis and infection, *J. Reticuloendothel. Soc.,* 20, 71, 1980.
140. **Skamene, E., Stevenson, M. M., and Kongshaven, P. A. L.,** Natural cell-mediated immunity against bacteria, in *NK Cells and Other Natural Effector Cells,* Herberman, R., Ed., Academic Press, New York, 1982, 1513.
141. **Cheers, C. and Macgeorge, J.,** Genetic and cellular mechanisms of natural resistance to intracellular bacteria, in *NK Cells and Other Natural Effector Cells,* Herberman, R., Ed., Academic Press, New York, 1982, 152.
142. **Tagliabue, A., Nencioni, L., Villa, L., and Boraschi, D.,** Natural and antibody-dependent cell-mediated activity against *Salmonella typhimuruim* by peripheral and intestinal lymphoid cells in mice, *Fed. Proc., Fed. Am. Soc. Exp. Biol.,* 42, 1338, 1983.
143. **Nencioni, L., Villa, L., Boraschi, D., Berti, B., and Tagliabue, A.,** Natural and antibody-dependent cell-mediated activity against salmonella typhimurium by peripheral and intestinal lymphoid cells in mice, *J. Immunol.,* 130, 903, 1983.
144. **Tagliabue, L., Nencioni, L., Villa, L., Keren, D. F., Lowell, G. H., and Boraschi, D.,** Antibody-dependent cell-mediated antibacterial activity of intestinal lymphocytes with secretory IgA, *Nature (London),* 306, 184, 1983.
145. **Kleinman, R. and Hunt, M. D.,** Characterization of lymphocyte subpopulation involved in spontaneous bactericidal reaction, *Fed. Proc., Fed. Am. Soc. Exp. Biol.,* 42, 5426, 1983.
146. **Eugui, E. and Allison, A. C.,** Natural and cell mediated immunity and interferon in malaria and babesia infection, in *NK Cells and Other Natural Effector Cells,* Herberman, R., Ed., Academic Press, New York, 1983, 1491.
147. **Eugui, E. M. and Allison, A. C.,** Differences in susceptibility of various mouse strains to haemoprotozoan infections: possible correlation with natural killer activity, *Parasite Immunol.,* 2, 277, 1980.
148. **Ruebush, M. J. and Burgess, D. E.,** Induction of natural killer cells and interferon production during infection of mice with *Babesia microti* of human origin, in *NK Cells and Other Natural Effector Cells,* Herberman, R., Ed., Academic Press, New York, 1982, 1483.
149. **Hunter, K. W., Folks, T. M., Sayles, P. C., and Strickland, G. T.,** Early enhancement followed by suppression of natural killer cell activity during murine malarial infections, *Immunol. Lett.,* 2, 209, 1981.
150. **Clark, I. A. and Allison, A. C.,** *Babesia microti* and *Plasmodium berghei yoelii* infections in nude mice, *Nature (London),* 252, 328.
151. **Hatcher, F. M., Kuhn, R. E., Cerrone, M. C., and Burton, R. C.,** Increased natural killer cell activity in experimental american trypanosomiasis, *J. Immunol.,* 127, 1126, 1981.
152. **Hatcher, F. M. and Kuhn, R. E.,** Destruction of *Trypanosoma cruzi* by natural killer cells, *Science,* 218, 295, 1982.
153. **Hatcher, F. M. and Kuhn, R. E.,** Spontaneous lytic activity against allogeneic tumor cells and depression of specific cytotoxic responses in mice infected with *Trypanosoma cruzi, J. Immunol.,* 126, 2436, 1981.
154. **Hatcher, F. M. and Kuhn, R. E.,** Natural killer (NK) cell activity against extracellular forms of *Trypanosoma cruzi,* in *NK Cells and Other Natural Effector Cells,* Herberman, R., Ed., Academic Press, New York, 1982, 1091.
155. **Hatcher, F. M., Cobbs, J. D., and Kuhn, R. E.,** Murine natural killer cell activity against blood-form trypomastigates of *Trypansoma cruzi, Fed. Proc., Fed. Am. Soc. Exp. Biol.,* 42, 1339, 1983.

156. **Albright, J. W., Huang, K.-Y., and Albright, J. F.,** Natural killer activity in mice infected with *Trypanosoma musculi, Infect. Immun.*, 40, 869, 1983.
157. **Murphy, J. W. and McDaniel, D. O.,** In vitro effects of natural killer (NK) cells in *Cryptococcus neoformans*, in *NK Cells and Other Natural Effector Cells*, Herberman, R., Ed., Academic Press, New York, 1982, 1105.
158. **Murphy, J. W. and McDaniel, D. O.,** In vitro reactivity of natural killer (NK) cells against *Cryptococcus neoformans, J. Immunol.*, 128, 1577, 1982.
159. **Cauley, L. K. and Murphy, J. W.,** Response of congenitally athymic (nude) and phenotypically normal mice to a *Cryptococcus neoformans* infection, *Infect. Immun.*, 23, 644, 1979.
160. **Graybill, J. R. and Mitchell, L.,** Cyclophosphamide effects on murine cryptococcus, *Infect. Immun.*, 21, 674, 1978.
161. **Cozad, G. C. and Lindsey, T. J.,** Effect of cyclophosphamide on *Histoplasma capsulatum* infections in mice, *Infect. Immun.*, 21, 674, 1974.
162. **Tewari, R. P., Mkwananzi, J. B., McConnachig, P., Von Behren, L. A., Eagleton, L., Kulkarni, P., and Bartlett, P. C.,** Natural and antibody dependent cellular cytotoxicity (ADCC) of human peripheral blood mononuclear cells (PBMC) to yeast cells of *Histoplasma capsulation* (HC) *ASM Abstracts (F66)*, p. 324, 1981.
163. **Allison, A. C.,** Interactions of antibodies, complement components, and various cell types in immunity against virus and pyogenic bacteria, *Transp. Rev.*, 19, 3, 1974.
164. **Fitzgerald, P. A. and Schindler, I.,** in preparation.
165. **Colmenares, et al.,** in preparation.
166. **Schindler, T. E., Fitzgerald, P. A., and Lopez, C.,** Distinguishing characteristics of the natural killer cells which lyse HSV-1 infected fibroblasts and K562 erythroleukemia cells, in *Natural Killer Activity and its Regulation*, Hoshino, T., Koren, H., and Uchida, A., Eds., Exerpta Medica, Amsterdam, 1984, 76.
167. **Messina, C., Kirkpatrick, D., Fitzgerald, P., O'Reilly, R., Siegal, F., Cunningham-Rundles, C., Blaese, M., Oleske, J., Pahwa, S., and Lopez, C.,** Natural killer cell function and interferon generation in patients with primary immunodeficiencies, submitted.
168. **Fitzgerald, P. A. et al.,** unpublished.
169. **Fitzgerald, P. and Lopez, C.,** in preparation.
170. **Zarling, J. M. et al.,** personal communication.
171. **Fitzgerald, P., Mendelsohn, M., and Lopez, C.,** Human mononuclear cells which produce interferon-alpha during NK(HSV-Fs) assays are distinct from cytolytic NK effector cells, submitted.
172. **Lopez, C. et al.,** unpublished.
173. **Lopez, C.,** unpublished.
174. **Fitzgerald, P. A., Mendelsohn, M., and Lopez, C.,** Human natural killer cells limit replication of Herpes Simplex Virus Type 1 in vitro, *J. Immunol.*, 134, 2666, 1985.

Chapter 8

CYTOKINE SECRETION AND NONCYTOTOXIC FUNCTIONS OF HUMAN LARGE GRANULAR LYMPHOCYTES

Giuseppe Scala, J. Y. Djeu, Paola Allavena, T. Kasahara, John R. Ortaldo, Ronald B. Herberman, and J. J. Oppenheim

TABLE OF CONTENTS

I. INTRODUCTION

The natural killer (NK) activity against tumor- and virus-infected cells is exerted by a distinct group of peripheral blood leukocytes (PBLs) with morphological characteristics of large granular lymphocytes (LGLs).[1,2] There is also considerable evidence that LGLs may play a critical role in the in vivo resistance against bone marrow allografts and primary oncogenesis as well as tumor metastases.[3-6]

Human LGLs show considerable surface marker heterogeneity with some of the cells expressing surface markers of T lymphocytes (OKT11, OKT10) and others of myelomonocytic cells (OKM1, DR).[7]

The NK activity of LGLs can be modulated by a variety of agents. Among these biological response modifiers, interferons (IFN) of all three types (α, β, γ) appear to be major regulators of NK cell activity in vivo as well as in vitro.[8,9] Moreover, interleukin-2 (IL-2) has been recently shown to support the continuous growth of LGLs[10] and to boost their NK activity alone[11] or in synergy with IFN and interleukin-1 (IL-1).[12]

Early observations by several investigators (referred to in detail later in the text) suggested the possibility that LGLs might themselves produce lymphokines such as IL-2 and IFN, which in turn modulate their NK function. Evidence has now been accumulated to indicate that LGLs, when appropriately stimulated, secrete a variety of cytokines such as IFN (α, γ), IL-2, B cell growth factor (BCGF), colony-stimulating factors (CSF), and IL-1.

II. IFN PRODUCTION BY LGLs

Trinchieri and co-workers[13] first reported in 1977 that human lymphocytes may be stimulated by some tumor cell lines to produce IFN. This initial observation was later extended by showing that production of IFN was also induced by virus-infected allogeneic fibroblasts.[14] In that study, the cell population responsible for the IFN production was identified as Fc-receptor (FcR) positive, surface immunoglobulin negative, non-T lymphocytes with functional activity of NK cells. In line with the above observations, Timonen et al.[15] reported some evidence that PBLs, possibly LGLs, might produce IFN during contact with the NK-susceptible target K562 tumor cells. Ratliff et al.[16] have reported that the polyclonal activator *Staphylococcus aureus* protein A activated null cells, which consist mainly of LGLs, to produce IFN-α. Moreover, Suzuki et al.[17] have recently reported that murine LGLs secrete IFN-γ during their proliferative response to IL-2. Similarly, Djeu et al.[18] found that human LGLs, purified by discontinuous Percoll density gradient centrifugation, could produce IFN-α as well as IFN-γ in response to polyclonal stimulants such as *Staphylococcus enterotoxin A* (SEA), concanavalin A (Con A), phytohemagglutinin (PHA), bacterial antigens (*Corynebacterium parvum*), and *Mycoplasma*-infected tumor cell lines such as K562 or Molt 4, whereas the same cell lines free of mycoplasma did not stimulate IFN secretion. In further studies,[19] purified LGLs were shown to secrete IFN-α and IFN-γ in response to influenza and herpes simplex viruses, with IFN-γ production dependent on previous exposure to the viruses. Recently, Kasahara et al.[20] have presented data showing that LGLs, depleted of Leu M1$^+$ monocytes (Mϕ) and OKT3$^+$ T lymphocytes, produced high levels of IFN-γ in response to the lectins PHA, Con A, and to phorbol myristic acetate (PMA).

In that study, however, the question of whether a specific subset of LGLs might be responsible for IFN production was not addressed. Trinchieri and Perussia[21] have recently reported that the major subset of PBLs which produced IFN-α in response to viruses co-purified with LGLs and was FcR and DR antigen positive, but lacked surface markers of NK active cells (B73.1$^-$, N901$^-$) as well as T, B, or myelomonocytic cells. Therefore, the above data suggested that IFN-α production and NK activity might be exerted by different subsets of LGL or that the IFN-producing cells were non-LGL in the same low density fractions of Percoll gradient.

Table 1
IL-2 AND IFN-γ PRODUCTION OF LGLs COCULTURED WITH TUMOR CELL LINES

	K562 (effector/target)					RL♂1 (effector/target)				
	—	4/1	8/1	16/1	32/1	—	4/1	8/1	16/1	32/1
IFN-γ[a]										
LGL	0	31,250	15,625	12,500	12,500	0	1887	1887	0	0
TLy	0	5	5	0	0	0	0	0	0	0
IL-2[b]										
LGL	8	15	32	50	40	8	5	0	0	0
TLy	0	3	0	0	0	0	5	0	0	0

Note: LGLs were isolated from PBLs by sequential elutriation, removal of adherent cells on a plastic surface and nylon wool columns, and centrifugation on a discontinuous Percoll density gradient.[39] LGLs were depleted of contaminant LeuM1$^+$ or OKT3$^+$ cells by treatment with αLeuM1 and αOKT3 MoAbs + C. LeuM1$^-$ OKT3$^-$ LGLs were cultured in RPMI 1640 medium (supplemented with 5% FCS 2.5 × 10^{-5} *M* 2 ME, 4 m*M* glutamine, 50 μg/mℓ gentamicin, 10 m*M* HEPES) at 1 × 10^6/mℓ cell concentration in the presence of the indicated concentrations of irradiated (10,000 rad) tumor cells. After LGL supernatants were collected and tested for IFN or IL-2 activity as described, T lymphocytes were recovered from high-density fractions of discontinuous Percoll density gradient and cocultured with tumor cells as described for LGL.

[a] IFN-γ activity is expressed as units per milliliter. Values of ≥10 U/mℓ are considered significant.
[b] IL-2 activity is expressed as units per milliliter. Values of ≥3 are considered significant.

In our studies to identify the cells responsible for IFN-γ production in response to PHA, we have obtained preliminary data indicating that OKT3$^-$ LGL and subsets with or without detectable reactivity with OKT11 or OKM1 and B73.1 monoclonal antibodies (MoAbs) were equally effective producers of IFN-γ (data not shown). Furthermore, in studies of lymphokine production by human LGLs upon interaction with tumor cell lines, we observed that Leu M1$^-$ OKT3$^-$ LGL consistently produced high levels of IFN-γ when cocultured with NK-sensitive targets (K562) while lower or no levels of IFN-γ were produced by LGLs when incubated with a non-NK-sensitive target (RL♂1). In the same studies, OKT3$^+$ T lymphocytes produced little or no IFN-γ when incubated with the same tumor cells (Table 1). Similar results were obtained when tumor membrane preparations were used as stimulants for lymphokine production (data not shown). The positive results with K562 cells could not be attributable to mycoplasma contamination of the cell line. The data suggest that LGLs may be selectively activated by tumor cells such as K562 which are also susceptible to their NK activity.

III. IL-2, BCGF, AND CSF PRODUCTION BY HUMAN LGLs

The possibility that human LGLs might secrete IL-2 was first addressed by Domzig and Stadler,[22] who showed that human LGLs enriched by removal of the E-rosetting cells at 29°C or by depletion of OKT3$^+$ cells produced appreciable levels of IL-2 activity in response to Con A and PMA. These results have been recently extended by Kasahara et al.,[20] who reported that LGLs enriched by discontinuous Percoll gradient centrifugation and depleted of OKT3$^+$ cells were the main producer cells within the PBL population in response to Con A and secreted levels of IL-2 in response to PHA that were comparable to those of unseparated PBL or T cells. In that study, the kinetics of IL-2 production by LGL differed from that of PBL, with similar levels of IL-2 produced from 24 through 96 hr. Moreover, while the IL-2 production by T cells was positively modulated by Mϕ or IL-1, the production of IL-2

Table 2
PRODUCTION OF IL-2 BY LGLs AND SUBSETS OF LGLs

	IL-2 (U/mℓ)	NK activity[a] (LU 30%/10^7)
Exp. a		
LGL[b]	68	222
LGL OKT11$^+$	96	225
LGL OKT11$^-$	14	166
Exp. b		
LGL[b]	125	188
LGL OKM1$^+$	100	481
LGL OKM1$^-$	122	112

[a] NK activity was measured against K562 cell line in a standard 4-hr ^{51}Cr-release assay at different effector to target ratios. Lytic units (LU) were calculated at 30% specific lysis per 10^7 effector cells.

[b] LGLs isolated by discontinuous Percoll density gradient centrifugation were depleted of LeuM1$^+$ or OKT3$^+$ cells by treatment with αLeuM1 and αOKT3 MoAb + C and separated by using an F(ab)$_2$ goat antimouse IgG immunoaffinity column as described elsewhere in this book. The negative fractions were further treated with αOKT11 or αOKM1 MoAb + C. Cells were cultured in RPMI 1640 with 5% heat-inactivated (56°C, 30 min) FCS, 2.5×10^{-5} *M* 2ME, 4 m*M* glutamine, 50 m*M* HEPES 50 μg/mℓ gentamicin, in the presence of 2.5 μg/mℓ phytohemagglutinin A (PHA). After 48 hr, supernatants were collected, dialyzed extensively, and tested for IL-2 as described.[40]

by LGL was not affected by addition of Mφ or IL-1, suggesting that different mechanisms may regulate this function in the LGL population.

By negative selection with MoAb + C treatment, the IL-2 production was attributable to OKT3$^-$, OKT11$^+$, DR$^+$ LGLs, while the question whether the OKT11$^+$ and/or DR$^+$ LGLs might also have regulatory functions on the IL-2 production was not resolved.

We recently addressed in more detail the issue of the phenotype of LGLs which produce IL-2 and whether the IL-2 producing LGLs might also have NK activity. LGLs depleted of any detectable OKT3$^+$ (T lymphocytes) or LeuM1$^+$ (monocytes) cells were separated by immunoaffinity column (as described in Chapter 2, Volume 1) or by fluorescence-activated cell sorter (FACS) into subsets according to their reactivity with OKT11, or α-OKM1 MoAbs. The IL-2 production by these LGL subsets in response to PHA was determined. As shown in Table 2, OKT11$^+$ LGLs were the main producers of IL-2, whereas NK activity was similar in both the OKT11$^+$ and OKT11$^-$ subsets. OKM1$^+$ as well as OKM1$^-$ LGLs produced equal levels of IL-2 activity, but as expected, the OKM1$^-$ LGLs had very low NK activity.

In other experiments, we tested whether highly purified LGLs might secrete IL-2 during the incubation with NK-sensitive targets. Preliminary results indicate that OKT3$^-$, LeuM1$^-$ LGLs consistently secreted significant levels of IL-2 when cultured with NK-sensitive target (K562) but not with NK-resistant targets (RL♂1). Similar results were obtained by using membrane preparations from K562 or RL♂1 tumor cells as stimulants (data not shown). Moreover, in these studies (see Table 1) purified T lymphocytes failed to secrete appreciable levels of IL-2 activity in response to either NK-sensitive (K562) or nonsensitive (RL♂1) targets. The results suggest that LGLs may be selectively stimulated by structures present on the surface of NK-sensitive targets such as K562 tumor cells to secrete IL-2 which in turn, as discussed above, can positively regulate their NK activity.

In addition to the ability of LGLs to secrete IFN, IL-1, and IL-2, LGLs have been shown to have the potential to either positively or negatively regulate B cells. Under some conditions, they can suppress B cell responses,[23] while on the other hand, they have the ability to secrete, in response to PHA, B cell growth factor (BCGF),[24] which appears to be the main proliferative signal for B cells.[27] However, there is as yet no indication as to whether the same or different subpopulation of LGLs is responsible for these divergent effects.

In addition to secretion of IL-2, LGLs purified by Percoll density gradient centrifugation have been shown to produce consistent levels of CSF as seen by promotion of colony and clusters formation in adherent cell-depleted human bone marrow cells.[20] The observed CSF activity was secreted in response to PHA or Con A. Moreover, in contrast with what was observed for IL-2 production, addition of PMA inhibited the CSF production by LGLs in response to PHA, suggesting either that CSF was produced by a subset of LGLs different from that producing IL-2 or that the cytokine secretory response of the same subset may vary with the stimulus.

IV. PRODUCTION OF IL-1 AND ANTIGEN-PRESENTATION FUNCTION BY LGLs

The observation that some LGLs react with OKM1 and DR MoAbs, which detect surface antigens usually associated with myelomonocytic cell types, led us to investigate whether LGLs that have been shown to secrete T cell-associated lymphokines such as IL-2 and IFN[20-22] might also secrete a myelomonocytic-associated cytokine such as IL-1. LGLs isolated by Percoll density gradient centrifugation were further depleted of any detectable T cells ($OKT3^+$ cells) or Mϕ ($LeuM1^+$ cells) and tested for the capacity to secrete IL-1. As shown in Table 3, endotoxin (LPS)-stimulated LGLs produced, on a per cell basis, levels of IL-1 activity that were higher than levels produced by adherent Mϕ. In these studies, removal of $OKT8^+$ cells increased the level of IL-1 secretion, suggesting that $OKT8^+$ suppressor T lymphocytes and/or $OKT8^+$ LGLs may negatively regulate IL-1 production by LGLs. By further separation of the cells by flow cytometry, the subset of LGLs secreting IL-1 was identified as $B73.1^+$,[26] $OKM1^+$, DR^+. In these studies, both $OKT11^+$ and $OKT11^-$ LGLs produced similar levels of IL-1 activity. The question of whether the IL-1-secreting LGLs may also have NK activity was addressed by comparing the levels of IL-1 activity with the level of NK activity of the LGL subsets. The results (see Table 3) showed that both activities were associated in the $OKM1^+$ subset of LGLs. The $B73.1^+$ LGL subset that accounted for virtually all of the NK activity[26] also was the main producer of IL-1. Furthermore, the IL-1-producing DR^+ subset of LGLs (as measured by reactivity with the AF10 MoAb[24]) showed NK activity which, however, was also present in the DR^- LGLs, as previously reported.[7] Both $OKT11^+$ and $OKT11^-$ LGLs exhibited similar levels of NK activity as well as IL-1 production. These results suggest that secretion of IL-1 and NK activity may be expressed by the same cell subset of LGLs. Further support for this possibility came from data obtained with clones of LGLs which showed both cytotoxic reactivity and IL-1 production (see below).

Functionally, the LGL-derived IL-1 was able to stimulate proliferation of human CRL 1445 fibroblasts and to sustain the response of T lymphocytes to phytohemagglutinin (PHA) in the apparent absence of Mϕ (data not shown), both of which are well-established properties of Mϕ-derived human IL-1.[28,29]

The biochemical characterization of the LGL-derived IL-1 revealed a molecular weight

Table 3
IDENTIFICATION OF THE SUBSET(S) OF LGLs PRODUCING IL-1

	Conditions	Percent recovery[a] LGL[d]	Percent recovery[a] Mφ[e]	IL-1 (units/mℓ)[b] LGL[d](p)[f]	IL-1 (units/mℓ)[b] Mφ[e]	NK activity[c] (LU 30%/10^7)
Exp. a	C	96	95	142 (−)	72	372
	LeuM1 + C	92	10	166 (>0.1)	<1	380
	OKT3 + C	88	86	164 (>0.1)	62	402
	OKT3 and LeuM1 + C	86	7	190 (<0.05)	<1	405
	LeuM1 and OKT4 + C	92	NT	145 (>0.1)	NT	390
	LeuM1 and OKT8 + C	90	NT	309 (<0.01)	NT	239
	OKM1 + C	48	30	60 (<0.01)	<1	13
	AF-10 + C	75	16	6 (<0.01)	24	174
Exp. b	LGL			102		222
	LGL OKT11$^+$			70		225
	LGL OKT11$^-$			103		166
	LGL B73.1$^+$			135		321
	LGL B73.1$^-$			15		6
	LGL			125		188
	LGL OKM1$^+$			168		481
	LGL OKM1$^-$			14		2
	LGL			156		240
	LGL DR$^+$			198		180
	LGL DR$^-$			2		215

[a] Final cell number/initial cell number × 100.

[b] IL-1 activity was determined as previously reported.[37]

[c] NK activity was measured against K562 cell line in a standard 4-hr ^{51}Cr-release assay at different effector to target ratios. Lytic units (LU) were calculated at 30% specific lysis per 10^7 effector cells.

[d] In exp. a, LGLs were isolated by discontinuous Percoll gradient (fraction 3) and washed 3× with RPMI 1640. Aliquots were treated with optimal cytotoxic concentrations of the indicated MoAb + complement (low Tox-H rabbit complement, Cedarlane) at 1:10 final dilution. Cells were washed 3× with RPMI 1640 and resuspended in HSA-supplemented medium at 1 × 10^6/mℓ of viable cells.

[e] Adherent monocytes (Mφ) were resuspended with cold PBS containing 10% FCS and treated with the MoAbs as indicated. Both LGL and Mφ populations were stimulated with 25 μg/mℓ LPS as described elsewhere.[35]

[f] The significance level of the data, related to C control, was calculated by Duncan's multiple range analysis of variance; *p* values of ≥0.1 were considered not significant. Data are expressed as the mean of six separate experiments.

In exp. b, LGLs from fraction 3 of discontinuous Percoll density gradient were treated with optimal cytotoxic concentrations of αOKT3 and αLeuM1 MoAb + C. The resulting OKT3$^-$ LeuM1$^-$ LGLs were treated with optimal concentrations of the listed MoAb (5 to 10 μg/mℓ) and then labeled with F(ab)$_2$ goat α-mouse fluoresceinated antibody (Cappel Labs.) at 1:10 final concentration. Cells were analyzed and sorted in positive and negative fractions by flow cytometry (Ortho Cytofluorograph). When reanalyzed, the positive fraction contained more than 98% positive cells. The negative fraction contained less than 2% positive cells. In all the experiments, the negative cell population was further treated with cytotoxic concentrations of the same MoAb + C. Cells were stimulated as described in experiment 2. This experiment was repeated two times with similar results.

of 15,000 on Sephacryl® S-200 gel filtration and charge heterogeneity on isoelectrofocusing, with a major peak at pI 6.8 and two others at pI 5.5 and 4.5 (Figure 1). These data are consistent with those reported for monocyte-derived human IL-1.[28]

A minimal estimate of the frequency of peripheral blood LGLs with the ability to secrete IL-1 was obtained by limiting dilution analysis.[30] OKT3$^-$ LeuM1$^-$ LGLs were cultured in serial twofold dilutions, with a minimum of 12 replicates for each concentration. A culture

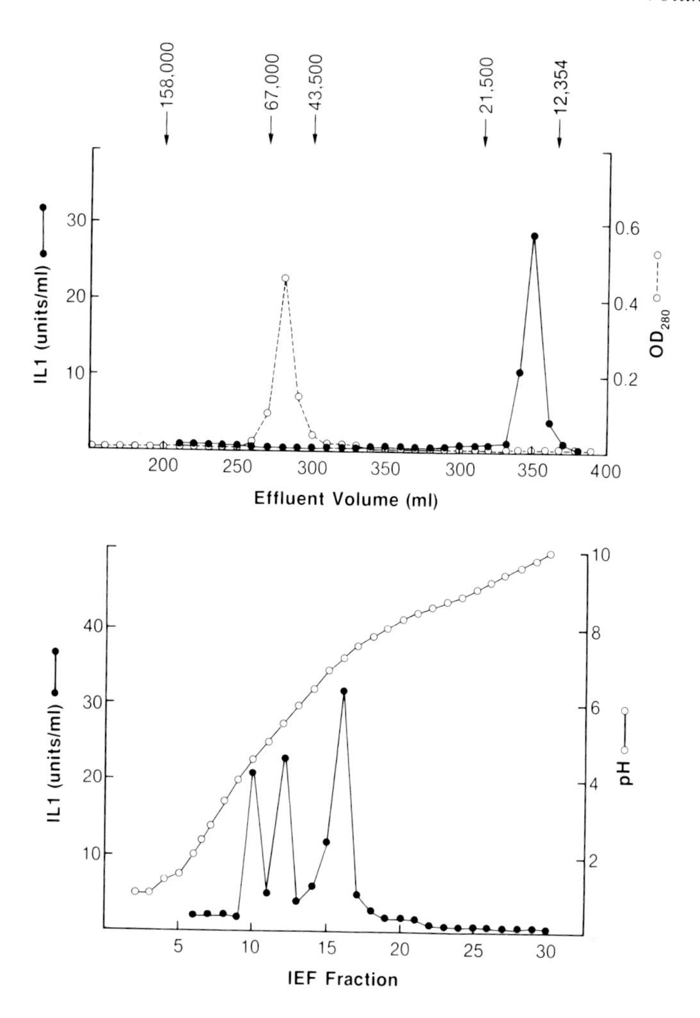

FIGURE 1. Biochemical characterization of LGL-derived IL-1. LGLs were cultured for 48 hr (5% CO_2, 37°C) in the presence of 25 μg/mℓ LPS at 2 × 10^6 cells per milliliter. Supernatants were harvested and utilized for the biochemical procedures; 47.6 g $(NH_4)_2SO_4$ per 100 mℓ were gradually added under gentle stirring to a final concentration of 75%. The precipitated proteins were collected by centrifugation at 5000 g for 10 min, resuspended in PBS, and dialyzed extensively against PBS (with 0.01% polyethylene glycol [PEG] and 50 μg/mℓ gentamicin). The sample was concentrated using Amicon® ultrafiltration unit with PM10 Diaflo® membrane (Amicon) and dialyzed against PBS (with 0.01% PEG and 50 μg/mℓ gentamicin). Aliquots of 2 mℓ were applied to a Sephacryl® S200 (Pharmacia) packed column (2.5 × 90 cm). The column was calibrated with the following markers: aldolase (158,000 mol wt), bovine serum albumin (67,000 mol wt), ovalbumin (43,500 mol wt), soybean trypsin inhibitor (21,500 mol wt), and cytochrome-*c* (12,354 mol wt). The sample was eluted at a flow rate of 20 mℓ/hr with PBS (0.01% PEG, 50 μg/mℓ gentamicin). Aliquots of 3 mℓ were collected, filtered, and tested for IL-1 activity as described.[40] The fractions active in the IL-1 assay (upper panel) were pooled, concentrated by Amicon® ultrafiltration unit as described above, and dialyzed extensively against PBS-0.01% PEG. The sample was loaded onto a preparative isoelectric focusing column (LKB) in a 100-mℓ 5 to 50% sucrose gradient with 0.01% PEG and 2% pH 3.5 to 10 ampholites (LKB). The pH gradient was formed over a period of 18 hr at 1600 V; 3-mℓ fractions were collected and the pH was determined (lower panel). Fractions were dialyzed extensively against PBS (0.01% PEC, 50 μg/mℓ gentamicin), filtered, and tested for IL-1 activity.

was considered positive when ^{3}H-TdR cpm incorporation was more than 3 SD above the mean background incorporation. Preliminary data showed a frequency of LGLs secreting IL-1 in response to LPS of 1/8420. In the case of the OKM1$^+$ subset of LGLs, the frequency of the IL-1-secreting cells was estimated to be 1/4277, while the OKM1$^-$ LGLs had an estimated frequency of 1/29644. These results are consistent with the previous data showing greater IL-1 production by OKM1$^+$ than OKM1$^-$ subsets of LGLs. Since the conditions of the assay, however, limit cell-cell interactions which may play a helper or suppressive role in IL-1 secretion by LGLs, it is very likely that much higher proportions of cells in a given population may actually produce IL-1.

IL-1 is produced by a variety of Ia-DR$^+$ cell types such as monocytes, dendritic cells, and some human B cell lines,[31-33] all of which are effective antigen-presenting cells (APCs). Therefore, it is generally accepted that Ia-DR$^+$ cells with the ability to secrete IL-1 are required as accessory cells for the activation of T lymphocytes. Since some LGLs are both DR$^+$ and secrete IL-1, we tested whether highly purified LGLs might also have antigen-presenting capabilities. As shown in Figure 2, LGLs could function as effective APCs for the proliferative responses of T lymphocytes to the soluble polyclonal stimulant *Staphylococcus aureus* protein A (SPA) or the antigen Streptolysin O (SLO) and for class II antigens in the autologous as well as allogeneic mixed leukocyte reaction (MLR). Further fractionation studies by immunoaffinity columns (see Chapter 2 in Volume 1) identified the subset(s) of LGLs exerting the APC function as OKM1$^+$ DR$^+$, while the OKM1$^-$ DR$^+$ LGLs were less effective and the OKM$^-$, DR$^-$ LGLs were ineffective.[34] As with the above data on IL-1 production, the phenotype of the APC differed from that of Mϕ, with OKT11$^+$ as well as the OKT11$^-$ LGLs in being effective as APC in MLRs for T lymphocyte response to SPA, SLO, or auto- and alloantigens (data not shown). These studies therefore have led to the identification of a nonadherent cell type distinct from monocytes, which has APC function and is a potential contaminant in many "purified" preparations of T lymphocytes.

V. PRODUCTION OF CYTOKINES BY CLONES OF LGLs

The recent finding that LGLs can be expanded in culture in IL-2-supplemented medium[10] has provided a means of obtaining a large number of LGLs with NK activity and to determine the association of surface markers and cytokine-producing capabilities of clones derived from individual LGLs. In preliminary experiments it was calculated that the median frequency of proliferation of LGL populations cultured in IL-2-containing medium was 1/55 (see Chapter 2 in Volume 1). In the experiments summarized in Table 4, purified OKT3$^-$ LGLs were cloned under limiting dilution (0.5 cells per well) conditions in gibbon IL-2-supplemented medium.[35] The resulting clones of LGLs were expanded for several weeks and retested for surface phenotype and NK activity, as well as production of cytokines. These cultured, cloned LGLs were 85% OKT3$^+$, 50% OKT8$^+$, 90% OKM1$^+$, and 30% B73.1$^+$. Results from several clones of LGLs tested showed that noncytotoxic as well as cytotoxic clones could produce IL-1, IL-2, and/or IFN-γ. Among these cytokines, IFN-γ was produced either spontaneously or after stimulation with PHA, by 86% of the clones, thus indicating the physiological relevance of production of this lymphokine for the whole LGL population. In contrast, IL-2 and IL-1 were produced by only 15 and 36% of the cytotoxic clones, respectively. Some clones were observed to produce both IFN-γ as well as IL-2 or IL-1. It was of interest that replicate cultures of one of the LPS-stimulated IL-1-secreting clones also produced low levels of IL-2 activity when stimulated with PHA. In addition, two clones, at different times of culture, produced IL-2 followed by IL-1, indicating that some LGL clones may have the capacity to sequentially express both functions.

In the above studies, no clear-cut dissociation was seen between surface marker phenotype (OKT3, OKT8, OKM1, B73.1) and the type of cytokine produced. This is in contrast with

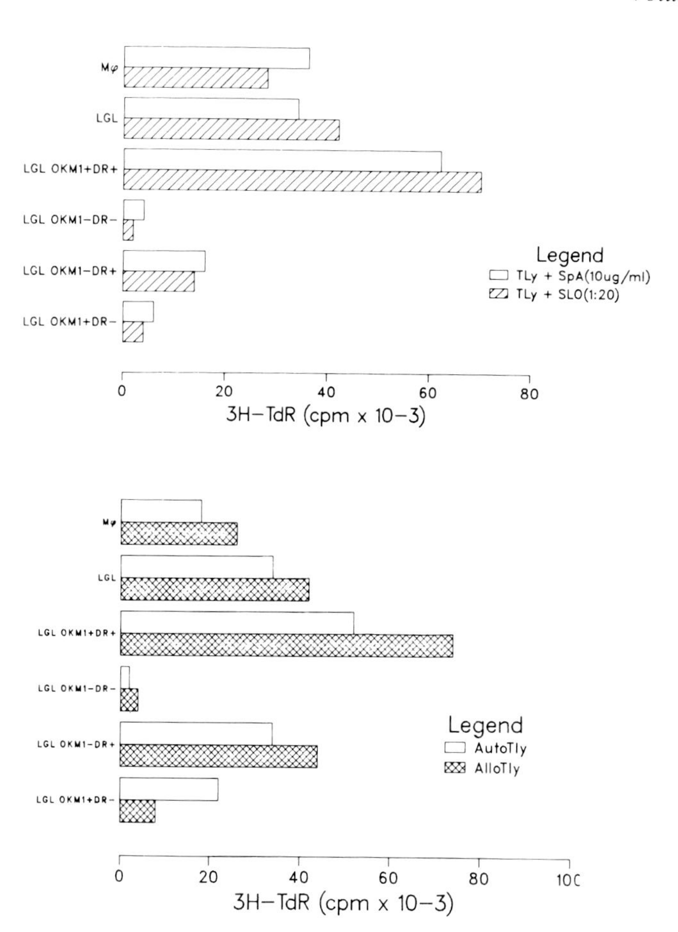

FIGURE 2. Antigen-presenting function of LGL and LGL subsets. LGLs isolated by discontinuous Percoll density gradients were depleted of $LeuM1^+$ (Mϕ) or $OKT3^+$ (T cells) cells by αLeuM1 and OKT3 MoAb + C and then separated according to their reactivity with OKM1 or α-DR MoAbs by using an immunoaffinity column as described elsewhere in this book. The resulting LGL population was cultured in 10% human serum and medium for 3 days (for SPA) or for 6 days (for SLO) with 2.5×10^5 purified T lymphocytes per well at 10% cell concentration in the presence of optimal concentrations of SPA or SLO. For mixed leukocyte reactions, LGL populations were irradiated (3000 rads) and cocultured with 2.5×10^5 autologous or allogeneic T lymphocytes for 2 days. Cultures were pulsed for the last 14 hr with 1 mCi ^{3}H-TdR (1.9 mCi/m*M*). Data are mean of triplicate cultures with the SEM $\leq$ 10% (not shown). Minimal values of background CPM were obtained throughout all the experiments (not shown).

what has been observed by us as well as by other with fresh LGLs, where the IL-1 and IL-2 were produced by phenotypically different subsets.[20,36] These data, however, confirm the general observation that cells cultured for 1 week or more may lose some surface markers and may express new ones, some of which may have been present intracellularly in an ''occult'' form.[37] Furthermore, the above results indicate that by cloning LGLs, we may have selected for a ''precursor'' subset of LGLs with the capacity to exert multiple functions which are usually associated with more differentiated subsets of peripheral LGLs with a more restricted range of functions.

Table 4
PRODUCTION OF CYTOKINES BY LGL CLONES

	Cytokine positive/tested (range of U/mℓ)			
	IFN-γ[a]	IFN-γ[b]	IL-1[c]	IL-2[d]
Total LGL clones	12/12 (10—125)	10/11 (10—625)	9/25 (20—85)	9/20 (3—165)
Cytotoxic LGL clones	5/5 (25—125)	2/2 (10—250)	2/5 (50—60)	2/7 (4—120)
Noncytotoxic LGL clones	7/7 (10—120)	8/9 (10—625)	7/20 (20—85)	7/13 (3—165)

Note: LGLs from low-density fractions of discontinuous Percoll density gradient were cultured under limiting dilution conditions (0.5 cell per well) in IL-2-containing medium.[35] The resulting cell clones were washed extensively and cultured overnight in IL-2-free medium. Cells were tested for cytotoxicity against NK-sensitive tumor cell lines and stimulated for cytokine production for 48 hr.

[a] Spontaneous production of IFN-γ.
[b] PHA (2.5 μg/mℓ)-stimulated production of IFN-γ.
[c] LPS (25 μg/mℓ)-stimulated production of IL-1.
[d] PHA (2.5 μg/mℓ)-stimulated production of IL-2.

VI. CONCLUDING REMARKS

The data briefly summarized in this review indicate that in addition to their cytotoxic activity, LGLs have secretory functions with production of a variety of cytokines such as IL-1,[36] IL-2,[20,22] BCGF,[24] CSF,[20] and IFN-α and IFN-γ.[19-21] For some of these soluble factors, a positive self-regulatory role on NK activity of LGLs has been proposed. All of the three types of NK (α, β, γ) are effective agents in boosting NK activity.[9,19] Recently, IL-2 has been shown to increase the NK activity of LGLs alone[11] and also synergistically with IFN.[12] Moreover, IL-2 may boost NK activity by stimulating LGLs to produce IFN-γ, which in turn may further increase their NK activity (see Chapter 9 in this volume). IL-1 has also been reported to participate in the augmentation of NK activity, synergizing with IL-2 and/or IFN.[12] The preliminary evidence that LGLs produce IL-2 and/or IFN when incubated with the NK-sensitive target K562 may indicate that during the binding and/or the killing phase of NK activity, LGLs may be stimulated to produce IL-2 and/or IFN, which in turn may augment their NK activity.

The positive self-regulatory role of the cytokine production by LGLs is further supported by data obtained with subsets of LGLs and with LGL clones,[35] suggesting that both NK activity and secretory functions may coexist in some individual cells. However, the data also indicate that noncytotoxic subsets and clones of LGLs could produce IL-2 and/or IFN-γ. This suggests that noncytotoxic LGL subsets may provide helper functions for the cytotoxic subsets of LGLs by their production of stimulatory cytokines. Furthermore, the production of cytokines by noncytotoxic LGLs as well as by LGLs with NK activity may be an indication that LGLs have a broader range of immunological functions than just NK activity. In line with this possibility, we have presented data showing that a OKT11$^+$ OKM1$^+$ DR$^+$ subset of IL-1-secreting LGLs exert an effective APC function for T lymphocyte activation.

Further studies will be needed to verify whether LGLs also participate in various immunological functions such as T lymphocyte cytotoxicity, delayed-type hypersensitivity, and helper function for antibody response, by their secretion of IL-1, IL-2, and IFN.[38] The available data strongly suggest that the noncytotoxic functions of LGLs may play a major role in immunoregulation.

REFERENCES

1. **Herberman, R. B. and Ortaldo, J. R.,** Natural killer cells: their role in defense against disease, *Science,* 214, 24, 1981.
2. **Timonen, T., Ortaldo, J. R., and Herberman, R. B.,** Characteristics of human large granular lymphocytes and relationship to natural killer and K cells, *J. Exp. Med.,* 153, 569, 1981.
3. **Kiessling, R., Hochmann, P. S., Häller, O., Shearer, G. M., Wigzell, H., and Cudkowicz, G.,** Evidence for a similar or common mechanism for natural killer cell activity and resistance to hemopoietic grafts, *Eur. J. Immunol.,* 7, 655, 1977.
4. **Warner, J. F. and Dennert, G.,** Effects of a cloned cell line with NK activity on bone marrow transplants, tumour development and metastasis *in vivo, Nature (London),* 300, 31, 1982.
5. **Lotzová, Savary, C. A., and Pollack, S. B.,** Prevention of rejection of allogeneic bone marrow transplants by NK 1.1 antiserum, *Transplantation,* 35, 490, 1983.
6. **Herberman, R. B.,** Lymphoid cells in immune surveillance against malignant transformation, in *Advances in Host Defense Mechanisms,* Vol. 2, Gallin, J. I. and Fauci, A. S., Eds., Raven Press, New York, 1983, 241.
7. **Ortaldo, J. R., Sharrow, S. O., Timonen, T., and Herberman, R. B.,** Determination of surface antigens on highly purified human NK cells by flow cytometry with monoclonal antibodies, *J. Immunol.,* 127, 2401, 1981.
8. **Herberman, R. B., Brunda, M. J., Cannon, G. B., Djeu, J. Y., Nunn-Hargrove, M. E., Jett, J. R., Ortaldo, J. R., Reynolds, C., Riccardi, C., and Santoni, A.,** Augmentation in natural killer (NK) cell activity by interferon and interferon inducers, in *Augmenting Agents in Cancer Therapy,* Hersh, E. M. et al., Eds., Raven Press, New York, 1981, 253.
9. **Ortaldo, J. R., Mason, A., Rehberg, E., Kelder, B., Harvey, C., Osheroff, P., Pestka, S., and Herberman, R. B.,** Augmentation of NK activity with recombinant and hybrid recombinant human leukocyte interferons, in *The Biology of the Interferon System,* De Maeyer, E. and Schellekens, H., Eds., Elsevier, Amsterdam, 1983, 353.
10. **Timonen, T., Ortaldo, J. R., Stadler, B. M., Bonnard, G. D., Sharrow, S., and Herberman, R. B.,** Cultures of purified human natural killer cells. Growth in the presence of Il-2, *Cell. Immunol.,* 72, 198, 1982.
11. **Domzig, W., Stadler, B. M., and Herberman, R. B.,** Interleukin 2 dependence of human natural killer (NK) cell activity, *J. Immunol.,* 130, 1970, 1983.
12. **Dempsey, R. A., Dinarello, C. A., Mier, J. W., Rosenwasser, L. J., Allegretta, J., Brown, T. E., and Parkinson, D. R.,** The differential effects of human leukocytic pyrogen/lymphocyte-activating factor, T cell growth factor, and interferon on human natural killer activity, *J. Immunol.,* 129, 2504, 1982.
13. **Trinchieri, G., Santoli, D., and Knowles, B. B.,** Tumour cell lines induce interferon in human lymphocytes, *Nature (London),* 270, 611, 1977.
14. **Trinchieri, G., Santoli, D., Dee, R. R., and Knowles, B. B.,** Anti-viral activity induced by culturing lymphocytes with tumor-derived or virus-transformed cells. Identification of the anti-viral activity as interferon and characterization of the human effector lymphocyte subpopulation, *J. Exp. Med.,* 147, 1299, 1978.
15. **Timonen, T., Saksela, E., Virtanen, I., and Cantell, K.,** Natural killer cells are responsible for the interferon production induced in human lymphocytes by tumor cell contact, *Eur. J. Immunol.,* 10, 422, 1980.
16. **Ratliff, T., MacDermott, R. P., and Poepping, N. P.,** Production of gamma interferon by human T and null cells and its regulation by macrophages, *Cell. Immunol.,* 74, 111, 1982.
17. **Suzuki, R., Handa, K., Itoh, K., and Kumagai, K.,** Natural killer (NK) cells as a responder to interleukin 2 (IL-2). I. Proliferative response and establishment of cloned cells. II. IL 2-induced interferon and production, *J. Immunol.,* 130, 981, 1983.
18. **Djeu, J. Y., Timonen, T., and Herberman, R. B.,** Production of interferon by human natural killer cells in response to mitogens, viruses, and bacteria, in *NK Cells and Other Natural Effector Cells,* Herberman, R. B., Ed., Academic Press, New York, 1982, 669.
19. **Djeu, J. Y., Stocks, N., Zoon, K., Stanton, G. J., Timonen, T., and Herberman, R. B.,** Positive self regulation of cytotoxicity in human natural killer cells by production of interferon upon exposure to influenza and herpes viruses, *J. Exp. Med.,* 156, 1222, 1982.
20. **Kasahara, T., Djeu, J. Y., Dougherty, S. F., and Oppenheim, J. J.,** Capacity of human large granular lymphocytes (LGL) to produce multiple lymphokines: interleukin 2, interferon, and colony stimulating factor, *J. Immunol.,* 131, 2379, 1983.
21. **Trinchieri, G. and Perussia, B.,** Characterization of interferon producing cells in human peripheral blood, in Proceedings of Symposium on Natural Killer Activity and Its Regulation, August 20—21, 1983, Kyoto, Japan.

22. **Domzig, W. and Stadler, B. M.,** The relation between human natural killer cells and interleukin 2, in *NK Cells and Other Natural Effector Cells,* Herberman, R. B., Ed., Academic Press, New York, 1982, 409.
23. **Arai, S., Yamamoto, H., Itoh, K., and Kumugai, K.,** Suppressive effect of human natural killer cells on pokeweed mitogen-induced B-cell differentiation, *J. Immunol.,* 131, 651, 1983.
24. **Herberman, R. B., Allavena, P., Scala, G., Djeu, J., Kasahara, T., Domzig, W., Procopio, A., Blanca, I., Ortaldo, J., and Oppenheim, J. J.,** Cytokine production by human large granular lymphocytes (LGL), in *Proc. Int. Symp. Natural Killer Activity and Its Regulation,* Excerpta Medica, Tokyo, 1983, in press.
25. **Muraguchi, A. and Fauci, A. S.,** Proliferative responses of normal human B lymphocytes. Development of an assay system for human B cell growth factor (BCGF), *J. Immunol.,* 129, 1104, 1982.
26. **Perussia, B., Starr, S., Abraham, S., Fanning, V., and Trinchieri, G.,** Human natural killer cells analyzed by B73.1, a monoclonal antibody blocking Fc receptor functions. I. Characterization of the lymphocyte subset reactive with B73.1, *J. Immunol.,* 130, 2133, 1983.
27. **Harada, H., Ogata, K., Kasahara, T., Shioiri-Nakano, K., and Kawai, T.,** Isolation of Ia positive human leukocytes by a direct rosette assay, *J. Immunol. Methods,* 59, 189, 1983.
28. **Schmidt, J. A., Mizel, S. B., Cohen, D., and Green, I.,** Interleukin-1, a potential regulator of fibroblast proliferation, *J. Immunol.,* 128, 2177, 1982.
29. **Gary, A. K., Daniele, R. P., and Nowell, P. C.,** A phorbol ester (TPA) can replace macrophages in human lymphocyte cultures stimulated with a mitogen but not with an antigen, *J. Immunol.,* 128, 1776, 1982.
30. **Taswell, C. A.,** Limiting dilution assays for the determination of immunocompetent cell frequencies. I. Data analysis, *J. Immunol.,* 126, 1614, 1981.
31. **Gery, L. and Waksman, B. H.,** Potentiation of the T-lymphocyte response to mitogens. II. The cellular source of potentiating mediator(s), *J. Exp. Med.,* 136, 143, 1972.
32. **Fisher, R. I., Bostick-Bruton, F., Sauder, D. N., Scala, G., and Diehl, V.,** Neoplastic cells obtained from Hodgkin's disease are potent stimulators of human primary mixed lymphocyte cultures, *J. Immunol.,* 130, 2666, 1983.
33. **Scala, G., Kuang, Y. D., Hall, R. E., Muchmore, A. V., and Oppenheim, J. J.,** Accessory cell function of human B cells. I. Production of both interleukin 1-like activity and an interleukin 1 inhibitory factor by an EBV-transformed human B-cell line, *J. Exp. Med.,* in press.
34. **Scala, G., Allavena, P., Ortaldo, J. R., Herberman, R. B., and Oppenheim, J. J.,** New functions of large granular lymphocytes (LGL). I. Accessory cell function by subsets of human LGL defined by monoclonal antibodies, submitted.
35. **Allavena, P. and Ortaldo, J. R.,** Characteristics of human NK clones: target specificity and phenotype, *J. Immunol.,* in press.
36. **Scala, G., Allavena, P., Djeu, J. Y., Kasahara, T., Ortaldo, J. R., Herberman, R. B., and Oppenheim, J. J.,** Human large granular lymphocytes (LGL) are potent producers of interleukin 1, *Nature (London),* in press.
37. **Morgan, A. C., Jr., Schroff, R. W., Klein, R. A., McIntyre, R. F., Mason, A., Herberman, R. B., and Ortaldo, J.,** Occult expression of T, B, and monocyte markers in human large granular lymphocytes, submitted.
38. **Farrar, J. J., Benjamin, W. R., Hilfiker, M. L., Howard, M., Farrar, W. L., and Fuller-Farrar, J.,** The biochemistry, biology and role of interleukin 2 in the induction of cytotoxic T cell and antibody-forming B cell responses, *Immunol. Rev.,* 63, 129, 1982.
39. **Timonen, T. and Saksela, E.,** Isolation of human natural killer cells by density gradient centrifugation, *J. Immunol. Methods,* 35, 285, 1980.
40. **Scala, G. and Oppenheim, J. J.,** Antigen presentation by human monocytes: evidence for stimulant processing and requirement for interleukin 1, *J. Immunol.,* 131, 1160, 1983.

Chapter 9

AUGMENTATION OF NATURAL KILLER ACTIVITY

John R. Ortaldo and Ronald R. Herberman

TABLE OF CONTENTS

I. INTRODUCTION

Natural killer (NK) cells have cytotoxic activity in vitro against a variety of tumor cells, against some microorganisms, and against cells which are infected with microbial agents.[1-11] In addition, there also are indications that NK cells serve as important effector cells in in vivo host resistance against disease.[8,12-14] NK cells are present in virtually all individuals, their activity can be augmented rapidly by a wide range of stimuli,[11,35] their activity does not depend on prior sensitization by antigens,[2,22,36] and NK cells have no major histocompatibility complex (MHC) recognition that is characteristic for cytotoxic T lymphocytes (CTLs).[3,21,22,36] Large granular lymphocytes (LGLs) mediate both NK and K cell (cells mediating antibody-dependent, cell-mediated cytotoxicity [CMC]) activity in mice, rats, and humans.[11,22,37-40] The role of NK cells in the immunoregulation of the immune system has been studied in several areas: (1) that NK cell activity can be positively or negatively regulated by a variety of signals;[11-20,23-35,41-67] (2) NK cells appear to have the ability to serve as immunoregulatory cells since they have been recently demonstrated to secrete a variety of soluble products upon stimulation with a variety of agents.[43,44,59]

The levels of NK activity in rodents have a characteristic age-related fluctuation.[1,3,6,22] In addition, there appear to be considerable differences in cytotoxic potential among various inbred strains of mice with genetically high and low strains with regard to NK function.[3,11,22,68,69] One example of genetic control of function is the C57BL6/beige mutation,[1,6,68] which has been demonstrated to have low NK activity in comparison to nonbeige littermates. In man, however, the characteristic age-related reactivity has not been seen.[22,40] Although normal donors have demonstrated variability, the levels of reactivity within an individual are relatively constant throughout its entire lifespan. However, there have been some reports that HLA phenotype influences the spontaneous level of NK activity.[11,22,54] In studying NK cells, one of the more important aspects of these age-related differences is the determination of the mechanisms responsible for basal levels of cytolytic activity.

Clues to understanding these mechanisms were first obtained when mice inoculated with a variety of viruses or immunoadjuvants such as BCG, *Corynebacterium parvum,* or tumor cells, were demonstrated to undergo a rapid and strong augmentation of NK activity.[2,3,7,8,10,11,18,22,25,31,69] This led to the observation that many agents augmented NK activity by the production of a potent mediator, interferon (IFN) (α, β, or γ).[7,8,11,18,22,25,70] However, to more definitely determine the role of IFN, a number of groups have recently performed experiments with a wide variety of species of IFN, most of which have been purified to homogeneity. With many of these IFNs, the proteins have potent antiviral activity and were produced by genetic engineering and recombinant DNA technology. In addition to examining the effects of these molecules on the cytolytic activity of NK, macrophages (Mϕ), and CTL, it has been possible to study the mechanism of action of IFN augmentation.[71-73] This has included the study of a variety of IFN-related pathways (as determined in the antiviral system), and determining whether these pathways were involved in the activation of NK cells (see Results).

In addition to agents which augment NK activity, a variety of agents have been shown to inhibit NK function. Some of the proposed mechanisms for negative regulation of NK function have been: (1) direct inhibition of functional NK cells, (2) the inhibition of the activity of accessory cells for NK activity, and (3) inhibition by suppressor cells. Although the inhibition of NK activity is not the topic of this review, it should be noted that NK is a highly regulated functional activity. One type of agent, which directly inhibits the function of NK cells and has been studied in detail[14,22,25-27,41,45,57] is the prostaglandins E_1 and E_2. Interestingly, the administration of inhibitors of prostaglandin synthesis (i.e., aspirin, indomethacin) have led to the partial restoration of NK activity in mice with depressed reactivity.[41,45,57] In studies with partially purified human NK cells, a variety of agents have been

Table 1
PROPERTIES OF NK CELLS

	Mouse	Rat	Human
Association with LGs	+	+	+
Adherence to plastic	−	−	−
Adherence to nylon	−	−	−
Fc_γ receptor	+ (weak)	+	+
C3 receptor	−	−	+
Surface Ig	−	−	−
Growth in IL-2	+	+	+
Major surface phenotype			
	NK 1.1,1.2$^+$	OX-8$^+$	B73.1 (Leu 11)$^+$
	Ly5$^+$	OX-1$^+$	OKT8 (Leu 3a,b)$^-$ (25%)
	Ly11$^+$	W3/25$^+$	OKT10$^+$
	Qa5$^+$	Asialo-GM1$^+$	OKM1$^+$
		Ia$^+$ (30%)	MO2 (LeuM1)$^-$
			OKT3 (Leu 1)$^-$
			DR$^+$ (25%)
			Asialo-GM1$^+$

demonstrated to inhibit NK activity, including prostaglandin, cyclic AMP, ATP, and cholera toxin.[11,14,21,22,25,26,45] These inhibitory effects have generally all been highly reversible. Regarding suppressor cells, the depression of NK activity and the induction of suppressor cells have been seen after administration (both in vitro and in vivo) with agents such as carrageenan, corticosteroids, adriamycin, *C. parvum,* etc.[11,22,27,34,55,56,74] The nature of these suppressor cells has not been totally defined; however, adherent cells have been responsible for a number of these inhibitory effects. However, in the *C. parvum*-elicited inhibition of NK cells, nonadherent lymphoid cells have been shown to be responsible for the majority of the suppressor activity induced.[34,74] These results are consistent with the reports of naturally occurring suppressor cells in multiple schlerosis patients, in newborn, and in aged mice.[1,3,12,22] In studies with A strain or SJL mice at various ages,[12,35] it has been noted that 4- to 6-week-old mice had similar levels of NK activity to other strains at the same age. However, by 8 weeks of age, their activity is substantially depressed. Adoptive transfer of adherent cells from SJL mice to high NK strains has been found to inhibit this NK activity.[12,22,25] Overall, the pattern of results has indicated that a number of mechanisms may have been involved in regulation of NK activity both in vivo and in vitro.

II. CHARACTERISTICS OF NK CELLS

NK cells have been associated with a morphological cell type, the LGLs, isolated from discontinuous Percoll gradients. Although some minor differences in properties exist between species, certain features (Table 1) have indicated that this unique cell type in the human, mouse, and rat is responsible for NK activity.[1-5,11,21,37-40,51,58,75-79] NK cells from all three species are nonadherent to both nylon and plastic, possess Fc_γ receptor, and lack complement receptors and surface immunoglobulin. NK cells express a variety of different surface markers. This is especially seen in humans, where LGLs share a number of monocyte- as well as T-related markers (OKM1, OKT8, OKT10, OKT11, respectively).[22,51,79] The ability of LGLs to bind the Fc proportion of the IgG and mediate antibody-dependent cytotoxicity (ADCC) has indicated that NK cells are synonymous with, or at least highly overlap with, killer (K) lymphocytes.[22,26,38,40]

Table 2
RELATIVE ACTIVITIES OF HUMAN LEUKOCYTE IFNs[a]

Species	Antiviral	Growth-inhibitory activity	NK
α_1	59	22	Low
α_2	68	12	Low
β_1	100	N.D.[b]	Low
β_2	45	100	High
β_3	68	6	High
γ_1	45	12	High
γ_2	34	47	Low
γ_3	3.4	16	Low
γ_4	91	5	Low
γ_5	0.45	75	Low

[a] Data were recalculated from Evinger et al.[84] and Ortaldo et al.[49] Antiviral and antiproliferative values are relative to 100% (best IFN); NK was rated high (requiring < 50 units) and low (> 50 units) for boosting.

[b] Not done.

III. AUGMENTATION OF NK ACTIVITY BY IFN

Animal studies examined the in vivo activation of NK activity by a variety of bacterial agents which included BCG and *C. parvum*, as well as synthetic agents such as poly IC and pyran copolymer.[2,3,11-17,21,29,30,34,80] A number of these studies[10,23-25,32,48,58] led to the direct observation that activity of NK cells could be augmented by IFN-α. These early results demonstrated that highly purified IFNs results in the dose-dependent activation of NK cells. A short period of exposure was required for maximal IFN-mediated NK activation, and augmentation had similar metabolic requirements to the antiviral systems.[7,8,11,18,42,50] The abrogation of RNA synthesis would inhibit NK boosting without any significant effect on basal NK activity.[52] Approximately 4 to 6 hr of exposure was required until insensitivity to RNA synthesis inhibitors was shown, which was parallel to the kinetics seen in the antiviral system. DNA synthesis, however, did not appear to be required for IFN-mediated NK boost, as shown by the lack of inhibition of augmentation by X-radiation. Details of the requirements and kinetics of IFN activation of NK cells have been described and reviewed in detail.[11,22,25]

The remainder of the present review will consider recent attempts to determine the structure-function relationship of a variety of different IFN molecules. These types of studies have only been possible because of the availability of recombinant cloned IFNs[23-25,32] especially IFN-α and IFN-γ, which allow testing of biological activity with IFN molecules of known biochemical structure. Since these clone IFN proteins have been shown to be potent activators of human NK cells, they have been purified to homogeneity and have been examined in great detail for their ability augment NK activity on the basis of antiviral units or micrograms of protein.

In recent studies using highly purified natural α-leukocyte IFNs,[25,32] the relative antiviral, antiproliferative, and NK stimulatory activity of these IFNs was studied. These results are summarized in Table 2. It is evident that there was no direct correlation between the antiviral, antiproliferative, and NK stimulatory activities of these various natural IFN-α. In some cases (e.g., IFN-αB_1), the antiviral activity was high and the NK-augmenting activity was low. However, in other cases (IFN-αB_2) the growth inhibitory activity was low and the antiviral and NK stimulatory activity was high. These results have suggested that these activities are

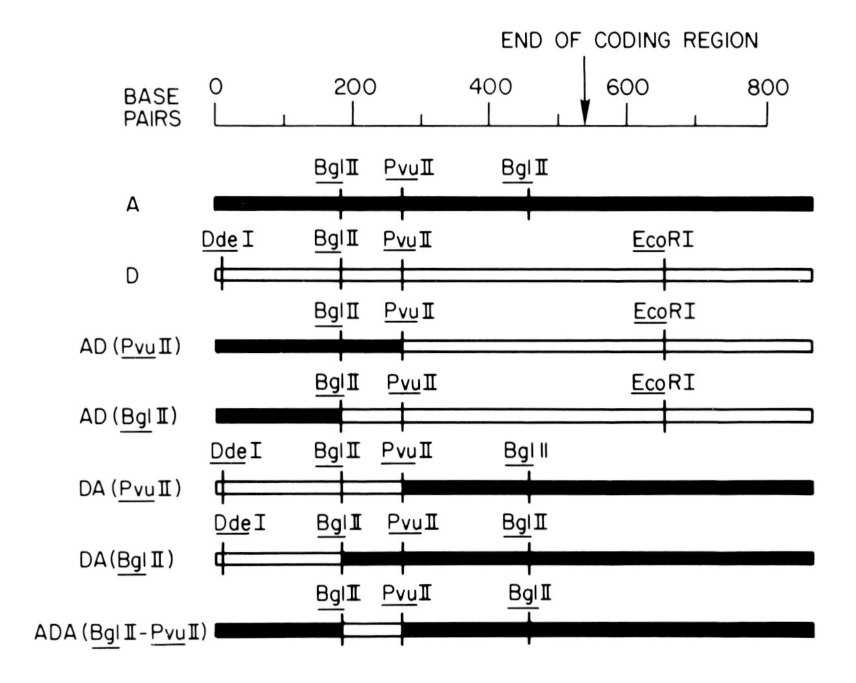

FIGURE 1. Schematic illustration and restriction maps of the coding regions for the mature proteins of IFN-αA, IFN-αD, and hybrids constructed from these two molecules.

independent of one another. Although the IFNs have other biological activities (e.g., the ability to modulate macrophage-mediated cytolysis and cytostasis of tumor cells), our initial studies have concentrated on these three relatively sensitive, as well as diverse, activities of IFN. Because of the ability to both purify and clone IFN-α, recombinant counterparts of the pure natural IFNs are available in pure, large quantities and have enabled us to study in detail their activation of various cellular functions. Because most of these IFNs were purified to homogeneity, we are able to determine their specific molecular activities in antiviral, antiproliferative, and stimulation of NK cell activity. In an attempt to evaluate the molecular nature of these IFNs, various recombinant human IFNs, IFN-αA, IFN-αD, and hybrid leukocyte IFNs,[32,49] were made as schematically illustrated in Figure 1. Comparison of the parental IFNs, IFNαA, IFNαD, as well as the hybrid IFNs (Table 3), demonstrated that an interesting pattern of activities was seen with the IFNs. Although the antiviral activities were essentially similar for all species on bovine cells, their activities on human and mouse cells differed markedly from the parental forms.[49] These various hybrid molecules demonstrated large quantitative differences in their ability to augment the reactivity of NK cells (Table 3). IFN-α A/D (Bgl) consistently gave high levels of augmentation. In addition, IFN-αD/A (Pvu), IFN-αD/A (Bgl) hybrids were quite efficient boosters (two- to sevenfold) compared to the less augmenting effects of the IFN-αA/D (Pvu) and IFN-αA/D/A molecules. Quite interestingly, the relative potency was quite similar between the IFN-αA and the IFN-αA/D (Bgl), since the hybrid was as potent as the parental species.

In addition to examining their activity on human cells, it was quite interesting (because the IFN-αD parental cross-reacted in the mouse system) to examine their possible cross-reactivities on rodent NK activity (Table 3). IFN-αA/D/A, which had no appreciable antiviral activity on mouse cells, demonstrated no augmentation of mouse NK activity. This was also seen with both D/A hybrids. In contrast, however, the A/D hybrids, A/D (Bgl) and A/D (Pvu), which have antiviral activity on mouse cells, demonstrated a strong augmentation of mouse NK activity. Because experimentation was performed with homogeneous material,

Table 3
ABILITY OF PURE RECOMBINANT AND HYBRID RECOMBINANT IFNs TO AUGMENT HUMAN AND MOUSE NK ACTIVITY

	Human NK[a]	Mouse NK[b]
	AD50[c]	
Species of IFN-α	Mean (range)	Mean (range)
A	1.5 (0.5—5)	>5,000[d]
D	7 (5—13)	66 (66)
A/D (Bgl)	1.3 (1—5)	150 (100—200)
A/D (Pvu)	40 (10—100)	450 (300—600)
D/A (Bgl)	20 (0.2—50)	>10,000[d]
D/A (Pvu)	10 (3—20)	>10,000[d]
A/D/A	70 (40—200)	>10,000[d]
Mouse α/β	— —	750 (500—1,000)

[a] Five experiments
[b] Two experiments
[c] Minimal IFN titer (antiviral units per milliliter) required for augmenting NK activity by 50%. All antiviral units for the human IFNs are expressed as the antiviral activity on AG1732 human fibroblasts.
[d] No boost at highest concentration of IFN tested.

this specific molar activity of IFN could be defined as the molecules per cell necessary to elicit a specific effect. This is an operational definition and is not dependent on knowledge of how much IFN protein is binding to the cells. Therefore, the comparison of specific molecular activities of the IFNs provides a useful way to compare the relative effects of IFNs on different cellular activities. However, it should be emphasized that the ultimate description of the ability of IFN to initiate a biological response must be correlated with the ability of IFN to bind to its receptor and its quantitation of specific molecular activity. Table 4 summarizes the results of these calculations in regard to the augmentation of mouse and human NK cells and the number of molecules of IFNs necessary for significant augmentation of human NK activity. With human cells, IFN-αA was a very potent augmentor of NK activity. In contrast, the parental IFN-αD molecule required approximately 300,000 molecules for stimulated NK activity. With the exception of the IFN-αA/D (Bg1), which had a potency similar to the parental IFN-αA, all of the hybrid molecules were less effective than the IFN-αD parental molecule. Therefore, the relative potency of the various IFNs for boosting of human NK activity on a molecular basis, was A/D (Bg1) ≥ A > A/D (Pvu) > A/D/A ≥ D/A (Pvu) > D/A (Bg1) ≥ D. If one ranks these using the antiviral units, although minor differences occur, the general ranking is quite similar. In contrast, substantial differences were seen with these IFNs with regard to the effects on mouse NK activity. The A/D hybrids were found to be considerably more potent than either of the two recombinant parental molecules, with the D molecules showing low-level cross-reactivity, and requiring large amounts of IFN. Efficacy of the IFN-αA/D (Bg1) and the IFN-αA/D (Pvu) species in inducing the mouse NK activity was similar to their potent antiviral effects on mouse cells. An examination of these data in relation to the structure of the hybrids provides some insight into the portion of the IFN molecules required for crossing the species barrier. Comparison of the data obtained with IFN-αA/D/A and the IFN-αA/D hybrids indicates that the C terminal portion of the D molecule is essential for biological activity on mouse NK cells. This conclusion also applies for the antiviral activities for these IFNs. Furthermore, comparison

Table 4
NUMBER OF MOLECULES OF THE VARIOUS RECOMBINANT IFNs REQUIRED FOR BOOSTING OF NK ACTIVITY

	Human cells			Mouse cells		
Species of IFN-α	Concentration of IFN at AD50 (pg/mℓ)	Molarity at AD50 (p*M*)	Required number of molecules per cell	Concentration of IFN at AD50 (pg/mℓ)	Molarity at AD50 (p*M*)	Required number of molecules per cell
A	9.4	0.48	120	$>3.1 \times 10^4$	$>1.6 \times 10^3$	$>3.9 \times 10^5$
D	2.3×10^4	1,172	2.8×10^5	2.3×10^5	1.2×10^4	$>2.8 \times 10^6$
A/D (Bgl)	4.6	0.24	58	535.7	27.6	6,700
A/D (Pvu)	105.2	5.41	1,300	1,184	61	1.4×10^4
D/A (Bgl)	2.0×10^4	1,041	2.5×10^5	$>1.0 \times 10^7$	$>5.2 \times 10^5$	$>1.2 \times 10^8$
D/A (Pvu)	3,703	193	4.6×10^4	$>3.7 \times 10^6$	$>1.9 \times 10^5$	$>4.6 \times 10^7$
A/D/A	1,628	84.7	2.0×10^4	$>2.3 \times 10^4$	$>1.2 \times 10^4$	$>2.9 \times 10^6$

Table 5
MOLECULES PER CELL FOR 50% EFFECT[49a]

IFN	AV[b]	AP	NK
A	4,900	13,000	120
D	360,000	450,000	2.8×10^5
A/D (Bgl)	5,500	9,300	58
A/D (Pvu)	4,100	30,000	1300
D/A (Bgl)	1.5×10^6	910,000	2.5×10^5
D/A (Pvu)	590,000	4.2×10^6	4.6×10^4
A/D/A	36,000	60,000	2.0×10^4

[a] Molecules refer to the minimal number of molecules of IFN required to induce each of the effects.
[b] AV, antiviral activity; AP, antiproliferative activity; NK, stimulation of NK cell activity.

of the data obtained with the IFN-α (Bg1) and the IFN-αA/D (Pvu) hybrids, which only differ in three amino acid substitutions (#69, #80, and #86), indicates that the IFN-αD form of the region conferred a twofold increase on a molecular basis.

With regard to the effects on human cells, molecular differences have not clearly correlated with variations in function and one might attribute the differences in the activity to confirmational changes, which may alter the binding affinity of the various hybrids to the cellular receptors for the IFNs. If comparisons of antiviral, antiproliferative, and NK stimulatory effects are performed based on the number of molecules that result in a 50% effect, some interesting differences in the IFN hybrids can be seen (Table 5). The quantity of each hybrid IFN that is necessary (to produce a 50% effect) is shown and it is evident that the antiviral potency does not directly correspond to the effects on other biological systems. The IFN-αA/D (Pvu), which demonstrates a relatively efficient antiviral effect, requiring only 4900 molecules, is relatively weak in its ability to augment NK activity or exert an antiproliferative effect. Conversely, some IFN species with potent stimulatory effects on antiproliferative and NK activities, e.g., IFN-αA/D (Bg1), do not stand out as being highly potent in inducing antiviral activity. These results indicate that IFNs with different structural configuration segregate independently regarding their efficiency in these biological systems.

In an attempt to directly compare the various biological assays, specific molecular ratios were calculated. These were the antiviral to proliferative ratio and the antiviral to NK ratio (Table 6). Examining the antiviral to NK ratios, as much as a 100-fold difference is seen with some IFNs. This is evident with the IFN-αD (parental molecule) and the IFN-αA/D (Bg1), which demonstrate 100-fold differences, based on their antiviral to NK ratio. In addition, other IFNs, such as the IFN-αA, also demonstrate similar 40- to 50-fold differences, indicating that on a molecular basis these molecules were more potent augmentors of NK than of antiviral effects. Similar types of differences, although quantitatively less marked, are also seen when one examines the antiviral to antiproliferative ratios where 10- to 20-fold differences are seen between IFN-αD/A (Bg1) and the IFN-αA/D (Pvu). Similar suggestions have been made previously when it was observed that individual natural purified human IFN-α exhibited different antiviral and antiproliferative as well as anti-NK stimulatory activity (See Table 2). The ability to clone and to express the gene for the various species of IFN has made it now feasible to produce even larger repertoires of IFNs. The ability now exists to select for IFN molecules that would vary at only one AA residue. These molecules would be useful to probe the structure-function relationship of the IFN sequence and determine if various biological activities would be regulated in parallel. The above results have

Table 6
RATIO OF SPECIFIC MOLECULAR ACTIVITIES[32,84]

IFN	AV/AP	AV/NK
A	0.38	41
D	0.80	1.3
A/D (Bgl)	0.59	95
A/D (Pvu)	0.14	3.2
D/A (Bgl)	1.7	6.0
D/A (Pvu)	0.14	13
A/D/A	0.60	1.8

Note: The AV, AP, and NK ratios were calculated from the data of Table 5.

Table 7
ABILITY OF RECOMBINANT IFNs TO AUGMENT HUMAN NK ACTIVITY

	Augmenting dose[a]; human NK[b]		
Species of IFN-α	Mean	Median	Range
A	1.5	0.5	(0.5—5)
B	1.1	0.1	(0.01—5)
C	1.8	1.0	(0.07—5)
D	7	7	(5—13)
F	89.2	80	(27—170)
I	10.7	8.2	(1.0—29)
J	>10,000	>10,000	(>10,000)[c]
K	29	23	(12—42)

[a] Minimal IFN titer (antiviral units per milliliter) required for augmenting NK activity.
[b] Five experiments.
[c] No boost at 10,000 U/mℓ.

indicated that the biological effects of IFN can be dissociated and support the possibility of different IFN receptors for each of these IFNs. Alternatively, one could postulate the IFN-receptor is a complex, and subtle molecular changes could result in differential activation of various molecular pathways.

In an attempt to more clearly determine the structure-function relationship of the IFN molecules and to understand better the identification of the portions in the sequences of the molecule responsible for the augmentation of NK activity, we have begun to examine a family of recombinant IFN-α species and compare their amino sequences with their ability to augment NK activity (Table 7). Recombinant leukocyte human IFN-αA, B, C, D, F, I, J, K with specific activities of preparations of $\leq 1 \times 10^8$ per milligram per protein (with the exception of IFN-αB, which was approximately 75% protein, and IFN-αF, which was a bacterial extract) were examined for their ability to augment NK activity. The recombinant species of human IFN-α also demonstrated biological diversity. The mean, the median, and the range of IFN activity required to produce significant augmentation of NK activity after a 2-hr incubation is shown. The rank order and potency of these IFNs for stimulating NK activity was $B \cong A \cong C > D > I > K > F > J$.

Table 8
COMPARISON OF AMINO ACIDS IN RECOMBINANT IFNs

IFN	Median concentration for NK cytolysis	Amino acid at position 10	35	40	46	116	132
IFN-αA	0.5	Gly	Asp	Gln	Asn	Ser	Lys
IFN-αB	0.1	Gly	Asp	Gln	Lys	Ser	Thr
IFN-αC	1.0	Gly	Asp	Gln	Asn	Ser	Ile
IFN-αD	7.0	Asp	Asp	Gln	Asn	Ser	Thr
IFN-αF	80.1	Gly	Asp	Gln	Asn	Ser	Thr
IFN-αH	—	Asn	Asp	Gln	Asn	Ser	**Met**
IFN-αI	8.2	Gly	Asp	Gln	Asn	Ser	Thr
IFN-αJ	>10,000	**Arg**	**Glu**	**Glu**	**His**	**Phe**	**Met**
IFN-αK	2.3	Gly	Asp	Gln	Asn	Ser	Thr
IFN-αL	—	**Arg**	Asp	Gln	Asn	Ser	Ile

Species IFN-αH and IFN-αL have not yet been expressed in *Escherichia coli*.

As seen with the natural IFNs, there was much diversity among these various IFNs in their ability to elicit augmentation of NK. IFN-αJ was the only preparation which did not boost the NK activity in a 2-hr pretreatment. IFN-αJ did have some ability to significantly augment NK activity but only upon exposure of cells for 18 hr to very high concentrations (greater than 1000 units) (data not shown). These results indicate that IFN-αJ is distinct from the other IFNs in its defective ability to augment NK activity (2 to 4 logs less than all of the other IFN-α species) despite its high antiviral activity. Preliminary attempts to determine the mechanism of this marked difference have indicated that IFN-αJ, when present together with other IFN-α species, inhibited augmentation in a dose-dependent fashion. Such inhibition did not appear to be due to toxicity, since augmentation of NK activity by pretreatment with IFN-αA or B was not inhibited by subsequent treatment with IFN-αJ. Further studies on the mechanism and the metabolic pathways involved in this blockade as well as binding studies with radiolabeled materials are presently underway.

Several different possibilities may be considered for the failure of IFN-αJ to boost NK activity in a 2-hr pretreatment. In addition, because IFN-αJ has been shown to retain its original level of antiviral activity, inactivation of IFN seems unlikely. From the blocking studies (above), it appears that IFN-αJ binds to receptors for NK cells but lacks the ability to activate the metabolic pathways required for stimulation. Studies in the antiviral system have indicated a number of enzyme pathways that are activated as the direct result of IFN exposure. One pathway, the induction of 2′-5′oligo-A synthetase,[71-73] has been implied in NK activation. It is unknown whether this pathway (or others) are able to be stimulated by IFN-αJ in NK cells.

In reviewing the reported sequences of the IFN leukocyte species, it is interesting to note that IFN-αJ differs significantly from the other leukocyte species at six different positions: #10, #35, #40, #46, #116, #32 (Table 8). For example, position 116, which generally has serine, is substituted by alanine in the IFN-αJ. The contribution of each of the amino acid substitutions in the stimulation of NK cells could be directly tested by introducing single alterations in the nucleotide sequence and testing the resulting mutant IFN molecules for their ability to stimulate NK cells. Because of its methionine substitution at position #132 (which is generally threonine or lysine in the IFN-α molecules), it would be of considerable interest to test the IFN-αH (which is presently unavailable).

The ability to identify leukocyte IFNs with antiviral activity but without appreciable NK-augmenting activity, provides an approach for the dissection of the relative importance of the various cell-mediated activities for in vivo antitumor effects. It would be of interest to explore the relative therapeutic efficacy of IFN-αJ in primates with human tumors shown to be responsive to IFN-αA. In the primate system, the antiproliferative and immunoenhancing effects might be dissected since the NK augmenting ability of the IFN is absent or diminished. In this situation, any results seen might be directly attributable to antiproliferative or antiviral effects and not to its immunoregulatory properties of NK cells.

IFN-γ and its ability to augment NK activity have been of considerable interest. One of the problems associated with testing IFN-γ has been the ability to obtain pure IFN which is devoid of IFN-α.[13,60,62,66,67] This is especially of concern since natural IFN-α species can result in augmentation of NK cells at very low titer (<10 units of antiviral activity). Recently several investigators[63,64] have demonstrated that highly purified IFN-γ or recombinant IFN-γ enhances the activity of NK cells. It is of interest that the major difference seen in the activation of IFN-γ augmentation of NK cells is the kinetics of effect. As discussed above, the activation process of NK cells by IFN-α requires only minutes of exposure to the antiviral agent. However, with IFN-γ maximal activation generally requires longer exposure times (2 to 8 hr),[63,66] with optimal augmentation of cytolysis not seen until 12 to 18 hr. However, this last issue needs further clarification using pure IFN-γ from several sources since most of the mentioned results are from nonglycosylated recombinant IFN.

IV. MECHANISM OF IFN-INDUCED AUGMENTATION OF NK ACTIVITY

The results of a number of laboratories support the basic concept that NK can be augmented by IFN at several distinct steps in the sequence of cytolysis.[25,56,81] The use of the single-cell assay[27,67,69] has allowed dissection of various events which occur in the activation processes of NK cells. In the augmentation of NK cells, several possibilities exist. First, the rate at which NK cells kill or their level of activity may be increased. Second, the number of effector cells which bind to target cells may be increased by induction of receptors for target cells. Third, nonlytic binders may be activated to develop lytic activity. Fourth, the rate of recycling of effector cells is increased. By use of combinations of the single-cell binding assay, the single-cell cytotoxicity assay, and the Cr-release cytotoxicity assay, one can dissect the effects of IFN on the activity of NK cells.[22,25,40,58] If these detailed studies are performed with a variety of NK-susceptible targets, all four effects can be seen with IFN-pretreated NK cells. With highly NK-susceptible targets such as K562, there is no detectable increase in the number of effector cells which bind.[55,56] In contrast, with low NK-susceptible targets IFN pretreatment of NK cells results in a significant increase in binders. In addition, significant increases in the number of lytic binders have been demonstrated as well as increases in the rate of lysis. Therefore, as previously reviewed,[25,36] the stimulation of NK cells by IFN appears to be at multiple levels: activation of pre-NK cells to bind and/or to become lytic, and stimulation of the levels of activity of NK cells. The overall effect is considerable augmentation in the cytolytic activity of these natural effector cells. In addition, recent results have indicated that IFN can also increase the recycling capacity of NK cells, therefore enabling the same effector cell to lyse more than one cell during the course of the assay.[21,22,58]

In addition to the augmentation of NK activity, IFN has been demonstrated to have a variety of other effects on LGLs (Table 9). IFN pretreatment of LGLs results in reduced DNA synthesis, reduced RNA synthesis, and reduced protein synthesis. Such effects, especially on RNA and protein synthesis, are similar to those associated with induction of the antiviral state. As indicated above, IFN enhances the binding capacity of NK cells to selected targets and also enhances their expression of FcR and of histocompatibility antigens.[64] It also has recently been shown that IFN enhances the ability of LGLs to grow in response to IL-2.[82]

Because of the considerable information on the metabolic pathways associated with in-

Table 9
RANGE OF EFFECTS OF IFN ON LGLs

Reduces DNA synthesis
Reduces RNA synthesis
Reduces protein synthesis
Induces 2′-5′ A synthetase
Induces protein kinase
Enhances binding of LGLs to some targets
Enhances Fc_γ receptor
Enhances histocompatibility antigens
Enhances the IL-2 response

Table 10
STIMULATION OF 2′-5′ A SYNTHETASE IN HUMAN LGLs BY IFN-αA

Treatment time	CPM (^{32}P) (2′-5′) oligo (A)/mg protein	Stimulation index
0	4,770	1.0
2	3,695	0.8
5	10,262	2.2
18	14,898	3.1

duction of the antiviral state,[71-73] it has been of interest to determine whether any of these pathways are involved in the activation of NK activity. Therefore, the importance of the 2′-5′ oligo-A synthetase pathway was examined by testing the ability of the 2′-5′ oligo-A to mimic the effects of IFN. When 2′-5′ pppApApA molecules were introduced into permeabilized cells, cellular ribonuclease activity, and inhibition of protein synthesis were observed.[1,46,76] Using this procedure, Schmidt et al.[85] demonstrated the ability of the 2′-5′ pppApApA to enhance NK activity, thereby implicating the 2′-5′ oligo-A synthetase pathway in the mechanism of NK augmentation by IFN. The activation of this pathway by IFN in LGLs was confirmed by direct measurements of 2′-5′ oligo-A synthetase activity using ^{32}P-labeled 2′-5′ oligo-A (Table 10). However, to directly examine the relationship of this pathway in cytolysis, the 2′-5′ pppA product (by-passing synthetase) was introduced into the cells by calcium chloride precipitation, which was required because of its impermeability of the intact cell membrane to this compound. As shown in Table 11, a significant increase in NK cytolysis was observed when increasing amounts of the material was introduced into the cells. These results indicate that not only is the increase in the activity of NK cells accompanied by an increase in 2′-5′ oligo-A synthetase, but introduction of the product of the enzyme into LGLs was able to mimic the effect of IFN and to augment cytolytic activity. Although it is possible that the enhancement of the NK activity by the 2′-5′ pppApApA-treated cells resulted from a non-IFN-related effect, the ability of the calcium-induced end product of the 2′-5′ A synthetase to increase cytolysis provides strong evidence for involvement of this biochemical pathway in IFN-induced augmentation of LGL killing. In addition, it should be noted that the level of the 2′-5′ oligo-A synthetase (see Table 10) in untreated LGLs is relatively high compared to the basal activity reported in most nonlymphoid cells.[71,72] This finding is in agreement with reports on the basal activity of enzyme in cells of the reticuloendothelial system and mouse splenic lymphocytes.[72] Although the mechanism of IFN-induced NK activation is still not precisely defined at the molecular level, the present results provide some insight into the mechanism of augmentation of NK activity after IFN binding.

Table 11
EFFECT OF 2′-5′ pppApApA ON NK ACTIVITY

NK cells	$CaCl_2$	$pppA_3$ (μM)	Percent cytolysis 17:1[a]	6:1
+	–	–	40	30
+	+	–	13	6
+	+	6.7	18[b]	6
+	+	16.7	26[b]	15[b]
+	+	33.3	27[b]	16[b]

[a] Effector to target ratio.
[b] Significant increase compared to $CaCl_2$ control ($p \leq 0.05$).

V. AUGMENTATION OF NK ACTIVITY BY AGENTS OTHER THAN IFN

Several agents have appeared to activate NK cells by non-IFN-mediated pathways. These have been recently reviewed[11,21,25] and include the treatment of NK cells with antibodies directed against H2, IA, or Thy-1 antigens or with lectins, such as phytohemagglutinin or wheat germ agglutinin or viral glycoproteins isolated from viruses such as mumps, measles, or Sendai. Generally, these agents result in augmentation of lysis against a variety of different targets within a few hours of treatment, without any detectable induction of IFN. However, one must question whether these are truly IFN-independent events or whether low levels of IFN production might be responsible for these events. Although some studies have shown that the augmentation occurred even after the inhibition of protein and RNA synthesis, which inhibits IFN-mediated augmentation, more detailed experiments are needed to eliminate the possibility that low levels of IFN may mediate augmentation through classical pathways.

One agent which recently has received a great deal of attention regarding its ability to augment mouse, rat, and human NK cells has been IL-2.[28,35,44,62,64,65,82,83] This lymphokine, which was first reported as a growth-promoting factor for T cells, has recently been shown to also affect growth of NK cells. In addition to its ability to promote the proliferation of NK cells, it has also been shown to augment NK activity. Recently, we have examined highly purified homogeneous preparations of IL-2 from the MLA 144 primate cell line.[83] This IL-2 preparation had the ability to enhance the NK activity of highly purified LGL after incubation for as little as 6 hr with effector cells. Maximal activation occurred (especially with low doses of IL-2) at 18 hr of preincubation (Table 12). This slower kinetics compared to that seen with IFN-α led to further examination into the mechanism of the IL-2 boosting. We found that IL-2 can act directly on LGLs, stimulating them to release IFN-γ.[62,64,65] The augmentation of cytolysis by LGL could be blocked, at least in part, by monoclonal antibodies (MoAbs) to IFN-γ (Table 12), indicating that this cytokine was the proximal activating factor. Thus, it appears that IL-2 binds to the LGL, resulting in the production of significant levels of IFN-γ, which in turn leads to the augmentation of NK activity. Previous reports indicating that IFN was not detected in the supernatants may have in fact (1) not significantly examined long-term incubations, (2) not used MoAbs directed against IFNs to rule out and elucidate the mechanism of augmentation, or (3) not employed sensitive assays to detect IFN-γ. The possibility of low levels of IFN-γ production being responsible for the augmenting effects of many agents must be considered in light of recent results[11,16] that a variety of stimuli can induce NK cells to produce IFN-γ as well as IFN-α and IFN-β.

Table 12
IL-2 BOOSTING OF NK CELLS: EFFECTS OF ANTI-IFN-γ

Treatment (18 hr)	LU (30%)		IFN-γ (U/mℓ)
None	32		<20
		} (36.1)[a]	
None	39		<20
IL-2 (MLA-144)	151		320
		} (145.5)	
IL-2 (MLA-144)	140		320
IL-2 + anti-IFN-γ (10^0)[b]	49		40
IL-2 + anti-IFN-γ (10^{-1})	72		40
IL-2 + anti-IFN-γ (10^{-2})	85		160

[a] Mean of duplicate negative or positive controls.
[b] Concentration of MoAb capable of neutralizing 1000 units of IFN-γ. Dilutions shown below are of this concentration (i.e., 1000, 100, 10 neutralizing units, respectively).

Note Added During Proof

In addition to data presented in Table 12, we recently have tested three purified Ig monoclonal antibodies to IFN-γ. These three antibodies to IFN-γ could not block the rIL-2 induction of NK activity, demonstrating that IFN-γ was not involved in the enhancement of NK activity by IL-2. The anti-IFN-γ antibody preparations (used in Table 12) showed significant inhibition of rIL-2-induced augmentation of NK activity, but the inhibition was found to be attributable to antibody-unrelated factors in the antiserum or ascites fluid.[86] In addition, several sources of recombinant IFN-γ were shown to have little or no ability to augment NK activity.[86] Our results now demonstrate that IFN-γ produced by rIL-2 treatment of human PBL does not play an essential role in increasing NK activity in most donors and that IL-2-induced augmentation of NK activity is due to the direct action of IL-2 on LGL.

VI. SUMMARY AND CONCLUSIONS

IFNs (α, β, and γ) have been shown to be very potent modulators of NK activity. Perhaps the most important question remaining is whether IFN is the sole positive regulator for NK activity or whether other factors may exist. However, as demonstrated, the IL-2-mediated mechanism of activation (previously thought to be independent of IFN), involves the production of IFN-γ and can be demonstrated by the neutralization of augmentation of NK activity by MoAbs to IFN-γ. It has also been recently reported that in addition to NK cells being responsive to IFN, they are a major producer of IFNs in response to various stimuli. Under a variety of conditions, highly purified LGLs have been shown to be able to produce substantial amounts of IFN[43,59] and also Il-1, Il-2, BGGF, CSF (see Chapter 8 in this volume) in response to a wide variety of stimuli. These have included tumor cell lines, viruses, BCG, *C. parvum,* and various mitogens and bacterial products. These observations of production of IFNs and other cytokines by highly enriched NK cell populations, have several important and interesting implications: (1) these results demonstrate that NK cells appear to be a major source of IFN production, which would allow them to function as immunoregulatory cells; (2) the ability of NK cells to produce IFN suggests that they have an alternative mechanism for host defense in addition to their direct cytotoxic activity; (3) they raise the interesting possibility that the effector cell population may be self-regulated in its ability to recognize and activate other populations of LGLs or themselves by the production of cytokines.

REFERENCES

1. **Clark, E. A., Russell, R. H., Egghart, M., and Horton, M. A.,** Characteristics and genetic control of NK-cell-mediated cytotoxicity by naturally acquired infection in the mouse, *Int. J. Cancer,* 24, 688, 1979.
2. **Henney, C. S., Tracey, D., Durdik, J. M., and Klimpel, G.,** Natural killer cells in vitro and in vivo, *Am. J. Pathol.,* 93, 459, 1978.
3. **Herberman, R. B. and Holden, H. T.,** Natural cell-mediated immunity, *Adv. Cancer Res.,* 27, 305, 1978.
4. **Herberman, R. B., Nunn, M. E., and Holden, H. T.,** Low density of thy 1 antigen on mouse effector cells mediating natural cytotoxicity against tumor cells, *J. Immunol.,* 121, 304, 1978.
5. **Reynolds, C. W., Timonen, T., and Herberman, R. B.,** Natural killer (NK) cell activity in the rat. I. Isolation and characterization of the effector cells, *J. Immunol.,* 127, 282, 1981.
6. **Roder, J. and Duwe, A.,** The beige mutation in the mouse selectively impairs natural killer cell function, *Nature (London),* 278, 451, 1979.
7. **Trinchieri, G. and Santoli, D.,** Anti-viral activity induced by culturing lymphocytes with tumor-derived or virus-transformed cells. Enhancement of natural killer activity by interferon and antagonistic inhibition of susceptibility of target cells to lysis, *J. Exp. Med.,* 147, 1314, 1978.
8. **Trinchieri, G., Santoli, D., Dee, R. R., and Knowles, B. B.,** Antiviral activity by culturing lymphocytes with tumor-derived or virus-transformed cells: identification of the antiviral activity as interferon and characterization of the human effector lymphocyte subpopulation, *J. Exp. Med.,* 147, 1229, 1978.
9. **Vose, B. M.,** Natural killers in human cancer: activity of tumor-infiltrating and draining node lymphocytes, in *Natural Cell-Mediated Immunity Against Tumors,* Herberman, R. B., Ed., Academic Press, New York, 1980, 1081.
10. **Welsh, R. M., Zinkernagel, R. M., and Hallenbeck, L. A.,** Cytotoxic cells induced during lymphocytic choriomeningitis virus infection of mice. II. Specificities of the natural killer cells, *J. Immunol.,* 122, 475, 1979.
11. **Welsh, R. M.,** Natural killer cells and interferon, in *CRC Crit. Rev. Immunol.,* 5(1), 55, 1984.
12. **Zarling, J. M., Eskra, L., Borden, E. C., Hooszewicz, J., and Carter, W. A.,** Activation of human natural killer cells cytotoxic for human cells by purified interferon, *J. Immunol.,* 123, 63, 1979.
13. **Wallach, D.,** Regulation of susceptibility to natural-killer cells cytotoxicity and regulation of HLA syntheses — differing efficacies of alpha-interferon, beta-interferon, and gamma-interferon, *J. Interferon Res.,* 2, 329, 1982.
14. **Lang, N. P., Ortaldo, J. R., Bonnard, G. D., and Herberman, R. B.,** Effects of interferon and prostaglandins on human natural and lectin-induced cytotoxicity, *J. Natl. Cancer Inst.,* 69, 339, 1982.
15. **Brunda, M. J., Herberman, R. B., and Holden, H. T.,** Interferon-independent activation of murine natural killer cell activity, in *Natural Cell-Mediated Immunity Against Tumors,* Herberman, R. B., Ed., Academic Press, New York, 1980, 525.
16. **Brunda, M. J., Herberman, R. B., and Holden, H. T.,** Antibody-induced augmentation of murine natural killer cell activity, *Int. J. Cancer,* 27, 205, 1981.
17. **Brunda, M. J., Varesio, L., Herberman, R. B., and Holden, H. T.,** Interferon-independent, lectin-induced augmentation of murine natural killer cell activity, *Int. J. Cancer,* 29, 299, 1982.
18. **Djeu, J. Y., Heinbaugh, J. A., Holden, H. T., and Herberman, R. B.,** Augmentation of mouse natural killer cell activity by interferon and interferon inducers, *J. Immunol.,* 122, 175, 1979.
19. **Gidlund, M., Örn, A., Wigzell, H., Senik, A., and Gresser, I.,** Enhanced NK cell activity in mice injected with interferon and interferon inducers, *Nature (London),* 223, 259, 1978.
20. **Goldfarb, R. H. and Herberman, R. B.,** Natural killer cell reactivity: regulatory interactions among phorbol ester, interferon, cholera toxin and retinoic acid, *J. Immunol.,* 126, 2129, 1981.
21. **Herberman, R. B., Ed.,** *Natural Cell-Mediated Immunity Against Tumors,* Academic Press, New York, 1980.
22. **Herberman, R. B. and Ortaldo, J. R.,** Natural killer cells: their role in defenses against disease, *Science,* 214, 24, 1981.
23. **Herberman, R. B., Ortaldo, J. R., Mantovani, A., Hobbs, D. S., Kung, H.-F., and Pestka, S.,** Effect of human recombinant interferon on cytotoxic activity of natural killer (NK) cells and monocytes, *Cell. Immunol.,* 67, 160, 1982.
24. **Herberman, R. B., Ortaldo, J. R., Rubinstein, M., and Pestka, S.,** Augmentation of natural and antibody-dependent cell-mediated cytotoxicity by pure human leukocyte interferon, *J. Clin. Immunol.,* 1, 149, 1981.
25. **Herberman, R. B., Ortaldo, J. R., Timonen, T., Reynolds, C. W., Djeu, J. Y., Pestka, S., and Stanton, J.,** Interferon and natural killer (NK) cells, in *The Interferon System: A Review of 1982. Texas Reports on Biology and Medicine,* Vol. 41, Baron, et al., Eds., University of Texas Medical Branch, Galveston, 1980, 590.

26. **Kendall, R. A. and Targan, S.,** The dual effect of prostaglandin (PGE2) and ethanol on the natural killer cytolytic process: effector activation and NK-target cell conjugate lytic inhibition, *J. Immunol.*, 125, 2770, 1981.
27. **Koren, H. S., Anderson, S. J., Fischer, D. G., Copeland, C. S., and Jensen, P. J.,** Regulation of human natural killing. I. Role of monocytes, interferon, and prostaglandins, *J. Immunol.*, 127, 2007, 1981.
28. **Kurabayashi, K., Gillis, S., Kern, D. E., and Henney, C. S.,** Murine NK cell cultures: effects of interleukin-2 and interferon on cell growth and cytotoxic reactivity, *J. Immunol.*, 126, 2321, 1981.
29. **Lotzová, E.,** *C. parvum*-mediated suppression of the phenomenon of natural killing and its analysis, in *Natural Cell-Mediated Immunity Against Tumors,* Herberman, R. B., Ed., Academic Press, New York, 1980, 735.
30. **Lotzová, E. and Gutterman, J. V.,** Effect of glucan on natural killer (NK) cells: further comparison between NK cell and bone marrow effector cell activities, *J. Immunol.*, 123, 607, 1979.
31. **Oehler, J. R., Lindsay, L. R., Nunn, M. E., Holden, H. T., and Herberman, R. B.,** Natural cell-mediated cytotoxicity in rats. II. In vivo augmentation of NK-cell activity, *Int. J. Cancer,* 21, 210, 1978.
32. **Ortaldo, J. R., Mantovani, A., Hobbs, D., Rubinstein, M., Pestka, S., and Herberman, R. B.,** Effects of several species of human leukocyte interferon on cytotoxic activity of NK cells and monocytes, *Int. J. Cancer,* 31, 285, 1983.
33. **Reynolds, C. W. and Herberman, R. B.,** In vitro augmentation of rat natural killer (NK) cell activity, *J. Immunol.*, 126, 1581, 1981.
34. **Riccardi, C., Barlozzari, T., Santoni, A., Cesarini, C., and Herberman, R. B.,** Regulation of in vivo reactivity of natural killer (NK) cells, in *NK Cells and Other Natural Effector Cells,* Herberman, R. B., Ed., Academic Press, New York, 1982, 549.
35. **Riccardi, C., Vose, B. M., and Herberman, R. B.,** Regulation by interferon and T cells of IL-2 dependent growth of NK progenitor cells: a limiting dilution analysis, in *NK Cells and Other Natural Effector Cells,* Herberman, R. B., Ed., Academic Press, New York, 1982, 909.
36. **Kärre, K., Klein, G. O., Kiessling, R., Klein, G., and Roder, J. C.,** Low natural in vivo resistance to syngeneic leukemias in natural killer-deficient mice, *Nature (London),* 284, 624, 1980.
37. **Herberman, R. B., Bartram, S., Haskill, J. S., Nunn, M., Holden, H. T., and West, W. H.,** Fc receptors on mouse effector cells mediating natural cytotoxicity against tumor cells, *J. Immunol.*, 119, 322, 1977.
38. **Oehler, J. R., Lindsay, L. R., Nunn, M. E., and Herberman, R. B.,** Natural cell-mediated cytotoxicity in rats. I. Tissue and strain distribution and demonstration of a membrane receptor for the Fc portion of IgG, *Int. J. Cancer,* 21, 204, 1978.
39. **Perlmann, H., Perlmann, P., Pape, D. R., and Halden, G.,** Purification fractionation and assay of antibody-dependent lymphocyte effector cells (K cells), *Scand. J. Immunol.*, 5, 5, 1976.
40. **Timonen, T., Ortaldo, J. R., and Herberman, R. B.,** Characteristics of human large granular lymphocytes and relationship to natural killer and K cells, *J. Exp. Med.*, 153, 569, 1981.
41. **Brunda, M. J., Herberman, R. B., and Holden, H. T.,** Inhibition of murine natural killer cell activity by prostaglandins, *J. Immunol.*, 124, 2682, 1980.
42. **Djeu, J. Y., Heinbaugh, J. A., Holden, H. T., and Herberman, R. B.,** Role of macrophages in the augmentation of mouse natural killer cell activity by poly I:C and interferon, *J. Immunol.*, 122, 182, 1979.
43. **Djeu, J. Y., Stocks, N., Zoon, K., Stanton, G. J., Timonen, T., and Herberman, R. B.,** Production of interferon by human large granular lymphocytes upon exposure to influenza and herpes viruses, *J. Exp. Med.*, 156, 1222, 1982.
44. **Domzig, W. and Stadler, B. M.,** The relation between human natural killer cells and interleukin 2, in *NK Cells and Other Natural Effector Cells,* Herberman, R. B., Ed., Academic Press, New York, 1982, 409.
45. **Droller, M. J., Schneider, M. V., and Perlmann, P.,** A possible role of prostaglandins in the inhibition of natural and antibody-dependent cell-mediated cytotoxicity against tumor cells, *Cell. Immunol.*, 39, 165, 1978.
46. **Einhorn, S., Blomgren, H., and Strander, H.,** Interferon and spontaneous cytotoxicity in man. I. Enhancement of the spontaneous cytotoxicity of peripheral lymphocytes by human leukocyte interferon, *Int. J. Cancer,* 22, 405, 1978.
47. **Farrar, W. L., Johnson, H. M., and Farrar, J. J.,** Regulation of the production of immune interferon and cytotoxic T lymphocytes by interleukin 2, *J. Immunol.*, 126, 1120, 1981.
48. **Herberman, R. B., Ortaldo, J. R., and Bonnard, G. D.,** Augmentation by interferon of human natural and antibody-dependent cell-mediated cytotoxicity, *Nature (London),* 277, 221, 1979.
49. **Ortaldo, J. R., Mason, A., Rehnbey, E., Moscheru, J., Kelder, B., Pestka, S., and Herberman, R. B.,** Effects of recombinant and hybrid recombinant human leukocyte interferons on cytotoxic activity of natural killer cells, *J. Biol. Chem.*, 258, 15,011, 1983.

50. **Ortaldo, J. R., Phillips, W., Wasserman, K., and Herberman, R. B.,** Effects of metabolic inhibitors on spontaneous and interferon-boosted natural killer cell activity, *J. Immunol.*, 125, 1839, 1980.
51. **Ortaldo, J. R., Sharrow, S. O., Timonen, T., and Herberman, R. B.,** Determination of surface antigens on highly purified human NK cells by flow cytometry with monoclonal antibodies, *J. Immunol.*, 121, 304, 1978.
52. **Reynolds, C. W., Brunda, M. J., Holden, H. T., and Herberman, R. B.,** Role of macrophages in in vitro augmentation of rat, mouse and human natural killer activities, *J. Natl. Cancer Inst.*, 66, 837, 1981.
53. **Riccardi, C., Santoni, A., Barlozzari, T., Cesarini, C., and Herberman, R. B.,** Suppression of natural killer (NK) activity by splenic adherent cells of low NK-reactive mice, *Int. J. Cancer*, 28, 811, 1981.
54. **Santoli, D., Trinchieri, G., Zmijewski, C. M., and Koprowski, H.,** HLA-related control of spontaneous and antibody-dependent cell-mediated cytotoxic activity in humans, *J. Immunol.*, 117, 765, 1976.
55. **Santoni, A., Riccardi, C., Barlozzari, T., and Herberman, R. B.,** Suppression of activity of mouse natural killer (NK) cells by activated macrophages from mice treated with pyran copolymer, *Int. J. Cancer*, 26, 837, 1980.
56. **Sulica, A., Gherman, M., Galatiuc, C., Manciulea, M., and Herberman, R. B.,** Inhibition of human natural killer cell activity by cytophilic immunoglobulin G, *J. Immunol.*, 128, 1031, 1982.
57. **Targan, S. R.,** The dual interaction of prostaglandin E_2 (PGE_2) and interferon (IFN) on NK lytic activation: enhanced capacity of effector-target lytic interactions (recycling) and blockage of pre-NK cell recruitment, *J. Immunol.*, 127, 1424, 1981.
58. **Timonen, T., Ortaldo, J. R., and Herberman, R. B.,** Analysis by a single cell cytotoxicity assay of natural killer (NK) cell frequencies among human large granular lymphocytes and of the effects of interferon on their activity, *J. Immunol.*, 128, 2514, 1982.
59. **Djeu, J. Y., Timonen, T., and Herberman, R. B.,** Production of interferon by humam natural killer cells in response to mitogens, viruses and bacteria, in *NK Cells and Other Natural Effector Cells*, Herberman, R. B., Ed., Academic Press, New York, 1982, 669.
60. **Saito, M., Yamaguchi, T., Aonuma, E., Noda, T., Edina, T., and Ishida, N.,** Antitumor effect of OK-432. I. Antitumor effect of OK-432 induced interferon-gamma, *Gan To Kagaku Ryoho*, 9, 2031, 1982.
61. **Kawase, I., Brooks, C. G., Kuribayashi, K., Olabuenaga, S., Newman, W., Gillis, S., and Henney, C. S.,** Interleukin 2 induces gamma-interferon production: participation of macrophages and NK-like cells, *J. Immunol.*, 131, 288, 1983.
62. **Weigent, D. A., Stanton, G. J., and Johnson, H. M.,** Interleukin-2 enhances natural-killer cell-activity through induction of gamma-interferon, *Infect. Immun.*, 41, 992, 1983.
63. **Weigent, D. A., Stanton, G. J., and Johnson, H. M.,** Recombinant gamma-interferon enhances natural-killer cell-activity similar to natural gamma-interferon, *Biochem. Biophys. Res. Commun.*, 111, 525, 1983.
64. **Weigent, D. A., Stanton, G. J., and Johnson, J. M.,** Interleukin-2 enhances natural-killer cell-activity through induction of gamma-interferon, *Fed. Proc., Fed. Am. Soc. Exp. Biol.*, 42, 1072, 1983.
65. **Handa, K., Suzuki, R., Matsui, H., Shimizu, Y., and Kumagai, K.,** Natural killer (NK) cells as a responder to interleukin-2 (IL-2), *J. Immunol.*, 130, 900, 1983.
66. **Platsoucas, C. D.,** Augmentation of human natural-killer cytotoxicity by alpha-interferon and inducers of gamma-interferon — an analysis by monoclonal antibodies, *Int. J. Immunopharmacol.*, 4, 255, 1982.
67. **Platsoucas, D. C.,** Augmentation of human natural killer cells by alpha-interferon, and gamma-interferon inducers — analysis by monoclonal antibodies, *Fed. Proc., Fed. Am. Soc. Exp. Biol.*, 41, 958, 1982.
68. **Talmadge, J. E., Meyers, K. M., Prieur, D. J., and Starkey, J. R.,** Role of NK cells in tumour growth and metastasis in beige mice, *Nature (London)*, 284, 622, 1980.
69. **Cudkowicz, G. and Hochman, P. S.,** Do natural killer cells engage in regulated reactions against self to ensure homeostasis?, *Immunol. Rev.*, 44, 13, 1979.
70. **Djeu, J. Y., Timonen, T., and Herberman, R. B.,** Augmentation of natural killer cell activity and induction of interferon by tumor cells and other biological response modifiers, in *Mediation of Cellular Immunity in Cancer by Immune Modifiers*, Progr. Cancer Res. Ther. Ser. Vol. 19, Chirigos, M. A. et al., Eds., Raven Press, New York, 1981, 161.
71. **Baglioni, C., Maroney, P. A., and West, K. K.,** 2′5′ Oligo (A) polymerase activity and inhibition of viral RNA synthesis in interferon-treated Hela cells, *Biochemistry*, 18, 1765, 1979.
72. **Minks, M. A., Benvin, S., Maroney, P. A., and Baglioni, C.,** Synthesis of 2′5′ oligo (A) in extracts of interferon-treated Hela cells, *J. Biol. Chem.*, 6, 767, 1979.
73. **Zilberstein, A., Kimchi, A., Schmidt, A., and Revel, M.,** Isolation of two interferon-induced translational inhibitors: a protein kinase and an oligoisoadenylate synthetase, *Proc. Natl. Acad. Sci. U.S.A.*, 75, 4734, 1978.
74. **Santoni, A., Riccardi, C., Barlozzari, T., and Herberman, R. B.,** Inhibition as well as augmentation of mouse NK activity by pyran copolymer and adriamycin, in *Natural Cell-Mediated Immunity Against Tumors*, Herberman, R. B., Ed., Academic Press, New York, 1980, 753.

75. **Burton, R. C.,** Alloantisera selectively reactive with NK cells: characterization and use in defining NK cell classes, in *Natural Cell-Mediated Immunity Against Tumors,* Herberman, R. B., Ed., Academic Press, New York, 1980, 19.
76. **Glimcher, L., Shen, F. W., and Cantor, H.,** Identification of a cell-surface antigen selectively expressed on the natural killer cell, *J. Exp. Med.,* 145, 1, 1977.
77. **Hansson, M., Kärre, K., Kiessling, R., Roder, J., Anderson, B., and Häyry, P.,** Natural NK-cell targets in the mouse thymus: characteristics of the sensitive cell population, *J. Immunol.,* 123, 765, 1979.
78. **Koo, G., Jacobson, J., Hammerling, G., and Hammerling, U.,** Antigenic profile of murine natural killer cells, *J. Immunol.,* 125, 1009, 1980.
79. **Zarling, J. and Kung, P. C.,** Monoclonal antibodies which distinguish between NK cells and cytotoxic T lymphocytes, *Nature (London),* 288, 394, 1980.
80. **Gerson, J. M., Varesio, L., and Herberman, R. B.,** Systemic and in situ natural killer and suppressor cell activities in mice bearing progressively growing murine sarcoma-virus-induced tumors, *Int. J. Cancer,* 27, 243, 1981.
81. **Lotzová, E. and Savary, C. A.,** Stimulation of NK cell cytotoxic potential of normal donors by two species of recombinant alpha interpheron, *J. Interferon Res.,* 4, 201, 1984.
82. **Timonen, T., Ortaldo, J. R., Stadler, B. M., Bonnard, G. D., Sharrow, S. O., and Herberman, R. B.,** Cultures of purified human natural killer cells: growth in the presence of interleukin 2, *Cell. Immunol.,* 72, 178, 1982.
83. **Ortaldo, J. R., Gerard, J. P., Henderson, L. E., Neubauer, R. H., and Rabin, H.,** Responsiveness of purified natural killer cells to pure interleukin-2 (IL-2), in *Interleukins, Lymphokines and Cytokines,* Oppenheim, J. J. and Rabin, H., Eds., Academic Press, New York, 1983, 63.
84. **Evinger, M., Maela, S., and Pestka, S.,** Recombinant human leukocyte interferon produced in bacteria has antiproliferative activity, *J. Biol. Chem.,* 256, 2113, 1981.
85. **Schmidt,** in preparation.
86. **Sayers, T., Mason, A. T., and Ortaldo, J. R.,** Regulation of human natural killer activity by interferon γ: lack of a role in interleukin 2-mediated augmentation, *J. Immunol.,* in press.

Chapter 10

REGULATION OF NK CELL ACTIVITY BY SUPPRESSOR CELLS

Eva Lotzová and Cherylyn A. Savary

TABLE OF CONTENTS

I. INTRODUCTION

As any other effector cell mechanisms, the natural immunity network does not represent an inert circuit, but is susceptible to a complex interplay of positive as well as negative regulatory influences. Both positive and negative regulation may be mediated by various biological materials (viruses, bacteria, tumor cells, virus-modified tumor cell extracts, lymphocyte and macrophage products),[1-10] chemicals,[11-15] as well as direct cell-to-cell communication.[2,4,16-21]

Of a compelling concern is the negative regulation of natural killer (NK) cells, especially in the light of an increasing evidence on the role of this branch of immunity in the defense against neoplasias.[8,10,22-24] This concern is even more substantiated by the experimental evidence demonstrating that NK cell antitumor activity can be regulated by suppressor cells of various histological types. These include macrophages,[20,25-28] T cells,[4,29-32] granulocytes,[26,33] and other cell types not belonging to any of the known lymphoid or myeloid cell classes.[16,34] Regulation of NK cell activity by suppressor cells was observed under both normal and pathological conditions. For instance, suppressor cells were detected in very young and old animals, in individuals treated with putative immunopotentiating agents, in tumor-bearing animals and cancer patients, and in several strains of mice exhibiting low natural immunity.[2,3,5,17-23,34] Concordant with the role of NK cells in resistance against tumors is the high incidence of neoplasias in strains of mice with low NK cell responder status.[22,35,36]

Even though the reviews concerned with positive regulation (stimulation) of natural immunity have been published quite frequently, no comprehensive review of negative regulation of NK cell function by suppressor cells is available today. This chapter is designed to bridge this gap. We trust that the awareness of the susceptibility of natural immune cells to regulatory activity of suppressor cells, together with the better understanding of the NK cell-suppressor cell relationships, will contribute to more sophisticated strategies for therapy of human cancer.

II. REGULATION OF NK CELL ACTIVITY BY SUPPRESSOR CELLS IN ANIMALS

Regulation of murine NK cell activity by suppressor cells was first observed in our laboratory in 1978 in several animal systems, including infant mice, *Corynebacterium parvum (C. parvum)*-treated mice, and F_1 hybrid mice made tolerant to parental bone marrow transplants.[2] Since these initial observations, studies on the regulation of NK cell functional activity by suppressor cells expanded quite rapidly, and NK cell-related suppressor cells were described by various other laboratories.[16,17,25-34]

A. Methods for Detection and Characterization of Suppressor Cells and their Limitations

1. Method for Detection of Suppressor Cells

The method routinely used for detection of suppressor cells involves mixing experiments, in which the tissue containing putative suppressor cells is mixed with highly NK cell-reactive tissue (such as spleen or peripheral blood) of syngeneic or allogeneic origin. A significant reduction in the NK cell cytotoxicity of mixtures, in comparison to that of cultures containing effector cells alone, is considered indicative of the presence of suppressor cells. To exclude the possibility that decreased activity in mixtures of effector and suppressor cells could be due to nonspecific factors, such as overcrowding or steric inhibition, NK cell-inactive, "filler" cell populations are routinely added to effector cells in the same ratios as suppressor cell-containing suspensions. Various populations have been used as "filler cells"; these include nylon wool (NW) or plastic adherent splenocytes of normal mice, frozen and thawed or heat-killed splenocytes, and splenocytes cultured for 24 hr at 37°C.[4,16,37,38] Although thymocytes have been used frequently as "fillers", we and other investigators have observed that this tissue may not be most suitable as a suppressor cell-lacking control, since thymocytes of certain strains of mice were shown to display suppression of splenic NK cell cytotoxicity.[31,39,74]

2. Methods for Characterization of Suppressor Cells

Various approaches have been used to characterize NK cell-directed suppressor cells. *The role of T cells in suppression* has been routinely assessed by using the specific monoclonal antibody (MoAb) directed against T cell-specific antigen, Thy-1, and by employment of congenitally athymic and/or thymectomized animals. *B cell involvement in suppression* has been tested by removal of surface immunoglobulin (Ig)-positive cells, or by passage of cell populations through NW columns. Under the latter conditions, most of the B cells exhibit adherent properties. *Involvement of macrophage/monocytes in suppression* has been evaluated by using glass or plastic adherence technique, NW and Sephadex G-10 columns, or carbonyl-iron ingestion method. However, it has to be emphasized that NW separation, which is quoted routinely to remove B cells and macrophage/monocytes series of cells, was described also to remove subpopulations of T cells.[40,41] Similarly, glass or plastic adherence and Sephadex G-10 column separation, as well as carbonyl iron ingestion technique, in addition to macrophages, deplete for other cell types.[37,42-44]

Since NK cells have been also implicated in suppression,[45-48] the antiasialo-GM1 antibody, which in a certain concentration selectively destroys NK cells,[49] has also been assessed in some experiments. Other parameters which have been examined in an attempt to characterize NK cell-related suppressor cells include sensitivity of suppressor cells to radiation, heat, cytotoxic drugs, and their physical properties, such as cell size and density.[4,31,34]

With the limitation of the current separation techniques in mind, we have briefly reviewed in this chapter the major findings concerning the characterization, and the role of suppressor cells in regulation of NK cell activity in normal animals and in those treated with various immunomodulating agents.

B. Naturally Occurring NK Cell-Directed Suppressor Cells

1. Suppressor Cells in Infant and Aged Animals

Low NK cell responsiveness of normal rodents is influenced by various factors, including the age of the animals. Specifically, NK cell lytic activity is virtually absent in infant mice, less than 2 to 3 weeks of age (depending on the strain of mice),[2,50-52] and is low in adult mice more than 10 to 14 weeks old.[23,53] We have studied the cause of low NK cell activity in infant (C57BL/6 × DBA/2)F_1 and (C57BL/6 × A)F_1 hybrid mice, and have shown in mixing experiments that splenic NK cell cytotoxic deficiency of these strains of mice was associated with the presence of inhibitory cells.[2] Characterization of suppressor cells in the spleens of infant mice indicated that they were not separable by plastic or NW adherence; specifically, suppression was displayed in both nonadherent and adherent populations of splenocytes following separation on plastic surfaces and NW columns.[74] Furthermore, suppressor cells were found to be nonphagocytic, as established by their failure to ingest carbonyl iron filings, and resistant to irradiation in a dose of 1000 to 3000 R.[74] However, importantly, we have shown that NK cell suppression in infant mice may be overcome by treatment with pyrimidinone molecules.[10,14]

Suppressor cells with similar characteristics were described by other laboratories in infant (C57BL/6 × C3H)F_1 hybrids and in athymic BALB/c mice.[16,54] The presence of suppressor cells in infant athymic mice indicates their T cell-independent nature. Similarly to mice, infant Rowett rats also display deficient splenic NK cell cytotoxic potential; however, in contrast to mice, their NK cell deficiency could be reversed by passage of splenocytes through NW columns.[55]

Although the splenic NK cell reactivity is reduced in aged mice, suppressor cells have not been detected in this specie.[54] In contrast, G-10 adherent population of splenocytes was shown to be responsible for low NK cell reactivity of aged F344 rats.[28] These regulatory cells were inhibited by antibody against prostaglandin E_2, suggesting that suppression was mediated by prostaglandins.[28] Importantly, the regulation of NK cell activity by suppressor cells in the latter strain of rats may be contributory to the increased incidence of malignancies shown in aged rats of this strain.[28]

The observations on the regulation of NK cell activity by suppressor cells in young and aged animals and its association with higher incidence of tumors deserves further investigation. This phenomenon may be clinically relevant to our understanding of high incidence of some types of tumors in aged humans and in children, and furthermore, the experimental animal model may be instrumental in designing new therapeutic strategies for depletion of suppressor cells.

2. *Suppressor Cells in Strains of Mice with Low and Normal NK Cell Responding Status*

Low splenic NK cell activity has been also associated with murine genetic background. Strains of mice, such as A, A.CA, ASW, SJL, and BPS-CI,[17,34] are invariably low NK cell responders, independently of their age. Analysis of low NK cell responder status of these strains of mice indicated that the NK cell cytotoxicity may be regulated by suppressor cells. Most exploratory studies were performed in SJL and BPS-CI mice. In the SJL strain, suppressor cells were characterized as plastic adherent and partially NW adherent, Thy-1.2 negative, and sensitive to carbonyl iron treatment, suggesting their macrophage/monocyte nature.[17] In BPS-CI mice, suppressor cells were less thoroughly characterized; these cells were found to be NW adherent and relatively dense as judged by their distribution on Ficoll-Hypaque gradient.[34]

Interestingly, macrophage-like (adherent to plastic, phagocytic, and esterase positive) suppressor cells directed against NK cells have also been detected in peritoneal exudate of CBA/J and C57BL/6 mice with normal levels of NK cell activity.[25,56] Furthermore, suppressor cells were detected in the spleen (tissue with high NK cell activity), lymph nodes, bone marrow, and thymus (tissues with low NK cell activity) of high NK cell responding CBA mice and BD$\tilde{X}$ rats after Percoll density gradient separation.[57] Even though the suppressor cells in these studies were not characterized thoroughly, their separation on Percoll density gradients indicated that they were of high density (1.077 to 1.121).[57]

More thorough investigation as to the characteristics of suppressor cells was performed with thymus tissue. For example, in rats, the thymus-associated inhibitory cells were found to be nonadherent to plastic, surface-Ig-negative, and Ly-1 and Ly-2 positive.[31] In the mouse, the suppressor cells in the thymus were positive for Thy-1.2 antigen and exhibited high sedimentation velocity and resistance to irradiation.[30,31] In both species, the inhibitory cells did not express Fc-receptor (FcR) for IgG, but expressed receptors for *Helix pomatia* A agglutinin, and were found to be resistant to cortisone treatment.[31] Thymus-related suppressive activity is compatible with the following observations: (1) suppression of splenic NK cells by thymocytes, when the latter cells were used as filler cells;[39,74] (2) higher NK cell cytotoxicity of congenitally athymic or thymectomized animals in comparison to their thymus-possessing littermates;[53] (3) decreased NK cell cytotoxic activity after implantation of thymus into thymectomized mice.[53]

C. Induction of NK Cell-Directed Suppressor Cells in Mice

It has been reported by various investigators that several agents and procedures could cause suppressor cell-related depression of NK cell cytotoxic activity. These are represented by Bacille Calmette-Guerin (BCG), *C. parvum,* pyran copolymer, adriamycin, β-estradiol, carrageenan, hydrocortisone, and irradiation.[2,4,16,37-39,58-63]

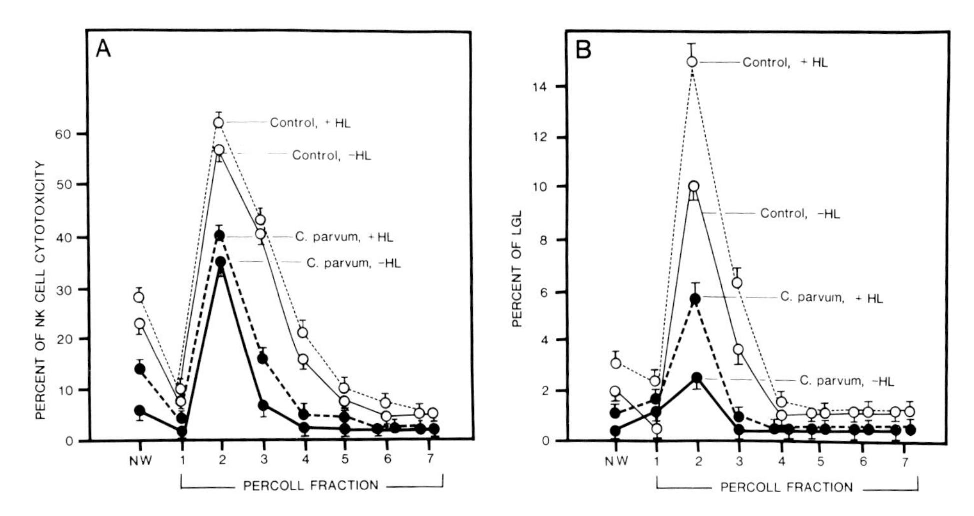

FIGURE 1. Percoll density gradient separation of splenic NK cells of control and *C. parvum*-treated B6D2F$_1$ mice. NW-filtered splenocytes were separated on discontinuous gradients of Percoll adjusted to 290 mOsm/kg H_2O. Gradients were prepared by layering 7 different concentrations of Percoll (38.6, 47.6, 52.1, 56.5, 61.1, 65.6, and 70.1%) in 1.5- to 2.5-mℓ volumes into 15-mℓ conical tubes; 50 million NW-filtered cells suspended in 1.5 mℓ RPMI 1640 were added to the top of the gradient, and the tubes were centrifuged at 550 × G for 30 min at room temperature. The cells were collected from the interfaces and washed in RPMI 1640. The recovery of the cells ranged from 70 to 85%. (A) NK cell cytotoxicity measured in a 4-hr ^{51}Cr-release assay against YAC-1 at 1:50 target to effector (T:E) cell ratio.[13,14] *C. parvum*-injected mice were tested 10 to 13 days after treatment. (B) LGL content was evaluated by analysis of May-Grünwald- and Giemsa-stained cytocentrifuge slides.[15,55] +HL, hypotonic lysis treatment of splenocytes; −HL, no treatment. Symbols represent mean percent ± S.E. of three experiments.

1. Studies on C. parvum-Mediated NK Cell Suppression

C. parvum was reported to augment substantially NK cell activity within a short time after injection into mice.[1,2,4] We found, however, for the first time that in the case of *C. parvum* this effect was of relatively short duration, and in fact, was followed by a severe and long-lasting depression of splenic NK cell activity.[2,4] *C. parvum*-induced NK cell depression was associated with the concomitant appearance of splenic cell population which inhibited NK cell cytotoxic potential of normal syngeneic mice. Attempts to characterize these suppressor cells indicated that more than one suppressor cell was involved, or that different mechanisms may operate in NK cell suppression in *C. parvum*-treated mice. This was exemplified by the presence of suppression in both nonadherent and adherent fractions following separation of splenocytes on plastic surface or NW and G-10 columns.[4,61,62] Furthermore, more detailed analysis of suppression by two different laboratories indicated that suppressor cells present in unseparated or NW-nonadherent population of splenocytes were resistant to carbonyl iron treatment;[4,62] however, it was reported by one group of investigators (but data were not shown) that the latter treatment removed the inhibitory cells from the plastic-adherent fraction.[61] We have demonstrated that NK cells and suppressor cells were separable on the basis of different densities after Ficoll-Hypaque gradient centrifugation, and that under these conditions NK cell activity of *C. parvum*-treated mice was partially recovered.[4] Specifically, suppressor cells were present in the denser fraction (>1.08), while NK cells were present in the lighter fraction (<1.08) following this separation procedure. Using the same approach, splenic suppressor cells with similar density characteristics were described later to inhibit NK cell cytotoxicity in low NK cell-responding BPS-CI mice.[34]

More recently, in agreement with our earlier observations, we found that the NK cell activity and large granular lymphocyte (LGL) content of *C. parvum*-treated mice was significantly enriched in light-density fraction 2 following separation of splenocytes on Percoll density gradient (Figure 1A and B). Mixing experiments indicated that Percoll density

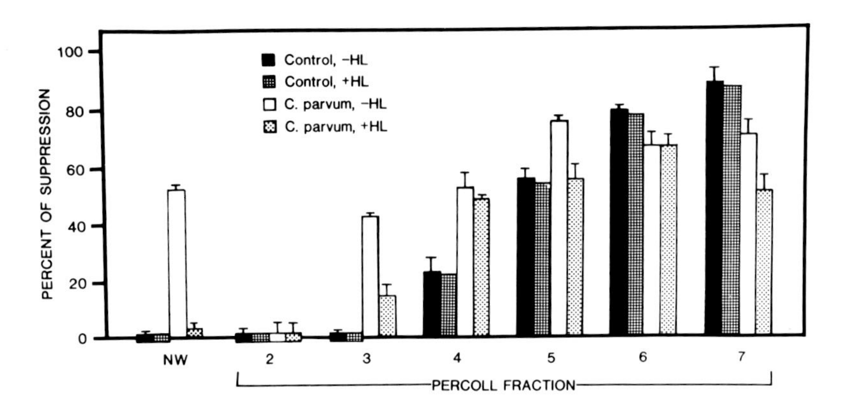

FIGURE 2. Separation of suppressor cells and NK cells of B6D2F$_1$ mice by Percoll density gradient. Splenocytes of control mice were mixed with *C. parvum*-treated or syngeneic spleen cells in a 1:2 effector to suppressor (E:S) cell ratio. T:E cell ratio was constant (1:50).[68] Cytotoxicity was evaluated against YAC-1 in a 4-hr ^{51}Cr-release assay.[68] Bars represent mean percent of suppression ± S.E. of two experiments. Bars without error represent one experiment.

gradient method was effective in separating the NK and suppressor cell activity; NK cells were recovered in the lighter-density fraction (fraction 2) and the suppressor cells were scattered within the higher-density fractions (3 to 7) after Percoll gradient separation (Figure 2).

That T cells may be involved, at least partially, in *C. parvum*-mediated suppression was suggested by our earlier findings indicating that inhibition of NK cell cytotoxicity could be partially removed following treatment with polyclonal anti-Thy-1.2 antibody and complement, and that NK cell depression was not generated following *C. parvum* treatment of congenitally athymic mice.[4,61] Some investigators, however, using the MoAb against the Thy-1.2 antigen were not able to fully remove suppression. Our more recent investigations (described below) shed some light on the complexity involved in defining the suppressor cells in *C. parvum*-treated mice.

The treatment of mice with *C. parvum* is accompanied by an increase in erythropoiesis within the spleen of conventional mice.[64] This is quite easily detectable by examination of the splenocytes on May-Grünwald- and Giemsa-stained cytocentrifuge slides. Using this technique, we detected an abundance of immature erythroid elements at the time of maximum NK cell suppression. This indicated to us that splenic megaloerythropoiesis may interfere with NK cell cytotoxic activity, perhaps through competitive binding of erythroid elements to the NK cell target. In an attempt to investigate this possibility, we studied in conjugate assay on cytocentrifuge slides, NK cell binding properties to YAC-1 in normal and *C. parvum*-treated mice, and in mixtures of both of these cell populations. We observed that in addition to lymphocytes and LGLs, erythroblasts avidly bound to YAC-1 target cells (Table 1). This resulted in an overall increase (3.3-fold) in the number of tumor-binding cells (TBCs) in *C. parvum*-treated mice in comparison to controls. Similarly, the analysis of TBCs in mixtures of normal and *C. parvum*-treated splenocytes demonstrated that approximately 60% of TBCs were of erythroid morphology (Table 2). We analyzed next whether NK cell activity of *C. parvum*-treated mice can be reconstituted and the suppression in mixtures removed by the hypotonic lysis treatment, which is known to lyse erythroid cells.[65] Tables 1 and 2 indicate that the latter treatment was efficient in depleting the erythroid cells, and consequently eliminating the erythroid cell-associated TBC. It therefore appeared

Table 1
MORPHOLOGY OF SPLENIC TBCs OF NORMAL AND *C. PARVUM*-TREATED B6D2F$_1$ MICE

	Control[b]		*C. parvum*[b]	
Type of TBC[a]	**−HL**[c]	**+HL**[c]	**−HL**	**+HL**
LGL	0.7 ± 0.1[d]	1.0 ± 0.2	0.2 ± 0.1	0.3 ± 0.2
Lymphocytes	4.9 ± 0.8	4.6 ± 0.5	5.7 ± 1.5	3.8 ± 1.3
Erythroblasts	1.0 ± 0.3	0.9 ± 0.2	16.7 ± 2.9	0.1 ± 0.1
Total % of TBC	6.6 ± 1.0	5.5 ± 0.8	22.0 ± 2.0	5.1 ± 1.2

[a] The morphology of splenic TBCs against YAC-1 was determined by analysis of May-Grünwald- and Giemsa-stained cytocentrifuge slides.[15,55]
[b] Percent of TBC was determined by mixing equal numbers of YAC-1 target and NW-filtered splenocytes (10^5 each) of control or *C. parvum*-treated mice, as described previously.[55]
[c] +HL, hypotonic lysis treatment of splenocytes; −HL, no treatment.
[d] Values indicate mean percent TBC ± standard error.

Table 2
MORPHOLOGY OF SPLENIC TBCs IN MIXTURES OF NORMAL AND *C. PARVUM*-TREATED B6D2F$_1$ MICE

	Control mixtures[b]		Experimental mixtures[b]	
Type of TBC[a]	**−HL**[c]	**+HL**[c]	**−HL**	**+HL**
LGLs	1.1 ± 0.4[d]	1.0± 0.1	0.5 ± 0.1	1.4 ± 0.4
Lymphocytes	4.9 ± 1.7	4.0 ± 0.1	4.9 ± 2.1	4.9 ± 1.6
Erythroblasts	1.0 ± 0.4	0	7.7 ± 1.8	1.2 ± 0.6
Total % of TBC	5.9 ± 1.7	5.0 ± 0.1	13.0 ± 1.7	7.2 ± 1.1

[a] The morphology of splenic TBCs against YAC-1 was determined by analyses of May-Grünwald- and Giemsa-stained cytocentrifuge slides.[15,55]
[b] Control mixtures were composed of 2×10^5 NW-filtered splenocytes and 10^5 YAC-1 target cells. Experimental mixtures consisted of 10^5 of control splenocytes, 10^5 of *C. parvum* splenocytes, and 10^5 of YAC-1 target cells.
[c] +HL, hypotonic lysis treatment of splenocytes; −HL, no treatment.
[d] Values indicate mean percent of TBC ± standard error.

that immature erythrocytes present in spleens of *C. parvum*-injected mice could be, at least in part, responsible for the inhibition of NK cell cytotoxicity in these animals. Compatible with this postulation was the observation that hypotonic lysis treatment resulted in removal of suppression of NK cell cytotoxicity in mixtures (Figure 3).

In spite of removal of suppression from mixtures of *C. parvum* and normal splenocytes, the NK cell activity of *C. parvum*-treated mice was not restored completely following hypotonic lysis treatment (Figure 3). This suggested that in addition to erythroid cells, suppressor cells could contribute to low NK cell activity in these mice. We argued that the effect of suppressor cells may not be readily observed in mixtures due to the contribution of NK cell activity present in the erythrocyte-depleted *C. parvum* splenocytes (Figure 3). Thus, in an attempt to uncover this putative suppressor cell population, we first depleted

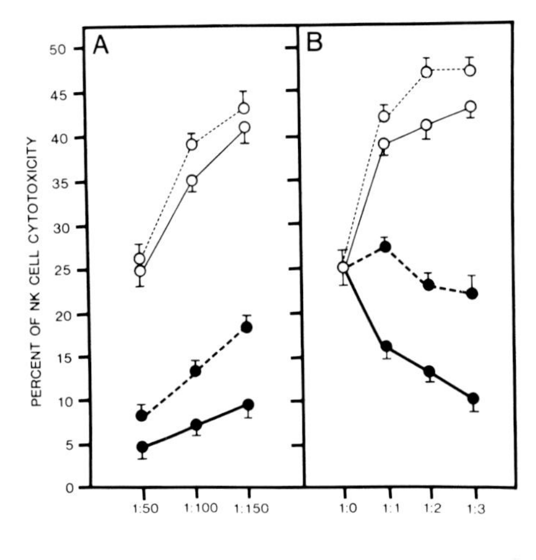

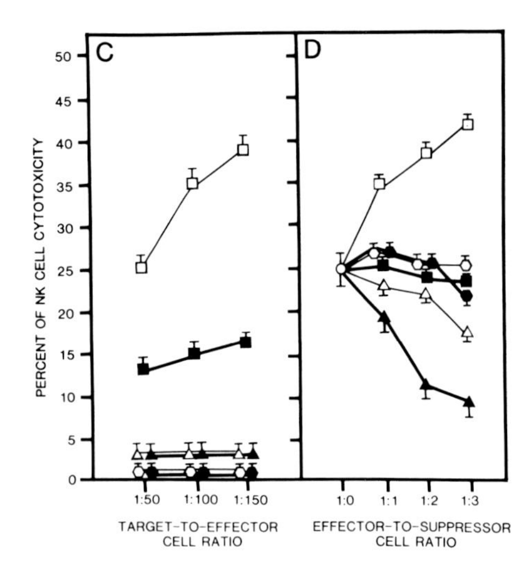

FIGURE 3. Effect of various treatments on suppressor cell activity of *C. parvum*-injected $B6D2F_1$ mice. Cytotoxicity of NW-filtered splenocytes against YAC-1 was tested at different T:E cell and E:S cell ratios in a 4-hr ^{51}Cr-release assay. T:E cell ratio of control splenocytes in mixtures was kept constant (1:50).[68] (A) NK cell cytotoxicity of HL-treated (---), or untreated (———), control (○), and *C. parvum*-injected (●) splenocytes. Significant increase in NK cell activity of *C. parvum* splenocytes was observed after HL treatment ($p<0.002$ to <0.01, as analyzed by a Student's *t*-test). (B) NK cell cytotoxicity of mixtures consisting of control and *C. parvum* splenocytes undergoing the same treatments as indicated in (A). Significant suppression of NK cell activity was observed in mixtures composed of control and *C. parvum*-injected, HL-untreated splenocytes ($p<0.001$), but not in those treated with HL. (C) NK cell cytotoxicity of HL and complement (C′)-treated control (□) and *C. parvum*-injected (■) splenocytes; HL, asialo-GM1 antibody and C′-treated control (△) and *C. parvum* (▲) splenocytes; HL, asialo-GM1 antibody, Thy-1.2 antibody, and C′-treated control (⬡) and *C. parvum* (⬢) splenocytes. (D) NK cell cytotoxicity of mixtures consisting of control and *C. parvum* splenocytes undergoing the same treatments as indicated in (C). Significant suppression of NK cell cytotoxicity was observed in mixtures of control and *C. parvum*-injected, HL and asialo-GM1, and C′-treated splenocytes ($p<0.001$ to <0.05). NK cell suppression was removed by Thy-1.2 treatment. Symbols represent mean percent of cytotoxicity ± S.E.

the *C. parvum* splenocytes of erythrocytes by hypotonic lysis, and then removed NK cell activity by treatment with asialo-GM1 antibody (Figure 3). When such treated *C. parvum* splenocytes were added to spleen cells from normal animals, suppression of NK cell activity in mixtures was once more detected, thereby indicating the presence of suppressor cells. To determine whether T cells were involved in suppression, we treated the *C. parvum*-injected, hypotonic lysis and asialo-GM1 antibody-treated splenocytes with anti-Thy-1.2 antibody and complement. Such treatment totally removed NK cell suppression in mixtures of *C. parvum*-treated and normal splenocytes. These data support our earlier findings that suppressor T cells operate in *C. parvum*-mediated NK cell suppression.[4] Preliminary analysis of the mechanism of NK cell suppression in *C. parvum*-treated mice indicated that suppression can be achieved by incubation of normal splenocytes with cell-free supernatants obtained from cultures of *C. parvum* splenocytes (Figure 4). It remains to be determined whether this factor can be obtained from a purified population of T cells.

Since NK cell activity is depleted in *C. parvum* splenocytes following asialo-GM1 treatment,[49] and is effected also by treatment with MoAb Thy-1.2,[66] it was not possible to determine if removal of suppressor T cells restores NK cell activity in *C. parvum*-treated mice. It appears, however, from Percoll density gradient separation studies, that lower LGL content in spleens of *C. parvum*-treated mice (in comparison to control animals) could be another factor underlying low NK cell activity in these mice (Figure 1). Also, the qualitative differences in the activity of these two LGL types remain to be determined.

Our studies demonstrate that the decline of NK cell activity following *C. parvum* treatment

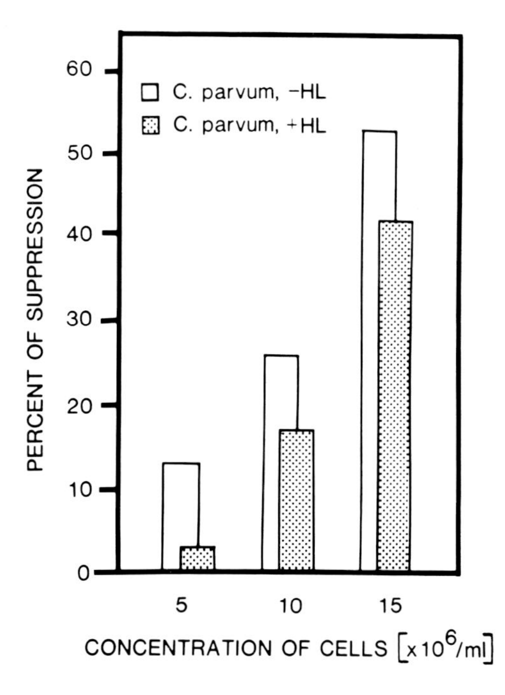

FIGURE 4. Suppression of NK cell cytotoxicity by soluble factor derived from NW-filtered splenocytes of *C. parvum*-treated B6D2F$_1$ mice. Control splenocytes were mixed with 150 μℓ of supernatants obtained from cultures consisting of different concentrations of *C. parvum* spleen cells (incubated for 4 hr in vitro). Cytotoxicity was tested in a 4-hr ^{51}Cr-release assay against YAC-1 at 1:50 T:E cell ratio. Significant suppression of NK cell activity was observed with supernatants containing 10×10^6 ($p<0.02$) and 15×10^6 ($p<0.001$) cells per milliliter.

is quite complex; this observation is not surprising considering the multitude of immunological, physiological, and hematological changes initiated by this agent.[64,67] The finding that erythroid cells interfere with NK cell lytic activity may be of relevance in normal and malignant hemopathies.

2. *NK Cell-Directed Suppressor Cells in Other Systems*

Treatment of mice with *β-estradiol* was also shown to result in reduction of splenic NK cell activity, which has been attributed to the generation of suppressor cells,[63] These cells were detected in both the plastic nonadherent and adherent fractions and were Thy-1.2, NK-1.1, Ia, and asialo-GM1 antigens negative. Since β-estradiol also induces increased erythropoiesis, some of the inhibitory activity may have been due to erythroid cells, as described by our studies in *C. parvum*-injected mice. In agreement with this postulation is an observation of Seaman et al.,[58] who failed to detect suppression in NK cell-deficient estradiol-treated mice in experiments in which ammonium chloride-treated splenocytes (the treatment removing erythrocytes) were used as a source of inhibitors.

Decreased splenic NK cell activity associated with suppressor cells has been described also 2 weeks after exposure of mice to a sublethal dose (700 R) of whole body *γ-irradiation*.[16] The splenic suppressor cells were NW and G-10 columns nonadherent and nonphagocytic. The fact that the inhibitory cells were also generated in thymectomized mice following irradiation indicates their thymic-independent nature. Irradiation of bone marrow by ^{89}Sr also has been reported to cause a severe and long-lasting (>3 months) decrease in murine splenic NK cell activity.[16,39] In one study this effect was attributed to splenic suppressor cells (similar to those described after sublethal γ-irradiation) detected 16 days after a single injection of this isotope. In contrast, another group of investigators was unable to demonstrate suppressor cell activity in spleens of mice treated with two injections of ^{89}Sr, 3 to 8 weeks previously.[39] The reasons for this discrepancy are not clear; while the dose and schedule of isotope administration could account for differences in the observed results, it is also possible that suppressor cell appearance may be a time-dependent phenomenon.

Some disagreement also exists concerning the presence of suppressor cells in cortisone-treated mice, which display deficient NK cell activity.[16,68] While one laboratory observed significant inhibition of normal NK cell activity by nonadherent, radioresistant, and phagocytic splenocytes,[16] we were unable to detect suppressor cell population in cortisone-treated mice.[68] In fact, our observation that NK cell activity was significantly depressed as soon as 3 hr after injection of the steroid suggested that NK cells may be directly affected by the treatment. It is possible, however, that different mechanisms may be involved in the NK cell decline of cortisone-treated mice, and that the discrepancies are due to the doses of the agent administered, or strains of mice tested, two parameters which differed in these experiments.

Suppressor cells have been also detected in the spleens of pyran and adriamycin-treated mice.[38,60] Macrophage-like suppressor cells appeared to be involved in pyran-treated mice, as judged by their plastic adherent, phagocytic, and radioresistant nature and the lack of expression of Thy-1.2 antigen.[38] Adriamycin-induced suppressor cells were found to be NW and plastic adherent.[60]

Regulatory cells with macrophage-like properties (radioresistant, glass and G-10 adherent, carbonyl iron ingesting, with negative Thy-1.2 and Ia cell surface phenotype) were described following in vivo treatment of mice with *carrageenan*.[16] In contrast, an in vitro carrageenan-induced suppressor cell population did not exhibit phagocytic and glass-adherent properties, but displayed G-10-adherent characteristics.

BCG is another agent reported to induce suppression of splenic NK cell cytotoxicity, as assessed in mixing experiments. The inhibitory cells in these studies were not characterized, with the exception that they did not display NW-adherent properties.

III. REGULATION OF NK CELL ACTIVITY BY SUPPRESSOR CELLS IN MAN

A. NK Cell-Directed Suppressor Cells of Monocyte-Macrophage Nature

Studies in humans also indicate that NK cell cytotoxic activity may be regulated by suppressor cells. For instance, suppressor cell-related decline of peripheral blood NK cell cytotoxic function directed against the K562 target cell line was found in patients with breast carcinoma after surgery.[69] Suppression was exhibited as early as 2 to 3 days postsurgery and persisted for 2 weeks. The suppressor cells in this system were identified as monocytes, based on their plastic- and Sephadex G-10 column-adherent properties and on positivity for nonspecific esterase staining. Suppressive effect was displayed across major histocompatibility complex (MHC) differences. Even though the exact mechanism of effect of suppressor cells on NK cell cytotoxicity was not delineated in these studies, a direct suppressor-effector cell contact (for 24 hr) was necessary for manifestation of suppression; serum from post-operative patients or supernatants from cultures of suppressor monocytes and effector cells did not mediate suppression.

It is possible that this long-lasting suppression of NK cell activity postsurgery may be one of the phenomena underlying increased incidence of metastasis shown in cancer patients undergoing surgical manipulation.[70]

Regulatory cells were also implicated in low NK cell cytotoxicity observed in carcinomatous pleural effusions of patients with lung cancer.[19] In a majority of these patients suppressor cells were identified as monocyte-macrophages using the similar techniques as those described above.[69] In agreement with previous studies,[69] manifestation of suppression in this system was dependent on direct cell-to-cell communication, since supernatants produced after coculture of suppressor cells and effector cells were ineffective to mediate suppression. Additionally, suppression was independent of prostaglandin production (indomethacin, an inhibitor of prostaglandin synthesis, did not affect the suppressive activity. Tumor-binding assay demonstrated that suppressor cells did not interfere with NK cell binding capacity, but operated at the lytic level of NK cell cytotoxic mechanism.

The observation that the NK cell activity of carcinomatous pleural effusions could be partially restored by removal of suppressor cells on G-10 columns, followed by 24 hr incubation in vitro, suggested that lung cancer patients were not totally deficient in NK cells. Interestingly, the low NK cell levels of pleural carcinomatous effusions could be augmented and suppressive activity abolished by intrapleural administration of OK432 (a heat and penicillin-treated, lyophilized powder of Su strain of *Streptococcus pyogenes* A3).[71] Interferon (IFN) did not exert such effect, suggesting that OK432 activity was not IFN-related.

In other study, macrophages (nonspecific esterase positive, phagocytic cells) obtained from bronchoalveolar washings of patients undergoing diagnostic bronchoscopy have been shown to inhibit autologous peripheral blood NK cells.[20] The suppressive activity was displayed against endogenous as well as IFN-stimulated NK cells. The mechanism by which alveolar macrophages displayed suppressive effect was not delineated in this study.

Autologous monocytes (based on plastic adherence properties) were implicated also in inhibition of Percoll gradient-enriched peripheral blood NK cell cytotoxicity.[27] Suppression was detected after coculture of NK cells with diffusates from plastic-adherent cells. Diffusate-mediated inhibitory effect was heat stable (it was not reduced after heating for 30 min at 60°C) and was found independent of prostaglandin E_2 or lysozymes. The lack of involvement of prostaglandin was suggested by failure of indomethacin to abolish diffusate-mediated suppression, and the effect of lysozymes was excluded by the observation that preincubation of monocytes with antilysozyme or treatment of NK cells with lysozymes did not affect cytotoxicity. Conjugate assay indicated that suppressive diffusates resulted in inhibition of binding of NK cells to the tumor. The role of monocytes-macrophages in suppression in this investigation was not conclusive, since the authors did not provide any evidence on the purity of the suppressor cell population.

Poly I:C-stimulated monocytes were reported also to display NK cell inhibitory effect.[5] Such inhibition was interpreted to be at least partly mediated by prostaglandins.

Suppression of autologous NK cell activity against K562 target was also demonstrated in long-term bone marrow cultures in vitro.[72] Inhibitory activity was attributed to plastic-adherent marrow cells, which after coculture with peripheral blood mononuclear lymphocytes or with nonadherent bone marrow cells, strongly inhibited NK cell cytotoxicity. Furthermore, treatment of adherent cells with OKM1 antibody and complement eliminated the suppressive effect. It thus appears that the suppressor cells belonged to monocyte-macrophage lineage.

B. NK Cell Suppression Mediated by T Cells and Other Lymphocytes

Involvement of T cells in the suppression of human autologous NK cell cytotoxicity of normal donors was also described. The suppressor cells in these studies were nonadherent to glass wool columns, and were identified as T cells on the basis of their adherence to bacterial monolayers.[29]

T cell-related NK cell suppression was reported later by another laboratory in three different experimental systems.[21,32,73] The suppressor cells were detected after separation on discontinuous Percoll density gradients in peripheral blood of normal donors and cancer patients, and in cord blood. The characterization studies showed that the cells were small- to medium-sized T lymphocytes of high density, expressing receptor for Fc portion of IgG and sheep erythrocytes, reactive with OKT3 MoAb, and exhibiting staining pattern of T cells with acid α-naphthyl acetate esterase.[21,32,73] Similar to other suppressor cells, cell-to-cell contact was required for exhibition of suppression. This was established by the lack of manifestation of suppression when the effector and suppressor cells were separated by Nucleopore® filters.[73] The suppressor cells were furthermore resistant to high doses of irradiation and their viability was not required for function.

Lymphocytes from ascitic tumors of some ovarian cancer patients, when mixed with allogeneic or autologous peripheral blood mononuclear cells, exhibited significant suppression of NK cell cytotoxicity.[18] Tumor-associated plastic-adherent cells did not display any inhibitory activity indicating that suppression was not mediated by macrophages. NW column separation demonstrated that suppression was mediated by both NW-adherent and -filtered suppressor cells. The exact nature of suppressor cells was not determined.

C. Granulocyte-Mediated NK Cell Suppression

Granulocytes represent another cell population implicated in NK cell suppression. For instance, granulocytes derived from normal donors or from patients with chronic granulatomatous disease suppressed activity of autologous and allogeneic NK cells.[33] Inhibition was also mediated by membrane fragments or extracts from sonicated granulocytes; however, the intact granulocytes were most effective. Inhibitory capacity was resistant to heat and appeared to affect both the binding and the postbinding step of NK cell cytotoxic mechanism. Negative regulation of NK cell activity by granulocytes was also described by Seaman et al.[26]

IV. CONCLUSION

Studies reviewed in this chapter indicate that NK cell cytotoxic activity may be regulated by suppressor cells in normal, clinically, surgically or biologically modulated, and pathological states. This review also shows that the suppressor cells do not represent a single cell type, but are quite heterogeneous and belong to different lineages of lymphoid and myeloid cells. Since NK cells are considered to be an important component of anticancer mechanism, such negative regulation of their tumor-associated functions may be responsible for a higher incidence of neoplasia in low-responding normal individuals, for metastatic spread after surgical procedure, and for inadequate antitumor immunity despite the immunomodulation of cancer patients. For these reasons, it is important to investigate the intimate NK cell-suppressor cell-relationships and to understand the mechanisms of suppressor cell-mediated NK cell regulation. Such knowledge may be instrumental in developing new protocols for treatment of malignancies.

ACKNOWLEDGMENT

The work from this laboratory was supported by Grant CA 31394 from the National Cancer Institute. The authors wish to express their thanks to Ann Childers for her excellent assistance in the preparation of this manuscript.

REFERENCES

1. **Herberman, R. B., Nunn, M. E., Holden, H. T., Staal, S., and Djeu, J. Y.,** Augmentation of natural cytotoxic reactivity of mouse lymphoid cells against syngeneic and allogeneic target cells, *Int. J. Cancer*, 19, 555, 1977.
2. **Savary, C. A. and Lotzová, E.,** Suppression of natural killer cell cytotoxicity by splenocytes from *Corynebacterium parvum*- injected, bone marrow-tolerant, and infant mice, *J. Immunol.*, 120, 239, 1978.
3. **Tracey, D. E., Wolfe, S. A., Durdik, J. M., and Henney, C. S.,** BCG-induced murine effector cells. I. Cytolytic activity in peritoneal exudates: an early response to BCG, *J. Immunol.*, 119, 1145, 1977.
4. **Lotzová, E.,** *C. parvum*-mediated suppression of the phenomenon of natural killing and its analysis, in *Natural Cell-Mediated Immunity Against Tumors*, Herberman, R. B., Ed., Academic Press, New York, 1980, 735.
5. **Koren, H. S., Anderson, S. J., Fischer, D. G., Copeland, C. S., and Jensen, P. J.,** Regulation of human natural killing. I. The role of monocytes, interferon and prostaglandins, *J. Immunol.*, 127, 2007, 1981.
6. **Lattime, E. C., Pecoraro, G. A., and Stutman, O.,** The activity of natural cytotoxic cells is augmented by interleukin 2 and interleukin 3, *J. Exp. Med.*, 157, 1070, 1983.
7. **Lotzová, E. and Savary, C. A.,** Stimulation of NK cell cytotoxic potential of normal donors by two species of recombinant alpha interferon, *J. Interferon Res.*, 4, 201, 1984.
8. **Lotzová, E.,** Function of natural killer cells in various biological phenomena. An overview, *Surv. Synth. Pathol.*, 2, 41, 1983.
9. **Lotzová, E., Savary, C. A., Freedman, R. S., and Bowen, J. M.,** Natural killer cell cytotoxic potential of patients with ovarian carcinoma and its modulation with virus-modified tumor cell extract, *Cancer Immunol. Immunother.*, 17, 124, 1984.
10. **Lotzová, E.,** The role of natural killer cells in immune surveillance against malignancies, *Cancer Bull.*, 36, 215, 1984.
11. **Puccetti, P., Santoni, A., Riccardi, C., Holden, H. T., and Herberman, R. B.,** Activation of mouse macrophages by pyran copolymer and role in augmentation of natural killer activity, *Int. J. Cancer*, 24, 819, 1979.
12. **Djeu, J. Y., Heinbaugh, J. A., Holden, H. T., and Herberman, R. B.,** Role of macrophages in the augmentation of mouse natural killer cell activity by Poly I:C and interferon, *J. Immunol.*, 122, 182, 1979.
13. **Lotzová, E., Savary, C. A., and Stringfellow, D. A.,** 5-Halo-6-phenyl pyrimidinones: new molecules with cancer therapeutic potential and interferon-inducing capacity are strong inducers of murine natural killer cells, *J. Immunol.*, 130, 965, 1983.
14. **Lotzová, E., Savary, C. A., and Stringfellow, D. A.,** Modulation of murine NK cell cytotoxicity *in vitro* and antitumor activity *in vivo* by low molecular weight interferon inducers, *Cancer: Etiology and Prevention*, Crispen, R. G., Ed., Elsevier, Amsterdam, 1983, 199.
15. **Lotzová, E., Savary, C. A., Khan, A., and Stringfellow, D. A.,** Stimulation of natural killer cells in two random-bred strains of athymic rats by interferon-inducing pyrimidinone, *J. Immunol.*, 132, 2566, 1984.
16. **Cudkowicz, G. and Hochman, P. S.,** Do natural killer cells engage in regulated reactions against self to ensure homeostasis?, *Immunol. Rev.*, 44, 13, 1979.
17. **Riccardi, C., Santoni, A., Barlozzari, T., Cesarini, C., and Herberman, R. B.,** Suppression of natural killer (NK) activity by splenic adherent cells of low NK-reactive mice, *Int. J. Cancer*, 28, 811, 1981.
18. **Allavena, P., Introna, M., Mangioni, C., and Mantovani, A.,** Inhibition of natural killer activity by tumor-associated lymphoid cells from ascites ovarian carcinomas, *J. Natl. Cancer Inst.*, 67, 319, 1981.
19. **Uchida, A. and Micksche, M.,** Suppressor cells for natural killer activity in carcinomatous pleural effusions of cancer patients, *Cancer Immunol. Immunother.*, 11, 255, 1981.
20. **Bordignon, C., Villa, F., Allavena, P., Introna, M., Biondi, A., Avallone, R., and Mantovani, A.,** Inhibition of natural killer activity by human bronchoalveolar macrophages, *J. Immunol.*, 129, 587, 1982.
21. **Tarkkanen, J., Saksela, E., and Paavolainen, M.,** Suppressor cells of natural killer activity in normal and tumor-bearing individuals, *Clin. Immunol. Immunopathol.*, 28, 29, 1983.
22. **Lotzová, E. and McCredie, K. B.,** Natural killer cells in mice and man and their possible biological significance, *Cancer Immunol. Immunother.*, 4, 215, 1978.
23. **Herberman, R. B. and Ortaldo, J. R.,** Natural killer cells: their role in defenses against disease, *Science*, 214, 24, 1981.
24. **Roder, J. C., Kärre, K., and Kiessling, R.,** Natural killer cells, *Prog. Allergy*, 28, 66, 1981.
25. **Brunda, M. J., Taramelli, D., Holden, H. T., and Varesio, L.,** Suppression of murine natural killer cell activity by normal peritoneal macrophages, in *NK Cells and Other Natural Effector Cells*, Herberman, R. B., Ed., Academic Press, New York, 1982, 535.
26. **Seaman, W. E., Gindhart, T. D., Blackman, M. A., Dalal, B., Talal, N., and Werb, Z.,** Suppression of natural killing in vitro by monocytes and polymorphonuclear leukocytes, *J. Clin. Invest.*, 69, 876, 1982.

27. **Yang, U. and Zucker, F. D.,** Modulation of natural killer (NK) cells by autologous neutrophils and monocytes, *Cell. Immunol.*, 86, 171, 1984.
28. **Bash, J. A. and Vogel, D.,** Cellular immunosenescence in F344 rats: decreased natural killer (NK) cell activity involves changes in regulatory interactions between NK cells, interferon, prostaglandin and macrophages, *Mech. Ageing Dev.*, 24, 49, 1984.
29. **DeBoer, K. P., Kleinman, R., and Teodorescu, J.,** Identification and separation by bacterial adherence of human lymphocytes that suppress natural cytotoxicity, *J. Immunol.*, 126, 276, 1976.
30. **Nair, M. P. N., Schwartz, S. A., Fernandes, G., Pahwa, R., Ikehara, S., and Good, R. A.,** Suppression of natural killer (NK) cell activity of spleen cells by thymocytes, *Cell. Immunol.*, 58, 9, 1981.
31. **Zöller, M. and Wigzell, H.,** Normally occurring inhibitory cells for natural killer cell activity. II. Characterization of the inhibitory cell, *Cell. Immunol.*, 74, 27, 1982.
32. **Tarkkanen, J., Saksela, E., von Willebrand, E., and Lehtonen, E.,** Suppressor cells of the human NK activity: characterization of the cells and mechanism of action, *Cell. Immunol.*, 79, 265, 1983.
33. **Kay, H. D. and Smith, D. L.,** Regulation of human lymphocyte-mediated natural killer (NK) cell activity. I. Inhibition *in vitro* by peripheral blood granulocytes, *J. Immunol.*, 130, 475, 1983.
34. **Blair, P. B., Staskawicz, M. O., and Sam, J. S.,** Inhibitor cells in spleens of mice with low natural killer activity, *J. Natl. Cancer Inst.*, 71, 571, 1983.
35. **Petrányi, G. G., Kiessling, R., Povey, S., Klein, G., Herzenberg, L., and Wigzell, H.,** The genetic control of natural killer cell activity and its association with *in vivo* resistance against a Moloney lymphoma isograft, *Immunogenetics*, 3, 15, 1976.
36. **Fitzgerald, K. L. and Ponzio, N. M.,** Natural killer cell activity in reticulum cell sarcomas (RCS) of SJL/J mice, *Cell. Immunol.*, 43, 185, 1979.
37. **Hochman, P. S. and Cudkowicz, G.,** Suppression of natural cytotoxicity by spleen cells of hydrocortisone-treated mice, *J. Immunol.*, 123, 968, 1979.
38. **Santoni, A., Riccardi, C., Barlozzari, T., and Herberman, R. B.,** Suppression of activity of mouse natural killer (NK) cells by activated macrophages from mice treated with pyran copolymer, *Int. J. Cancer*, 26, 837, 1980.
39. **Kumar, V., Ben-Ezra, J., Bennett, M., and Sonnenfeld, G.,** Natural killer cells in mice treated with ^{89}strontium: normal target-binding cell numbers but inability to kill even after interferon administration, *J. Immunol.*, 123, 1832, 1979.
40. **Stutman, O.,** Humoral thymic factors influencing postthymic cells, *Ann. N.Y. Acad. Sci.*, 249, 89, 1975.
41. **Toda, T., Takemori, T., Okumura, K., Nonaka, M., and Tokuhisa, T.,** Two distinct types of helper T cells involved in the secondary antibody response: independent and synergistic effects of Ia^- and Ia^+ helper T cells, *J. Exp. Med.*, 147, 446, 1978.
42. **Ly, I. A. and Mishell, R. I.,** Separation of mouse spleen cells by passage through columns of Sephadex G-10, *J. Immunol. Methods*, 5, 239, 1974.
43. **Hathcock, K. S., Singer, A., and Hodes, R. J.,** Obtaining adherent cells from the spleen, in *Methods for Studying Mononuclear Phagocytes*, Adams, D. O., Edelson, D., and Koren, H. S., Eds., Academic Press, New York, 1981, 89.
44. **Fernandez, L. A. and Macsween, J. M.,** Effect of removal of monocytes by iron filing phagocytosis on mononuclear subpopulations, *J. Immunol. Methods*, 18, 193, 1977.
45. **Nabel, G., Allard, W. J., and Cantor, H.,** A cloned cell line mediating natural killer cell function inhibits immunoglobulin secretion, *J. Exp. Med.*, 156, 658, 1982.
46. **Tilden, A. B., Abo, T., and Balch, C. M.,** Suppressor cell function of human granular lymphocytes identified by the HNK-1 (Leu 7) monoclonal antibody, *J. Immunol.*, 130, 1171, 1983.
47. **Arai, S., Yamamoto, H., Itoh, K., and Kumagai, K.,** Suppressive effect of human natural killer cells on pokeweed mitogen-induced B cell differentiation, *J. Immunol.*, 131, 651, 1983.
48. **Abruzzio, L. V. and Rowley, D. A.,** Homeostasis of the antibody response: immunoregulation by NK cells, *Science*, 222, 581, 1983.
49. **Kasai, M., Yoneda, T., Habu, S., Maruyama, Y., Okumura, K., and Tokunaga, T.,** In vivo effect of anti-asialo GM-1 antibody on natural killer activity, *Nature (London)*, 291, 334, 1981.
50. **Lotzová, E. and Savary, C. A.** Possible involvement of natural killer cells in bone marrow graft rejection, *Biomedicine*, 27, 341, 1977.
51. **Lotzová, E.,** Hemopoietic histocompatibility: genetic and immunological aspects, in *Compendium of Immunology*, Vol. III, Schwartz, L. M., Ed., Van Nostrand Reinhold, New York, 1983, 468.
52. **Koo, G. C., Peppard, J. R., and Hatzfeld, A.,** Ontogeny of NK-1$^+$ natural killer cells. I. Proportion of NK-1$^+$ cells in fetal, baby and old mice, *J. Immunol.*, 129, 867, 1982.
53. **Herberman, R. B. and Holden, H. T.,** Natural cell mediated immunity, *Adv. Cancer Res.*, 27, 305, 1978.
54. **Santoni, A., Riccardi, C., Barlozzari, T., and Herberman, R. B.,** Natural suppressor cells for murine NK activity, in *NK Cells and Other Natural Effector Cells*, Herberman, R. B., Ed., Academic Press, New York, 1982, 527.

55. **Lotzová, E., Savary, C. A., Gray, K. N., Raulston, G. L., and Jardine, J. H.,** Natural killer cell profile of two random-bred strains of athymic rats, *Exp. Hematol.*, 12, 633, 1984.
56. **Brunda, M. J., Taramelli, D., Holden, H. T., and Varesio, L.,** Suppression in in vitro maintenance and interferon-mediated augmentation of natural killer cell activity by adherent peritoneal cells from normal mice, *J. Immunol.*, 130, 1974, 1983.
57. **Zöller, M. and Wigzell, H.,** Normally occurring inhibitory cells for natural killer cell activity. I. Organ distribution, *Cell. Immunol.*, 74, 14, 1982.
58. **Seaman, W. E., Merigan, T. C., and Talal, N.,** Natural killing in estrogen-treated mice responds poorly to poly I:C despite normal stimulation of circulating interferon, *J. Immunol.*, 123, 2903, 1979.
59. **Ito, M., Ralph, P., and Moore, M. A. S.,** Suppression of spleen natural killing activity induced by BCG, *Clin. Immunol. Immunopathol.*, 16, 30, 1980.
60. **Santoni, A., Riccardi, C., Sorci, V., and Herberman, R. B.,** Effects of adriamycin on the activity of mouse natural killer cells, *J. Immunol.*, 124, 2329, 1980.
61. **Santoni, A., Riccardi, C., Barlozzari, T., and Herberman, R. B.,** *C. parvum*-induced suppressor cells for mouse NK activity, in *NK cells and Other Natural Effector Cells*, Herberman, R. B., Ed., Academic Press, New York, 1982, 519.
62. **Milisauskas, V. K., Cudkowicz, G., and Nakamura, I.,** Cellular suppression of murine ADCC and NK activities induced by *Corynebacterium parvum, Cancer Immunol. Immunother.*, 15, 149, 1983.
63. **Milisaukas, V. K., Cudkowicz, G., and Nakamura, I.,** Role of suppressor cells in the decline of natural killer cell activity in estrogen-treated mice, *Cancer Res.*, 43, 5240, 1983.
64. **Milas, L. and Scott, M. T.,** Antitumor activity of *Corynebacterium parvum, Adv. Cancer Res.*, 26, 257, 1978.
65. **Mishell, B. B., Shiigi, S. M., Henry, C., Chan, E. L., North, J., Gallily, R., Slomich, M., Miller, K., Marbrook, J., Parks, D., and Good, A. H.,** Preparation of mouse cell suspensions, in *Selected Methods in Cellular Immunology*, Mishell, B. B. and Shiigi, S. M., Eds., W. H. Freeman, San Francisco, 1980, 3.
66. **Mattes, M. J., Sharrow, S. O., Herberman, R. B., and Holden, H. T.,** Identification and separation of Thy-1 positive mouse spleen cells active in natural cytotoxicity and antibody-dependent cell-mediated cytotoxicity, *J. Immunol.*, 123, 2851, 1979.
67. **Adlam, C. and Scott, M. T.,** Lympho-reticular stimulatory properties of *Corynebacterium parvum* and related bacteria, *J. Med. Microbiol.*, 6, 261, 1973.
68. **Lotzová, E. and Savary, C. A.,** Parallelism between the effect of cortisone acetate on hybrid resistance and natural killing, *Exp. Hematol.*, 9, 766, 1981.
69. **Uchida, A., Kolb, R., and Micksche, M.,** Generation of suppressor cells for natural killer activity in cancer patients after surgery, *J. Natl. Cancer Inst.*, 68, 735, 1982.
70. **El Rifi, K., Bacon, B., Methigan, J., Hope, E., and Cole, W. H.,** Increased incidence of pulmonary metastasis after celeotomy: counteraction by heparin, *Arch. Surg.*, 91, 625, 1965.
71. **Uchida, A. and Micksche, M.,** Intrapleural administration of OK432 in cancer patients: activation of NK cells and reduction of suppressor cells, *Int. J. Cancer*, 31, 1, 1983.
72. **Punjabi, C. J., Moore, M. A. S., and Ralph, P.,** Suppression of natural killer activity in human blood and bone marrow cultures by bone marrow-adherent OKM1-positive cells, *Cell. Immunol.*, 77, 13, 1983.
73. **Tarkkanen, J. and Saksela, E.,** Umbilical-cord-blood-derived suppressor cells of the human natural killer cell activity are inhibited by interferon, *Scand. J. Immunol.*, 15, 149, 1982.
74. **Lotzová, E. and Savary, C. A.,** unpublished.

Chapter 11

NK CELL CLONING TECHNOLOGY AND CHARACTERISTICS OF NK CELL CLONES

Colin G. Brooks

TABLE OF CONTENTS

I. INTRODUCTION

A major impediment to our progress in research on natural killer (NK) cells has been the difficulty of obtaining large numbers of highly purified cells. Indeed, for many years following the discovery of this cell population, no specific markers or characteristics of these cells were known which could facilitate cell separation procedures. Even with the description of relatively specific NK cell markers, such as NK alloantigens in the mouse,[1,2] a series of markers recognized by monoclonal antibodies (MoAbs) in man,[3-6] and the realization that NK cells in many species have a lower density than most lymphoid cells,[7-9] it has still proved impossible to obtain highly purified populations of NK cells in sufficient numbers to permit, for example, biochemical analysis of their function and regulation. Two factors mitigate against success using these conventional approaches: the intrinsic low frequency of NK cells in the lymphoid organs (frequency estimates are of the order of 1%) and the possible heterogeneity of this class of effectors.[5,10-12]

Clearly an alternative strategy was required. About 4 years ago a number of laboratories began investigating the possibility of expanding NK cell populations by culture in lymphokine-rich media. Considerable encouragement was derived from the observation that interleukin-2 (IL-2), which had played a central role in the development of similar techniques for expansion of T cell populations,[13-14] was a potent regulator of NK activity.[15] Two outcomes of this new strategy could be envisioned. On the one hand, if NK cells were end cells, then attempts to propagate them in vitro were probably doomed to failure. On the other hand, if these cells retained the potential for replication, then by use of the correct growth factors it would be possible to maintain and clone these cells at will.

As is often the case in science, neither initial hypothesis proved correct. Considerable evidence now indicates that mature NK cells, i.e., the majority of cells responsible for the rapid lysis of prototype NK targets (YAC-1 in the mouse and K562 in humans), are incapable of sustained cell division in vitro, at least under the culture conditions that immunologists have currently engineered. Yet long-term cell lines, and indeed clones, displaying NK-like reactivity can be readily obtained. A considerable accumulation of circumstantial evidence in a variety of systems, together with some direct evidence obtained in the mouse, indicates that in a large proportion of cases such NK-like cell lines are derived by activation or differentiation of cells within the cytotoxic T lymphocyte (CTL) lineage. Indeed, it has been shown that the lymphokines primarily responsible for the positive regulation of NK activity in vivo, namely IL-2 and interferon (IFN), are capable of inducing, in a reversible manner, the expression of classical NK activity in monoclonal CTL cell lines. Thus, by a somewhat circuitous route, the important goal of establishing monoclonal cell lines with NK activity has been achieved and exploration of some of the major issues confronting NK cell biologists, such as the biochemical pathways involved in regulating NK activity, the nature of the receptors and recognition structures involved in NK-target cell interaction, the biochemistry of the cytolytic process, and definitive analysis of the role of cells with NK activity in vivo, can now be approached in a novel manner. In the next few years major advances in these areas of research can be expected. In this review, I would like to summarize the various technologies and lines of experimentation which have led to our ability to study NK activity at the clonal level in vitro, and describe some of the important advances in our understanding of NK cells which have already been generated by this approach.

Before beginning, it is important to have some understanding of what is meant by an NK cell. Currently, it is extremely difficult to formalate a comprehensive definition. At the present time, a definition in terms of function is the most appropriate. Thus, an NK cell will be considered to be a cell present in lymphoid tissues, which can lyse prototype NK targets (e.g., YAC-1 in the mouse, K562 in humans) in a short-term Cr-release assay without apparent prior sensitization. The term "NK-like" will be used to describe cultured cell lines which lyse YAC-1 and K562 tumor cell targets, but whose exact relationship to NK cells in vivo is unclear.

In this review, most emphasis will be given to the results and experience obtained with cloned cell lines. This is not to say that interesting findings have not been obtained with uncloned lines and, where relevant, these will be included. However, the real center of interest is in dissecting the NK system down to the simplest level and examining the physiology, biochemistry, and cell biology of cell populations assuredly derived from a single progenitor.

II. A GENERAL OVERVIEW OF THE TECHNOLOGY

The majority of protocols which have been used for the generation of cloned cell lines displaying NK-like activity have been variants on a common theme, and can be considered as comprising three basic steps: the selection of a starting population, the placing of this population in culture medium containing appropriate growth factors, and the cloning of the culture. The simplest procedure, and one of the most successful, is that used by Dennert[16] in the first description of the production of clones with NK activity. Unfractionated mouse spleen cells were placed directly into culture medium supplemented with 40% supernatant obtained from Concanavalin A (Con A)-stimulated spleen cells. Cell proliferation occurred and cultures were maintained by splitting and/or feeding as appropriate. The uncloned cultures (cell lines) displayed potent cytolytic activity against prototype NK targets (e.g., YAC-1) and could be maintained in continuous growth indefinitely. After about 4 months, cultures were cloned by limiting dilution in microplate wells, with feeding every 3 to 4 days. Wells containing growing colonies were identified by microscope and, as they approached confluency, were transferred to successively larger vessels. Recloning of such clones provided additional assurance of monoclonality.

Essentially identical procedures were used by Kedar et al.[17] and Riccardi et al.[18] to obtain NK-like clones from murine spleen cells and by Lagarde and Florian[19] to prepare NK-like clones from murine spleen and bone marrow cells. Conscious of the possibility that the use of unselected populations might lead to the outgrowth of undesired cell types, several workers chose to initiate cultures with partially purified NK cells. Of particular concern was the presence of residual mitogen in the growth factor preparations; this could cause polyclonal activation of T cells which would then be driven to rapid proliferation by the IL-2 present in the growth medium. Thus, Nabel et al.[20] passed mouse spleen cells over nylon wool columns to deplete B cells and macrophages, then treated them with anti-Thy-1 antibody and complement (C) to deplete T cells, and finally positively selected for Ly5 positive cells using a panning technique. Brooks et al.[21] treated spleen cells with anti-Thy-1 and C, and cultured them for 24 hr with polyinosinic-polycytidylic acid (poly I:C), prior to placing them in medium with growth factors. It was reasoned that activation of NK cells with poly I:C (which occurs via the release of IFN)[22] might favor their proliferation. Suzuki et al.[23] used the carbonyl iron/magnet technique to remove macrophages, nylon wool columns to remove B cells, and then purified low-density cells (which are enriched for NK activity) on Percoll gradients.

The extent to which any of these selection procedures were advantageous is unclear. As will be discussed extensively below, it has now been shown that factors present in mitogen-induced spleen cell supernatants can induce the expression of NK activity in CTLs and, following prolonged exposure, can cause CTLs to differentiate into cells which are morphologically, phenotypically, and functionally extremely similar to the NK-like clones generated using the empirical procedures. The implication is that the NK-like clones obtained in the earlier studies arose, at least in part, from polyclonal activation of contamininating cells within the CTL lineage. Because it is currently unclear whether cells other than T cells can generate long-term cell lines expressing NK-like activity (see below), removal of T cells could in fact be counterproductive.

The nature of the medium used for the propagation of the chosen starting population is presumably critical to the overall success of the procedure. However, very little information is available as to what medium components are essential. Most workers have chosen to use RPMI-1640 medium supplemented with 10% fetal bovine serum (FBS) and 2-mercaptoethanol (usually 5×10^{-5} *M*) for mouse cells and RPMI-1640 supplemented with 10 to 20% FBS or human serum for human cells. Mercaptoethanol has generally not been used in human studies, but there is evidence that it is essential for the growth of murine NK-like cells.[19] More enriched media, such as Click's medium, may offer some advantages in terms of overall cell viability and maximal cell densities.

Of paramount importance is the inclusion in the medium of an appropriate source of growth factors. In the absence of any knowledge as to the growth factor requirements of NK cells, the pragmatic approach has been to use crude growth factor preparations, usually obtained as supernatants from lectin-stimulated spleen cells or blood mononuclear cells (MNCs). Supernatant prepared by Con A stimulation of mouse or rat spleen cells has invariably been used as the source of factors for growing murine NK-like cell lines. In one case, the IL-2-containing fraction obtained by Sephacryl® S200 chromatography of such supernatant was used successfully to establish murine NK-like cells lines.[23] Such material, however, undoubtedly contained many cytokines.

The majority of studies with human cells have employed supernatant from phytohemagglutinin (PHA)-stimulated pooled blood MNCs as a source of growth factors. In some cases, phorbol-myristate acetate and Epstein-Barr virus (EBV)-transformed B lymphocyte cell lines (LCLs) have been added together with PHA as supplementary stimulates. In many cases the growth factor preparation has been obtained commercially. Two alternative sources of growth factor have been employed. Krensky et al.[24] maintained uncloned CTLs and NK-like cell lines in lectin-depleted supernatant obtained by PHA stimulation of the human lymphoma cell line, Jurkat. Allavena and Ortaldo[25] used supenatant from the MLA-144 monkey cell line which constitutively secretes lymphokines, obviating the use of lectins. These supernatants contain IL-2 but otherwise constitute a very restricted spectrum of lymphokines and growth factors compared with similar supernatants prepared from blood MNCs. Unfortunately, a danger in the use of such cell lines is that they are often contaminated with mycoplasma, and unless precautions are taken to remove the organisms from the growth factor-containing supenatants, rapid transfer of infection to the recipient cell lines would ensue.

It is interesting to note that in every case where NK-like cell lines have been established, mitogen or antigenic stimulation has been either deliberately or inadvertently applied to the starting population. Thus, in the mouse, all experiments have been performed using as growth factor, high concentrations (10 to 50%) of supernatant from Con A-stimulated spleen cells. In some cases, a simple fractionation has been performed to remove mitogen,[17,23] or α-methyl-D-mannoside has been added to inhibit mitogen binding,[17,26] but it is unlikely that these procedures completely abrogated mitogen interaction with effectors. In the studies of Benson et al.,[26] spleen cells were stimulated with allogeneic cells prior to placement in medium with growth factor. In man, NK-like clones or cell lines have been obtained from cultures stimulated with allogeneic cells, B lymphocyte cell lines, or with PHA. The apparent requirement for mitogenic or antigenic stimulation for the establishment of NK-like cell lines was confirmed directly by Abo and colleagues[27,28] using purified HNK-1$^+$ cells, but this study contrasted with some reports that low-density blood mononuclear cells could form colonies in the absence of mitogen.[29,30] These results have been reconciled by the finding that very low concentrations of mitogen are both necessary and sufficient to induce proliferation of human NK-like cells.[95]

It is often presumed that IL-2 is the critical factor required for the growth of cell lines with NK activity. Indeed, such is the current preeminence of this lymphokine, that crude supernatants of lectin-stimulated lymphocytes, which probably contain tens if not hundreds of biologically active molecules, are often referred to as IL-2 preparations. The important role of IL-2 as a second signal promoting the proliferation of antigen (or mitogen)-triggered T cells is well established, but the extent to which this lymphokine is sufficient for the long-term proliferation of T cell lines is unclear. In the case of CTLs, evidence has been presented that additional factors are required for optimal proliferation and/or expression of cytolytic function.[31-33] The growth requirements of other classes of T cells are even less clear. It is therefore regrettable that such a restricted source of growth factors, with emphasis on IL-2 content alone, has been used in attempts to promote clonal growth of NK cells. In the study of cultured human cell lines with NK activity, a major problem has been their short lifespan (usually only a few weeks). It is conceivable that supplementation of media with other sources of growth factors may extend the longevity of these cells or promote the growth of classes of NK cells capable of greater proliferative expansion.

A further consideration regarding the growth requirements of cell lines is the use of "feeder cells". In studies with human NK-like cell lines, autologous or allogeneic blood MNC, or EBV-transformed B LCL have usually been used as feeder cells. In murine studies, virus-transformed 3T3 cells, thioglyollate-induced peritoneal exudate cells, and a variety of tissue-derived cells have been used. Feeder cells are irradiated with 1000 to 5000 R to inhibit their replication, the larger radiation doses being applied to the cell lines, such as virus-transformed 3T3 cells or B LCL, because of their greater resistance to radiation than freshly obtained lymphoid cells. Feeder cells may function in three capacities: (1) as providers of an antigenic stimulus, (2) as secretors of undefined growth factors, (3) as nonspecific promoters of a favorable microenvironment (e.g., they might secrete enzymes which modify or activate other growth factors, absorb or degrade growth inhibitory substances, provide an essential nutrient, etc.). In all studies reported to date, feeder cells have been used during the cloning of human NK-like cell lines, and usually also for their subsequent maintenance. In at least one case, continuous use of feeder cells was found to be essential,[34] but in another study no feeders were added after cloning.[35] With mouse NK-like cell lines, feeders have been employed only at the cloning stage, and in many studies cloning has also been performed without feeders. The use of feeder cells should certainly be avoided unless essential, because there are some important disadvantages. Thus, when tissue culture cells are used as feeders, there is a high risk of transmitting mycoplasmal and/or viral infection to the cloned lines. Furthermore, even if it is assumed that the irradiation completely abrogates any sustained proliferation by the feeder cells, small numbers of functional feeder cells may persist for some time. In those cases where continuous periodic addition of feeder cells is necessary, the purity of the cloned cell lines could be significantly compromised.

The third aspect of procedures for producing cloned NK cell lines which needs some consideration is the cloning procedure itself. Most workers have used the limiting dilution method of cloning, but some have also used agar/agarose cloning[17,26,36] or micromanipulation.[20,36] The different cloning procedures have various advantages and disadvantages which were recently discussed by Bach.[37] The limiting dilution method has the advantage of simplicity but its effectiveness is limited first by the constraints of Poisson statistics and second, and more seriously, by the fact that, unless the starting cell population is composed entirely of single cells and has a cloning efficiency of close to 100%, it is difficult or impossible to state the probability that any given colony arose from a single precursor. Cloning in semisolid medium is also relatively simple but is associated with numerous interpretational problems. The extremely low cloning efficiencies usually obtained with semisolid media raise concerns over the single cell nature of the colony-forming unit (CFU) and over the possibility that rare variants, capable of growth in soft agar, are selected.

Furthermore, various hematopoietic elements are capable of migration through agar and may be "recruited" into growing colonies. At the time of colony excision from the agar it is always possible that noncolony cells, which remained viable but did not form visible colonies in the agar, will also be withdrawn and subsequently proliferate in liquid medium. Clearly, the most rigorous cloning technique, at least if performed with skill and patience, is micromanipulation. While the precision of this technique is theoretically independent of the cloning efficiency of the starting population, in practice it is only realistically feasible to employ this method when the cloning efficiency is reasonably high. Hence, its greatest value is as a recloning method for colonies isolated by limiting dilution or from agar.

When clones have been obtained in a manner which ensures, to a high level of probability, their origin from a single cell, it is generally assumed that the expanded clone represents a uniform population of cells. While it is certainly true that clones are relatively homogenous compared with uncloned populations, two factors continuously operate to ensure that the cloned cell line does not consist of an array of identical cells. First, and most obvious, a proliferating clone contains cells at each stage of the cell cycle. Second, stochastic events ensure that no uniform population of cells can ever exist. In practical terms, the most serious consequence is that variants, caused by both genetic and epigenetic changes, are continuously arising. A clone, in essence, represents a microcosm of Darwinian evolution, and the longer it exists the more diverse it becomes. The reality of this generation of diversity is strikingly apparent upon recloning any cloned cell population: morphological and proliferative (colony size) variants are readily observed, and what is seen in the microscope is presumably only the tip of the biochemical iceberg. The purpose of this digression is not to deny that cloning is an important approach (indeed it is one of the most powerful techniques yet devised for analyzing the complexity of the immune system), but to encourage some vigilance of this problem. In some cases, recloning of clones, followed by selection for the trait of interest, represents a partial solution. For example, in our initial studies, cloned murine NK-like cell lines consistently lost cytolytic activity over a period of months, presumably due to overgrowth of the clones by variants with lower cytolytic activity.[38] Upon recloning, clones displaying very high (similar to the original parent) and very low cytolytic activity could be recovered. Selection for highly cytotoxic subclones at regular intervals would thus permit an analysis of cytolytic mechanisms at the clonal level.

III. THE NATURE OF NK-LIKE CELL LINES

A. Do Mature NK Cells Proliferate?

A basic assumption implicit in all attempts to generate NK cell clones is that NK cells themselves can proliferate. Some evidence to suggest that NK cells may divide in vivo has in fact been described by Biron et al.[39] Following infection of mice with lymphocyte choriomeningitis virus, a significant proportion of the enhanced splenic NK activity resided in large cells, whereas in normal mice all NK activity was confined to small-medium sized cells. If the spleen cells were labeled in vitro with ^{3}H-thymidine, the blast cells became radioactive and, in an autoradiographic single cell cytotoxicity assay, a proportion of the cells lysing YAC-1 targets were labeled. The large size cells which lysed YAC-1 cells were at least partially sensitive to lysis by anti-NK-alloantiserum or antiasialo-GM$_1$ serum and complement.

More directly relevant to this present chapter is the issue of whether NK cells can be induced to proliferate in vitro. The discovery that treatment of mouse spleen cells with IL-2 strongly potentiated NK activity (for review see Reference 40), provided a considerable impetus for the development of NK cell lines using IL-2-containing growth factors. However, despite the fact that numerous cell lines and clones displaying NK-like reactivities have been obtained by such procedures, the evidence that classical NK cells proliferate under the culture conditions used is weak.

The ability of IL-2 to augment NK activity has often been considered as evidence for the existence of IL-2 receptors on NK cells. Recent studies by Kawase et al.[41] demonstrated, however, that the mechanism of NK potentiation is probably an indirect one, involving the IL-2-induced production of IFN-γ. Because IFNs, including those of type γ, are potent stimulators of NK activity (for review see Welsh[42]), the NK boosting by IL-2 can be explained, at least in part, by the action of the induced IFN-γ on NK cells. The ability of IL-2 to induce IFN-γ has been confirmed in both murine and human systems,[43-45] and Weigent et al.[44] showed that an anti-IFN-γ serum blocked IL-2-induced NK potentiation. Somewhat surprisingly, further studies revealed that the induction of IFN by IL-2 occurred by a complex mechanism which did not require mature T cells, but rather an interaction between adherent cells and NK cells themselves.[41] The cooperation between splenic adherent cells and NK cells was apparently mediated by a soluble factor released when adherent cells were treated with IL-2-containing preparations. Whether this factor acted directly on NK cells to induce IFN or required the further participation of IL-2 was not determined. Thus, the question of whether IL-2 interacts with NK cells in this system has not been fully resolved.

The issue of whether human NK cells express IL-2 receptors has recently been directly addressed by Abo et al.[28] They have made use of two MoAbs, one directed against the HNK-1 antigen which is present on virtually all NK cells, and one directed against the Tac-1 antigen. This latter antigen is believed to be a determinant on the IL-2 receptor because (1) it is present on antigen- or mitogen-activated T cells but not on unstimulated T cells or resting or activated B cells, (2) it inhibits the proliferation of IL-2-dependent T cell lines, (3) it inhibits the binding of highly purified IL-2 to such cell lines.[46,47] Abo et al. showed by fluoromicrocytometry that freshly isolated blood MNC, whether HNK-1$^-$ or HNK-1$^+$, contained no detectable Tac-1$^+$ cells. Thus, if the Tac-1 antigen is indeed an integral and unconcealable component of the IL-2 receptor, it can be concluded that resting NK cells lack IL-2 receptors, at least of the type found on activated T cells. This conclusion is compatible with the observation that HNK-1$^+$ cells fail to proliferate when cultured with lectin-free IL-2.[27]

Abo et al.[28] went on to examine whether the Tac-1 antigen could be induced during culture of NK cells. Within a few hours of culture of blood mononuclear cells with mitogens or allogeneic cells, a large proportion of T cells acquired the Tac-1 antigen. In addition, about 25% of HNK-1$^+$ cells became Tac-1$^+$. However, the Tac-1$^+$ HNK-1$^+$ cells belonged entirely to the T cell-like subset of HNK-1$^+$ cells. These cells express the E receptor and OKT3 antigen and have low NK activity.[12,48] The HNK-1$^+$ subset which lacks T cell markers, expresses the NK (and myeloid) marker OKM1, and which contains the bulk of blood NK activity,[12,48] did not acquire the Tac-1 antigen. Thus, the current indications are that the majority of blood NK cells do not express the T cell IL-2 receptor when freshly isolated, nor upon subsequent culture.

As already discussed, the presumption that IL-2 is a growth factor utilized by NK cells may be erroneous. Hence, it is important to examine whether there is any evidence that NK cells can proliferate in vitro. Two approaches have been taken. The first is to investigate whether purified NK cells can be propagated. Timonen et al.[49] and Ortaldo et al.[29] cultured NK cells and small T cells, isolated by Percoll density gradient centrifugation, in crude supernatant from PHA-stimulated blood mononuclear cells. Both sets of cultures could be maintained, with proliferation, for several weeks. The T cell cultures consisted predominantly of agranular blast cells with little cytotoxic activity. Cultures containing NK cells retained their large granular morphology and NK and antibody-dependent cell-mediated cytotoxic (ADCC) activity. However, the surface marker profile of the cultures containing NK cells changed dramatically within the first few days: loss of OKT10, OKM1, and Fc receptors, and gain of E receptor, Ia, and OKT3.[29] Indeed, after 2 weeks, the surface phenotype of the cultures containing NK cells was identical to that of the T cell culture. Two explanations of this result are possible: either NK cells undergo a radical change in surface glycoprotein expression during culture or the cultures become overgrown by a minor subpopulation of T cells present in the initial inoculum.

This latter explanation is supported by the studies of Abo and Balch,[27] who purified NK cells from human blood by use of the HNK-1 marker and cell sorting. When these cells were cultured with PHA + mitogen-stimulated leukocyte supernatant, there was an initial phase of cell death followed by slow proliferation. The cells which grew were large and granular and had NK-like cytolytic activity and a marker profile similar to that of the cultured cells studied by Ortaldo et al.[29] Fractionation of the HNK-1^+ cells prior to culture showed that the proliferating cells resided entirely in the minor subpopulation bearing the E receptor. The marker profile of this subpopulation prior to culture is very similar (e.g., OKT3^+, OKM1^-) to that predominating after culture of unfractionated HNK-1^+ cells for several weeks. In addition, this is the same subpopulation of HNK-1^+ cells which acquire the Tac-1 antigen after culture with PHA.[28]

The second approach which has been used to determine whether mature NK cells proliferate in vitro is limiting dilution analysis (LDA). Riccardi et al.[50,51] studied the development of colonies with anti-YAC-1 activity following the limiting dilution of mouse spleen cells into microplate wells containing syngeneic irradiated feeder cells and partially purified IL-2. Conventional Poisson analysis of cytotoxic colony distribution gave a precursor frequency of about 1 in 5×10^4 spleen cells. Pretreatment of spleen cells with IFN increased the colony frequency to about 1 in 5×10^3 cells. However, this figure is still well below the frequency of NK cells in mouse spleen, estimated morphologically or by single cell cytotoxicity assays to be of the order of 1 to 7%.[9,39] Thus, under the culture conditions used, partially purified IL-2 either induced the proliferation of NK cells at very low efficiency or, alternatively, the progenitor cell was not a typical NK cell. In support of the latter conclusion, spleen cells from BALB/c nu/nu mice, which contain a higher proportion of NK cells than do spleen cells from euthymic mice, gave very low frequencies of cytotoxic colonies, of the order of 1 per 10^6 spleen cells without IFN pretreatment and 1 per 10^5 spleen cells with IFN pretreatment. These results in fact suggest either that a thymus-dependent cell is the progenitor of the vast majority of colonies with anti-YAC-1 activity or that NK cells will not grow autonomously in the absence of thymus-dependent cells.

Similar studies were performed in the human by Vose and Bonnard[30] and Vose et al.[52] NK cells were highly purified by successive incubation on plastic, passage through nylon wool columns, density gradient centrifugation and depletion of E-rosette forming cells. When such cells (termed LGL) were studied in LDA, using crude or partially purified IL-2, an average of 1/200 cells was capable of cytotoxic colony formation. Pretreatment with IFN increased this figure slightly, but it was clear that the vast majority of cells in these highly purified NK cell fractions were unable to form cytotoxic colonies. Pretreatment with anti-OKM1 + complement, if anything, slightly enhanced the frequency of such colonies. Because the majority of blood NK cells are OKM1^+, this provides direct evidence that NK cells are in general unable to develop into cytotoxic colonies. Pretreatment with anti-OKT3 + complement had no effect on cytotoxic colony frequency, suggesting that the precursor of these colonies is an OKT3^- cell. Somewhat similar observations were made by Grimm et al.,[53] who studied the development of NK-like cytotoxic activity in unfractionated blood mononuclear cells incubated for several days with partially purified IL-2. The precursor cells were found to be of low density but could not be lysed by MoAbs which react with NK cells, such as OKM1 and HNK-1. Indeed, assuming that the cells were not simply resistant to complement-mediated lysis, they lacked all markers that were tested, including E receptor, OKT3, OKT8, OKT11, and Leu-1.

Up to 70% of the cells in LGL populations of the type used by Vose and colleagues[52] are capable of lysing K562 cells in single cell assays.[53a] Still further purification of such

LGL populations, using MoAbs reactive with NK cells and cell sorting, and their subsequent cloning has been described by Allavena and Ortaldo.[25] This study represents the most concerted attempt to date to clone NK cells directly, but whether the clones obtained were indeed derived from NK cells themselves was not entirely clear. As in other studies, the cloning efficiency was disappointingly low: generally only 3 to 10% of plated cells formed cytotoxic colonies. Also, although the MoAbs used (OKTI0, OKMI, B73.1) are selective for NK cells, they are not absolutely specific and, in addition, the sorted populations may have contained up to 5% contaminating cells, which may have included activated T cells. These reservations are of particular concern because the purified cells were precultured for 1 week prior to cloning. This would have provided strong selection for the more vigorously proliferating cells and, coupled with the low cloning efficiency, raises considerable uncertainty as to whether the precursors of the cytotoxic colonies were NK cells. Furthermore, most of the clones displayed the T cell markers OKT3 and/or OKT4, which have not been detected on mature NK cells.

Thus, although a variety of systems have been examined, no compelling evidence to indicate that mature NK cells can form clones in vitro has been obtained. The possibility that such clones will be obtained in the future cannot, of course, be ruled out. However, the weight of evidence indicates that the cloned cell lines with NK-like activity which have been studied to date are derived either from mature T cells (mainly CTL) or from precursor cells with a null phenotype and of unknown nature. Because some subpopulations of T cells probably lack the capacity to develop into cells displaying NK-like activity, the failure in some instances of cultures of purified T cells to develop NK activity could be caused by the purification and/or culture procedures favoring the growth of, for example, helper T cells. Studies of the surface markers of NK-like cell lines and with T cell clones, to be described in the next two sections, support these general conclusions.

B. Surface Markers on NK-Like Clones

The issue of whether the spectrum of surface markers displayed on a cell tells us anything of its origin is most controversial, not least within the field of study of NK cells. With regard to cultured cell lines, the major question centers on the stability of expression of membrane glycoproteins during culture. On the one hand there are those who will argue that prolonged maintenance of cells in vitro may cause instabilities or abnormalities in surface antigen display. There is no doubt that loss and gain of antigens from cloned cell lines has been observed, but whether this occurs frequently enough to cause a serious problem is questionable. On the other hand, some will argue that the combination of surface antigens observed on a cloned cell line is reflective of the origin of that line from a cell of the same, possibly extremely rare, phenotype in vivo. Given the immense effort expended in analyzing surface antigens on cloned NK-like cell lines, it would appear that most workers ascribe to the latter philosophy.

In the half dozen or so independent reports of cloned human cell lines with NK-like activity, a large array of MoAbs have been employed. Table 1 summarizes the results obtained with the most commonly used reagents. The most consistent findings have been the presence of the E receptor/OKT11 structure, the presence of OKT10, the absence or only weak display of OKM1, the absence of HNK-1, and the presence of Ia. Because the majority of blood NK cells are OKT11$^+$, OKT10$^+$, OKM1$^+$, HNK-1$^+$, Ia$^-$, the NK-like clones differ from fresh NK cells in expression of the latter three markers.

With regard to other markers, the clones appear to fall into two classes: those which display markers of mature T cells, such as OKT3, OKT4, and OKT8, and those which lack such markers. With the exception of weak staining of some NK cells with OKT8,[59] these markers are absent from blood NK cells. The difference between the two sets of clones was most apparent in the study of Hercend et al.[56] NK-like cell lines obtained by cloning

Table 1
SURFACE MARKERS DETECTED ON HUMAN NK-LIKE CLONES

No. of clones	4	6	6	8	1	3	1
OKT1/Leu-1		+			−	−	
OKT3/Leu-4			+	+ (MNC) − (NK)	−	−	+
OKT4/Leu-3a	3/4 $T4^-/T8^+$	−	3/6 $T4^-/T8^+$	1/4 (MNC) 0/4 (NK)	−	−	−
OKT8/Leu-2a	1/4 $T4^-/T8^-$	+	3/6 $T4^+/T8^-$	3/4 (MNC) 0/4 (NK)	−	−	−
OKT10				+	+	+	+
OKT11/Leu 5/Lyt-3/E recep	+		+	+ (7/8)	+	+	+
OKM1			±		−	−	−
HNK-1/Leu-7				− (1/8)	−	−	
HLA-DR/Ia	+		+	+	+		+
FcγR	−				±		
Ref.	54	55	34	56[a]	35	57	58

[a] Clones were derived from either unfractionated MNC or from an NK cell-enriched fraction.

unfractionated blood MNC generally possessed T cell markers, whereas clones prepared from MNC treated with anti-T3, anti-B1, and anti-Mo2 and complement lacked these markers. Although these latter clones generally lacked the NK marker HNK-1, and similar clones prepared by Kornbluth et al.[36] and Flomenberg et al.[57] also lacked OKM1, they reacted with a newly obtained, apparently NK-specific antibody, N901.[6] It is interesting to note that the two types of NK-like clones correspond phenotypically to the cell types identified by Abo and Balch[27] ($HNK\text{-}1^+$, $OKT3^+$, $OKM1^-$, with eventual loss of HNK-1) and Vose and Bonnard[30] ($OKM1^-$, $OKT3^-$) which can proliferate to form NK-like cell lines or colonies, respectively. It should also be noted that considerable instability of T cell markers on cloned cell lines has been reported by Zagury et al.[59a]

The existence of NK-like clones displaying either a CTL or a non-CTL phenotype has been described, perhaps rather more succinctly, in the mouse. With some minor variations, the phenotype of all mouse NK-like clones is Ig^-, $Thy\text{-}1^+$, $Ly\text{-}1^-$, Ly5 $(T200)^+$, asialo-$GM1^+$, $Mac\text{-}1^-$, FcR^-. Various workers have reported reactivity of the clones with NK alloantisera,[20,21,26] but the staining is usually weak, and in one case was not seen.[60] The most important variable has been in the expression of the cytotoxic/suppressor T cell marker Ly-2, some clones being strongly positive, some totally negative.[17,18,21,60] Because loss of Ly-2 from $Ly\text{-}2^+$ CTL clones has been observed,[61,62] it could be argued that $Ly\text{-}2^-$ NK-like clones have deleted the antigen. However, Suzuki et al.[23] showed that the colony-forming cells from which their $Ly\text{-}2^-$ NK-like clones were derived were predominately asialo-$GM1^+$, $Ly\text{-}2^-$.

C. CTL with NK Activity

The similarity in phenotype between many human and mouse NK-like clones and their corresponding CTL clones is striking. Particularly intriguing was the discovery that some mouse NK-like clones simultaneously displayed a CTL-specific marker, Ly-2, and NK-alloantigens.[21] This suggested that CTL and NK cells may be closely related, and that the culture conditions employed had either captured or induced cells which displayed a mixed phenotype.

To explore this relationship further, the issue of whether antigen-specific CTL could be induced to express NK activity was addressed directly.[63,64] CTL clones were generated by limiting dilution following mixed lymphocyte culture and maintained in medium containing low concentrations of Con A-induced supernatant. Many of the clones were recloned to ensure monoclonality. The lines were clearly CTL by the following criteria: (1) they expressed Thy-1 and Ly-2 antigens; (2) their proliferation was antigen- and IL-2-dependent; (3) they displayed exquisite antigen-specific cytolysis towards lymphoblast targets.

It was readily determined that these antigen-specific CTL lines expressed low quantities of the appropriate NK alloantigens.[65] Most interestingly, it was observed that, in addition to their antigen-specific cytolytic activity, about half of the clones displayed cytotoxic activity towards YAC-1. Employment of CTL clones raised in various allogeneic combinations ruled out the possiblity that this reactivity against YAC-1 was due to antigen cross-reactivity. The specificity of this additional cytotoxic function of CTL was, in some cases, similar to the promiscuous cytotoxicity displayed by most NK-like clones (see below). However, in many cases, it was identical to that of splenic NK cells.

When CTL clones were transferred into medium containing high concentrations of crude Con A-induced supernatant, a series of remarkable changes occurred. First, the cells went through a phase of rapid proliferation and became somewhat enlarged and more rounded. During this period there was a small increase in antigen-specific cytolytic activity, but a spectacular increase in NK activity. Indeed, even CTL clones which were initially devoid of NK function acquired it. The induced NK activity was initially identical in specificity to that of splenic NK cells. However, after a certain period of time (which varied from a few days to a few weeks, depending on the particular clone) the specificity degenerated towards promiscuous cytotoxicity, as manifested by the acquisition of lytic activity against NK-resistant targets. At least over the period during which the CTL expressed true NK specificity, the changes were reversible; after transfer back to medium containing low concentrations of IL-2-containing supernatant, the cells ceased to divide, gradually (over a period of several days) lost NK activity, and reverted back to small spindle-shaped cells. On the other hand, if the cells were kept in high concentrations of IL-2-containing supernatant, the rate of division slowed and sometimes the cells went through a crisis period, but no loss of cytolytic activity occurred. Eventually, such cultures became overgrown with large, highly granular cells which were able to proliferate indefinitely in the absence of antigen, lacked antigen-specific cytolytic activity, had a potent promiscuous cytotoxic activity, and, indeed, were identical by morphology, by surface markers, and by function to the NK-like clones studied previously.[21] During the latter stages of the lymphokine-induced differentiation of CTL, profound changes in cell surface glycolipids and glycoproteins were observed.

These studies have established unequivocally that NK activity can reside in cells of T cell (CTL) lineage, and that CTL are not, as had been prviously believed, restricted to antigen-specific cytotoxic activity. These findings have provided direct confirmation, at the clonal level, of the hypothesis of Klein,[66,67] that NK and CTL activity may reside in the same cell. A number of other reports have confirmed these findings. Acha-Orbea et al.[68] observed that I-2^b-restricted CTL clones, grown in an antigen-independent manner, gradually lost specific cytolytic activity but displayed NK-like or promiscuous cytotoxicity. In a series of elegant experiments, Binz et al.[69] observed that certain rat CTL clones displayed both antigen-specific and NK-like cytotoxicity, but that only the antigen-specific reactivity was inhibitable by specific anti-idiotype antibodies. This provides compelling evidence that the two types of cytotoxic reactivity are mediated via distinct receptor systems. Heuer et al.[70] have reported that suppressor T cells may also express NK-like function. They isolated a T cell clone from CBA/J mice tolerized to BSA which secreted a BSA-specific suppressor factor, displayed antigen-specific cytolytic activity, and also lysed YAC-1 cells.

NK activity is an inducible, rather than constitutive, function of CTL. All CTL clones which have been examined can be induced, although the kinetics of induction vary considerably from clone to clone. Provided the cells are not left in high concentrations of Con A-induced supernatant for too long, the induction of NK activity is fully reversible. Although the initial induction experiments were performed using crude supernatant, we have now shown that both highly purified mouse and human IL-2, and various IFNs, including a cloned recombinant IFN, are effective (References 64 and 96). The most spectacular inductions have been observed with mixtures of IL-2 and IFN. Such synergism between these mediators in potentiating NK activity in unfractionated mouse spleen cells has been documented.[15] One possible explanation of this effect, suggested by previous data,[15] is that IFN can promote expression of IL-2 receptors.

As noted, prolonged exposure of antigen-dependent cloned CTL lines to high concentrations of growth factors leads to the appearance of cells which are morphologically, biochemically, and functionally very different to the initial CTL cells, but apparently identical to many Ly-2^+ NK-like clones previously described by ourselves and others. There is thus strong circumstantial evidence that these NK-like clones arose from CTL. Despite numerous efforts, we have been unable to reverse the changes that led to the formation of these cells. High concentrations of growth factor are not essential for their appearance, since morphologically similar cells, displaying broad NK-like reactivity, lacking antigen-dependent proliferative responses, and bearing the marker asialo-GM2 have occasionally appeared in cloned CTL cultures maintained in low concentrations of growth factor.[97] It appears that such variant cells may continuously be thrown off at very low frequency by antigen-dependent CTL, but are selected against by the use of antigenic stimulation and low concentrations of growth factor. When CTL clones are placed in high concentrations of growth factor in the absence of antigen, such variants, once they arise (during which interval the culture may pass through a "crisis period"), grow to dominate the culture. Whether they develop through a process of differentiation, dedifferentiation, or even malignant transformation is uncertain.

Two studies performed using limiting dilution analysis have suggested that a large proportion of CTL or CTL precursors in human blood and mouse spleen are capable of expressing an NK-like reactivity. Thus, Moretta et al.[71] observed that virtually every human peripheral blood T cell could form a colony when plated in medium containing PHA and IL-2, and that about 30% of these colonies displayed lectin-dependent cytotoxic activity, and were therefore presumably of the CTL lineage. Of these colonies, about half displayed lytic activity towards K562. In limiting dilution cultures of mouse spleen cells containing Con A and growth factors, Shortman et al.[72] found that colonies with promiscuous cytolytic activity and large granular morphology arose with very high frequency; indeed, virtually every Ly-2 positive spleen cell could generate such a colony. The cytotoxicity was apparently lectin-independent, because it was still observable when 100 m*M* α-methyl-D-mannoside (a potent inhibitor of Con A binding) was added to the assay system. These colonies presumably contain CTL, activated by Con A, together with endogenously and exogenously supplied lymphokines, to the point where they express promiscuous lytic activity.

Even at this level of activation, some target cell selectivity is still apparent. This was most clearly documented using a mouse NK-like clone, which exerted marked cytolytic activity against a spectrum of NK-sensitive and NK-resistant mouse lymphoid tumor cells, but had much lower reactivity towards xenogenic lymphoid tumor cells and towards mouse solid tumor-derived targets.[21] A similar species restricted cytolytic activity was observed by Kedar et al.[17] and has been noted in some human NK-like clones.[55] Interestingly, Galili et al.[73] have reported that mouse thymocytes, or mature T cells treated with neuraminidase, spontaneously bind to a variety of mouse, but not xenogeneic targets. It may be speculated that during activation of CTL selective enhancement of the avidity of this type of interaction occurs, leading eventually to effective cytolytic interaction. Activated killer cells with a broad specificity have been observed in a number of situations in vivo.[74,75]

IV. NEW INFORMATION GAINED FROM THE STUDY OF NK-LIKE CELL LINES

A. The Origin of NK Cells

Ever since their discovery, the exact nature and origin of NK cells has been a subject of enormous controversy. The simultaneous expression on NK cells of both T cell markers such as Thy-1 and E receptor/OKT11 and myeloid markers such as Mac-1 and OKM1 is enigmatic. As discussed extensively above, studies with NK-like cell lines have provided unambiguous evidence that T cells, and particularly cells of CTL lineage, can express NK activity. Under the correct culture conditions, the NK specificity of CTL is identical to that of fresh NK cells. The finding that the induction of NK activity in CTL can be mediated by the two previously identified major regulators of NK activity, IFN and IL-2, strongly supports the notion that this pathway is physiologically relevant, and that at least some NK cells are closely related to CTL. It is interesting to note that the thymus, which lacks NK activity, contains cells which bind to NK-sensitive, but not to NK-resistant, targets.[76] However, the glycoprotein profile of induced CTL is not identical to that of fresh NK cells, e.g., Ly-2$^+$, Mac-1$^-$ for CTL and Ly-2$^-$, Mac-1$^+$ for NK cells. Clearly, if NK cells are related to CTL, some steps in the process have not yet been reproduced in vitro. A variety of schemes in which NK cells arise from differentiation or dedifferentiation of CTL, from prethymic CTL, or as a branch in the CTL pathway, can be constructed, but there is insufficient evidence for a meaningful discussion. The reason why some NK-like clones in the mouse lack the Ly-2 marker and some NK-like clones in the human lack the mature T cell markers OKT3, OKT4, and OKT8 is unclear. It would be important to determine whether these are also derived from cells in the CTL lineage or from a distinct source. The possibility exists that more than one cell type may contribute to the NK compartment. Piontek et al.[76] observed that peritoneal macrophages could display NK-patterned binding, and suggested that any cell with such binding specificity which acquired a cytolytic apparatus would be a functional NK cell.

B. The Specificity of NK Cells

Another issue of considerable controversy has been the mechanism of determination of specificity in NK cells. Two principal models have been considered: one in which NK effector cells bear clonally distributed receptors — here, the overall specificity of an NK population is largely determined by the frequency of NK cells which can recognize each given target cell; and one in which all NK cells bear the same receptor — specificity is determined principally by the affinity of interaction between NK cells and the potential target. The general finding that NK target cells show extensive cross-inhibition in cold target competition experiments argues strongly against the existence of a single clonally distributed receptor on NK cells, and has led to the visualization of hybrid models in which NK cells bear multiple receptors, some or all or none of which may be clonally distributed.

The results obtained with cloned cell lines have effectively ruled out models which propose clonal variation in specificity. The clearest results have been obtained in the mouse. Dennert et al.[16,77] found that cultured cell lines obtained from normal or nu/nu BALB/c mice showed the same specificity as fresh BALB/c spleen cells on a panel of nine target cells. Each of five clones obtained from a normal BALB/c cell line again showed identical specificity to unfractionated spleen cells. Similar results were obtained in the CTL NK induction system. Provided the CTL were not exposed to high concentrations of lymphokines for too long, the acquired NK-like activity was identical in specificity to that of fresh splenic NK cells.[63] Paradoxically, although NK cytotoxicity itself is thus mediated via a receptor system which lacks clonal variation, NK cells may still bear clonally restricted receptors. This was suggested by Klein,[66] and is clearly the case for antigen-specific CTL which acquire NK activity in vitro. As demonstrated convincingly by Binz et al.,[69] the clonally distributed receptors on CTL play no role in the NK-like cytotoxicity which may be expressed by these cells.

It is clear, however, that many NK-like cell lines display a broader or promiscuous lytic specificity, killing various NK-resistant target cells in addition to NK-sensitive target cells. The overwhelming impression from a large number of studies, particularly those where several such lines have been compared,[17-19,21,23,26] is that the specificities of each cell line are very similar, although occasionally some minor variations are seen. As has been noted, this promiscuous pattern of cytolytic activity inevitably develops when cloned CTL are exposed to high levels of Con A-induced spleen cell supernatant for prolonged periods. The kinetics of induction and sensitivity to the inducing factors varies between clones. Given that many NK-like cell lines are probably antigen-independent derivatives of conventional CTL (see above), the occasional variations in specificity are most likely attributable to clonal variation in responsiveness to the factors responsible for the shift from true NK specificity to promiscuous reactivity. It is relevant to note that activation of normal spleen cells with IFN or IFN inducers, either in vivo or in vitro, causes a broadening of specificity. The very broad specificity of many NK-like cell lines may simply represent ''ultimate activation''.

In the human, the situation is rather less clear. Variation in the specificity of NK-like clones has been the exception rather than the rule. Sugamara et al.[55] studied a large series of clones derived following culture of blood MNC from an EBV-seropositive donor with autologous EBV-transformed LCL. Three types of cytotoxic clone were produced: a few rare ''specific'' clones which killed autologous LCL but not K562; clones which killed LCL and K562; and clones which killed K562 but not LCL. Subclones derived from a killer clone of the second type all retained the ability to kill both targets, indicating that the two reactivities resided in the same cell and that the original clone was indeed monoclonal. However, the killing of autologous LCL was not a specific cytolytic reactivity because allogeneic LCL and indeed a wide spectrum of NK sensitive and NK resistant human targets were lysed. Further analysis of a clone which lysed K562 but not LCL showed lysis also of the NK-sensitive targets Molt 4 and Daudi.

NK-like clones isolated from conventional MLC by Pawelec et al.[78] showed even greater variation in specificity. Of six clones tested on a panel of eight targets, one lysed only HSB2, one lysed only K562, while the other four lysed K562 together with some but not all of the other targets. None of the clones lysed blood MNC derived from either the responder or stimulator in the original MLC. Given the ease with which murine MLC-derived CTL can acquire NK-like reactivity and still retain antigen-specific cytotoxicity, the absence of such clones in the human studies is noteworthy. This might be because human CTL lose antigen-specific reactivity more rapidly than murine CTL when cultured under conditions which promote the acquisition of NK function, or that the human NK-like clones are derived from precursors which lack antigen-specific responsiveness.

Hercend et al.[56] also reported that NK-like clones derived from ''null cells'' or whole blood MNC stimulated with PHA or EBV-transformed LCL varied in specificity. All eight clones were strongly lytic against K562 and, with one exception, weakly or noncytolytic towards LCL. Variable lytic activity was seen on the tumor targets Molt 4, HL60, and U937. Allavena and Ortaldo[25] studied 44 cytolytic clones derived by PHA stimulation of purified NK cells. Most clones with high cytolytic activity lysed all NK-sensitive targets tested, but three clones were lytic for K562 but not for Molt 4. Some weakly cytolytic clones showed evidence of selective specificity towards targets other than K562.

Taken at face value, these studies suggest that human NK cells display extensive variation in specificity at the clonal level. However, a number of technical considerations raise doubts about the validity of this conclusion. First, the results with mouse CTL clones show that, consequent to the induction of an NK specificity identical to that of splenic NK cells, there is a degeneration towards promiscuous lytic activity. Because the rate at which this process occurs varies from clone to clone, variation in specificity could be caused by variable rates of clonal evolution and/or variation between clones in their sensitivity to factors which induce NK reactivity and promiscuous killing. Second, Ortaldo et al.[29] reported that if uncloned NK-like cell lines with NK-like reactivity were "rested" for 24 hr by placement in medium lacking the PHA-induced growth factor preparation, cytotoxicity against some target cells was selectively lost. Whether this was caused by loss of lectin from the effector cells, loss of lymphokine-dependent cytotoxicity, or selective death of some effector cells was not investigated, although in a later study Spits et al.[79] showed clearly that minute amounts of PHA in cytotoxicity assays could augment the lytic activity of NK-like cells. Regardless of mechanism, variation in the rate at which different clones enter the resting state could be an important factor in determining specificity. A third problem is the short lifespan and limited proliferative vigor of human NK-like clones. Sometimes even repeat testing of specificity patterns on multiple targets has been difficult, and recloning to establish monoclonality has rarely been possible. In essence, many of the studies have been peformed with cells displaying varying degrees of senescence. Lastly, and in support of these concerns, is the documented evidence of unexpected variation in cultures of cloned human NK-like cells. Thus Pawelec et al.[78] found that, upon repeated testing of an NK-like clone, the ratio of killing on K562 to that on JM cells was, 2.6, 1.3, 6.6, 6.6, and 0.3 — a variation in specificity of 20-fold in five tests. Allavena and Ortaldo[25] observed an NK-like clone which on one test caused 62, 56, and 33% killing of K562, Molt4, nd Alab, respectively, and on a second test caused 75, 0, and 43% killing — a selective loss of activity against Molt 4. Even more dramatic is the extensive variation in surface marker profile seen on NK-like clones displaying differences in specificity.[25,56] This observation alone provides evidence that specificity variation of cells in human NK-like clones is determined in a fundamentally different manner from that in conventional B and T cells.

C. ADCC and NK Activity

It has been generally found that in human blood MNC and mouse spleen which mediate ADCC copurify with NK cells, although there have been some exceptions. Unambiguous evidence that cells with NK-like reactivity can also have ADCC activity has been obtained using cloned cell lines.[17,20,25,35,36,58] However, the two reactivities are not inevitably linked. Clones displaying ADCC but not lysis of K562 and clones lysing K562 but lacking ADCC have been described.[25,54] A curious observation is that in vitually every study where ADCC activity was found in cloned cells, xenogeneic antiserum was used to sensitize the targets (the exception is the study of Nabel et al.),[20] whereas in studies reporting negative results alloantiserum was used.[21,23,26,77] This raises the possibility that cytotoxic cells bearing receptors for certain classes/species of immunoglobulin, or perhaps such receptors themselves, are selectively lost during culture.

D. Studies of Morphology and Cell Chemistry

Cloned human and mouse NK-like cells are large and contain prominent granules, although some clones prepared from SJL mice,[18] and, in one study, clones of human NK-like cells were reported to be agranular.[78] No ultrastructural studies of the human cells have yet been published and only one human NK-like clone has been studied cytochemically. Kornbluth et al.[36] found it to contain acid phosphatase and nonspecific esterase, and to lack periodic acid-Schiff (PAS)-staining material and peroxidase.

Electron microscopy revealed the granules of murine NK-like cells to have a complex and characteristic structure.[21] The granules, 1 to 2 μm in diameter, were membrane bound and usually contained a central core of homogeneous or fine granular osmiophilic material surrounded by numerous microvesicles or microgranules. The relative proportions of core and microvesicular material varied, and some granules were composed entirely of core material. Similar results were obtained with several other NK-like clones.[60,80,81] Furthermore, an Ly2^{+}3^{+} cytotoxic/suppressor clone,[81] a CTL clone,[82] CTL clones which have lost antigen-specific cytotoxicity and display NK-like activity,[68] an antigen-specific suppressor clone with NK-like activity,[70] and antigen-specific CTL clones induced to express an antigen independent NK-like phenotype,[97] possess granules with similar ultrastructure. Such granules are absent from helper T cell clones.[81] Dvorak and colleagues have pointed out that these granules are similar to those of basophils.[80,81] Most interestingly, the NK-like clone described by Nabel et al.[20] was found by Galli et al.[80] to express IgE Fc receptors (FcR) of similar high affinity to those of basophils and mast cells. However, to date, subsequent examination of several other NK-like clones has failed to reveal further examples of clones displaying high-affinity IgE receptors.[26,60]

Using conventional cytochemical techniques, the granules appear to contain acid phophatase but to lack peroxidase.[20,21,23,60,68] This would suggest that NK lysis is not mediated by a H_2O_2/peroxidase system. Chloroacetate esterase activity has been observed in granules,[60,68] and at the electron microscope level the peripheral area of some granules is seen to contain nonspecific esterase activity,[81] which is also present in small cytoplasmic vesicles and on the cell membranes.[21,60,81] The nonspecific esterase in these cells was fluoride sensitive,[60,82] a characteristic normally associated with the myeloid rather than the lymphocytic version of the enzymic activity. However, it should be noted that following activation, the histochemistry of lymphocytes can change radically.[83] PAS positive material, presumably glycogen, has been observed in a number of NK-like clones[21,60] and, using electron microscopy, the osmium-potassium ferrocyanide technique revealed abundant cytoplasmic deposits of particulate glycogen in an NK-like clone and in a cytotoxic/suppressor clone, but not in a helper clone.[81] Glycogen deposits, frequently present in various types of granulocytes, have not been previously observed by ultrastructure in lymphocytes.

Intriguingly, both an NK-like clone and a cytotoxic/suppressor clone, but not a helper clone, incorporated $^{35}SO_4$ into the granules as chondroitin sulfates A and C (NK-like clones) or A, B, and C (cytotoxic/suppressor clone), but not into heparin.[81] The same cells could also actively sequester 5-hydroxytryptamine (serotonin) from the culture medium, whereas helper T cells could not. Both these biochemical processes have been previously associated with basophils, mast cells, and platelets (see Dvorak et al.[81] for references). However, NK-like clones, unlike basophils and mast cells, do not synthesize or store histamine.[21,80] These studies with cloned cell lines have thus provided new information on the selective sharing of genetic programs and biochemical processes between cells of different lineages.

E. Growth Requirements of NK-Like Cells

Present evidence suggests that IL-2 is necessary but not sufficient for the growth of these cells. Olabuenaga et al.[84] observed that in a 24-hr thymidine uptake assay, cloned mouse NK-like cells proliferated equally well in medium supplemented with either crude Con A-induced spleen cell supernatant or mouse IL-2 purified from LBRM-33 tumor cells by sequential ammonium sulfate precipitation, G100 chromatography, and isoelectric focusing. Similar findings have been reported for mouse NK-like clones by Suzuki et al.[23] and for uncloned cultures of NK-like cells by Ortaldo et al.[29] and Flomenberg et al.[57] Olabuenaga et al. went on to show that NK-like cells could absorb IL-2 activity from medium at 4°C and deplete IL-2 from medium during growth at 37°C. However, IL-2-containing fractions obtained from LBRM-33 cells as described above, or from Con A-induced spleen cell supernatant, were unable to support long-term (>2 days) growth of the cells. Supplementation of the partially purified IL-2 with IFN or Con A was without effect. With human NK-like cells, Pawelec et al.[34] reported that both crude mitogen-induced growth factor and irradiated feeder cells were essential for growth. These results are reminiscent of those of Lutz et al.,[31] which showed that IL-2 was not sufficient for the growth of antigen-specific CTL clones.

F. Cytolytic Mechanisms

A common approach for examining lytic processes in cytotoxic cells has been to determine, using antibody blocking, which cell surface glycoproteins may be involved. Antibodies to Ly-2, Ly-5, and LFA-1 can block lysis by cloned mouse NK-like cells.[21,26,68,70] In the case of Ly-2, clones which fail to express this antigen cannot be blocked by antibodies to Ly-2,[21] and even some clones which are Ly-2 positive are unaffected.[26,68] Similar variable results have been obtained with classical CTL, and it has been suggested that the Ly-2 molecules may strengthen adhesion between some CTL effectors and target cells, perhaps via a contribution of Ly-2 to the binding affinity of the antigen-specific receptor.[85] Given the lack of evidence for participation of a clonally distributed antigen-specific receptor in lysis by cloned NK-like cells, involvement of Ly-2 as a component of such a receptor would seem less likely. However, the ability of antibodies to Ly-2 to inhibit NK-like lysis by cloned cell lines is paradoxical because the absence of Ly-2 from splenic NK cells demonstrates that Ly-2 plays no role in NK function.

Inhibition of the lysis mediated by NK-like clones by antibodies to Ly-5[21] is consistent with a number of studies showing inhibition of splenic NK activity, but not CTL activity, by anti-Ly-5.[86,87] Although Ly-5 is present on most lymphoid cells, the inhibition studies suggest that the molecule bearing this determinant plays a special function in NK-lysis. It would be interesting to know whether anti-Ly-5 antibodies would inhibit antigen-specific cytolysis by CTL clones before and/or after induction of NK activity. In a further study, Krensky and colleagues[88] showed that antibodies to OKT3, LFA-2, and LFA-3 blocked lysis by a human CTL line but not by an NK-like cell line. Antibodies to LFA-1 blocked lysis by both lines. These studies collectively suggest that a different, but overlapping, set of surface molecules are required for NK lysis and CTL lysis.

At the electron microscope level, Dennert[89] observed that interaction between a mouse NK-like clone and YAC-1 cells, caused the appearance of circular "lesions" in the target membrane, similar (but not necessarily identical) to those formed by complement and cloned CTL (for short review see Lachman[90]). Such findings indicate that a colloid-osmotic lytic mechanism is utilized by both CTL and NK cells, although at least in the case of CTL there is evidence to the contrary.[91] Kedar et al.[17] reported that cloned mouse NK-like cells secreted a factor (NKCF) cytotoxic to NK-sensitive, but not to NK-resistant, targets. However, studies in this laboratory have so far failed to reproduce these results.[98] Indeed, the observation that NKCF production in mixed cultures of splenic NK cells and tumor targets is dependent upon the tumor cells being mycoplasma infected[92] casts some doubt on the physiological significance of this mediator.

G. NK Function In Vivo

Undoubtedly, the most important question of all relating to NK cells is that of the role of these cells in vivo. The need to answer this question was a principal motivating force in the development of techniques for cloning NK cells. To date, only two studies have been reported but the results are so spectacular as to command attention, and will undoubtedly lead to a complete investigation of this area.

Nabel et al.[93] showed that an NK-like clone would, at low concentrations, inhibit secretion of T cell-dependent immunoglobulin by B cells in vitro. As few as 1×10^3 cloned NK-like cells, injected into 700 R irradiated mice at about the same time as normal B cells and antigen (but not simultaneously), inhibited the plaque response to TNP-Ficoll measured 7 days later. Furthermore, if irradiated mice were reconstituted with normal T cells and cloned NK-like cells, spleen cells removed 7 days later and mixed with normal spleen cells and sheep red blood cells inhibited the PFC response. This demonstration that an NK-like clone has suppressor activity in vivo fits nicely with the finding of a suppressor T cell clone which displays NK-like lytic activity.[70]

Even more dramatic results were reported by Warner and Dennert.[94] C57BL/6 bg/bg or immunosuppressed normal C57BL/6 mice, which have poor NK activity, fail to reject allogeneic bone-marrow following lethal irradiation. However, if such mice were given 2 $\times$ 10^6 syngeneic cloned NK-like cells, rejection responses were fully restored despite the fact that splenic NK activity remained low. Remarkably, the adoptive in vivo transfer was effective if the NK-like cells were given up to 30 days prior to transplantation. Thus, not only are the effects of the in vivo transfer of NK-like cells long lasting, but they also resist the 850 to 950 R given prior to bone marrow transplantation. The apparent display of specific allorejection by the NK-like cells in vivo is curious as such specificities are not seen in vitro. It is conceivable that the cloned NK cells acted as antibody-dependent killer cells in conjunction with host antibody, or amplified host radiation-resistant specific responses via the secretion of lymphokines.

Transfer of cloned NK-like cells into bg/bg or cyclophosphamide-treated mice suppressed lung colony formation and metastasis of subsequently injected B16 melanoma cells. Transfer of control cultured cells lacking NK activity had no effect. In further experiments it was observed that administration of cloned NK-like cells following a split dose irradiation treatment of C57BL/6 mice reduced the development of thymomas 3 to 5 months later by greater than 90%. These results provide the strongest evidence obtained so far that cells with NK activity are involved in both graft rejection and the inhibition of tumor growth.

ACKNOWLEDGMENTS

I would like to thank the many colleagues who supplied me with reprints and preprints of their work. In particular, I thank Dr. Elizabeth Benson, Massachusetts General Hospital, Boston; Dr. Stephen Galli, Department of Pathology, Beth Israel Hospital, Boston; Dr. Alain Lagarde, Cancer Research Laboratories, Department of Pathology, Queen's University, Kingston, Ontario, Canada; Dr. John Ortaldo, Biological Response Modifiers Program, National Cancer Institute, NCI-Frederick Cancer Research Facility, Frederick, Md. for giving me access to their unpublished work. I am grateful to Ms. Kathy Eichinger for her careful typing of the manuscript. This work was supported by grant AI-15384 from the National Institutes of Health.

REFERENCES

1. **Glimcher, L., Shen, F. W., and Cantor, H.,** Identification of a cell surface antigen selectively expressed on the natural killer cell, *J. Exp. Med.*, 145, 1, 1977.
2. **Burton, R. C. and Winn, H. J.,** Studies on natural killer (NK) cells. I. NK cell specific antibodies in CE anti-CBA serum, *J. Immunol.*, 126, 1945, 1981.
3. **Abo, T. and Balch, C. M.,** A differentiation antigen of human NK and K cells identified by a monoclonal antibody (HNK-1), *J. Immunol.*, 127, 1024, 1981.
4. **Perussia, B., Starr, S., Abraham, S., Fanning, V., and Trinchieri, G.,** Human natural killer cells analyzed by B73.1, a monoclonal antibody blocking Fc receptor functions. I. Characterization of the lymphocyte subset reactive with B73.1, *J. Immunol.*, 130, 2133, 1983.
5. **Lanier, L. L., Le, A.-M., Phillips, J. H., Warner, N. L., and Babcock, G. F.,** Subpopulations of human natural killer cells defined by expression of the Leu-7 (HNK-1) and Leu-11 (NK-15) antigens, *J. Immunol.*, 131, 1789, 1983.
6. **Griffin, J. D., Hercend, T., Beveridge, R., and Schlossman, S. F.,** Characterization of an antigen expressed by human natural killer cells, *J. Immunol.*, 130, 2947, 1983.
7. **Timonen, T. and Saksela, E.,** Isolation of human natural killer cells by density gradient centrifugation, *J. Immunol. Methods*, 36, 285, 1980.
8. **Reynolds, C. W., Timonen, T., and Herberman, R. B.,** Natural killer (NK) cell activity in the rat. I. Isolation and characterization of the effector cells, *J. Immunol.*, 127, 282, 1982.

9. **Kumagai, K., Itoh, K., Suzuki, R., Hinuma, S., and Saitoh, F.,** Studies of murine large granular lymphocytes. I. Identification as effector cells in NK and K cytotoxicities, *J. Immunol.*, 129, 388, 1982.
10. **Paige, C. J., Figarella, E. F., Cuttito, J. J., and Stutman, O.,** Natural cytotoxic cells against solid tumors in mice. II. Some characteristics of the effector cell, *J. Immunol.*, 121, 1827, 1978.
11. **Kumar, V., Luevano, E., and Bennett, M.,** Hybrid resistance to EL4 lymphoma cells. I. Characterization of natural killer cells that lyse EL4 cells and their distinction from marrow-dependent natural killer cells, *J. Exp. Med.*, 150, 531, 1979.
12. **Abo, T., Cooper, M. D., and Balch, C. M.,** Characterization of HNK-1$^+$ (Leu-7) human lymphocytes. I. Two distinct phenotypes of human NK cells with different cytotoxic capability, *J. Immunol.*, 129, 1752, 1982.
13. **Moller, G., Ed.,** T cell clones, *Immunol. Rev.*, 54, 1981.
14. **Fathman, C. G. and Fitch, W. W., Eds.,** *Isolation, Characterization, and Utilization of T Lymphocyte Clones*, Academic Press, New York, 1982.
15. **Kuribayashi, K., Gillis, S., Kern, D. E., and Henney, C. S.,** Murine NK cell cultures: effects of interleukin-2 and interferon on cell growth and cytotoxic reactivity, *J. Immunol.*, 26, 2321, 1981.
16. **Dennert, G.,** Cloned lines of natural killer cells, *Nature (London)*, 287, 47, 1980.
17. **Kedar, E., Ikejiri, B. L., Sredni, B., Bonavida, B., and Herberman, R. B.,** Propagation of mouse cytotoxic clones with characteristics of natural killer (NK) cells, *Cell. Immunol.*, 69, 305, 1982.
18. **Riccardi, C., Allavena, P., Ortaldo, J., and Herberman, R. B.,** Cloned lines of SJL/J spleen cells with cytotoxic reactivity, *Int. J. Cancer*, 31, 345, 1983.
19. **Lagarde, A. E. and Florian, M.,** Spleen- and bone-marrow-derived murine cloned cell lines mediating natural killer activity. I. Establishment and functional characteristics, submitted.
20. **Nabel, G., Bucalo, L. R., Allard, J., Wigzell, H., and Cantor, H.,** Multiple activities of a cloned cell line mediating natural killer function, *J. Exp. Med.*, 153, 1582, 1982.
21. **Brooks, C. G., Kuribayashi, K., Sale, G. E., and Henney, C. S.,** Characterization of five cloned murine cell lines showing high cytolytic activity against YAC-1 cells, *J. Immunol.*, 128, 2326, 1982.
22. **Djeu, J. Y., Heinbaugh, J. A., Holden, H. J., and Herberman, R. B.,** Augmentation of mouse natural killer activity by interferon and interferon inducers, *J. Immunol.*, 122, 181, 1979.
23. **Suzuki, R., Handa, K., Itoh, K., and Kumagai, K.,** Natural killer (NK) cells as a responder to interleukin 2 (IL-2). I. Proliferative response and establishment of cloned cells, *J. Immunol.*, 130, 981, 1983.
24. **Krensky, A. M., Sanchez-Madrid, F., Robbins, E., Nagy, J. A., Springer, T. A., and Burakoff, S. J.,** The functional significance, distribution, and structure of LFA-1, LFA-2, and LFA-3: cell surface antigens associated with CTL-target interactions, *J. Immunol.*, 131, 611, 1983.
25. **Allavena, P. and Ortaldo, J. R.,** Characteristics of human NK clones: target specificity and phenotype, submitted.
26. **Benson, E., Giorgi, J., Dvorak, A., and Russell, P.,** "Activated killer" clones derived from MLC. Function, morphology and phenotype, submitted.
27. **Abo, T. and Balch, C. M.,** *In vitro* propagation of cultured human natural killer cells expressing the HNK-1 differentiation antigen and spontaneous cytotoxic function, *Eur. J. Immunol.*, 13, 383, 1983.
28. **Abo, T., Miller, C. A., Balch, C. M., and Cooper, M. D.,** Interleukin 2 receptor expression by activated HNK-1$^+$ granular lymphocytes: a requirement for their proliferation, *J. Immunol.*, 131, 1822, 1983.
29. **Ortaldo, J. R., Timonen, T. T., Vose, B. M., and Alvarez, J. A.,** Human natural killer cells as well as T cells maintained in continuous cultures with IL-2, in *The Potential Role of T Cells in Cancer Therapy*, Fefer, A. and Goldstein, A., Eds., Raven Press, New York, 1982, 191.
30. **Vose, B. M. and Bonnard, G. D.,** Limiting dilution analysis of the frequency of human T cells and large granular lymphocytes proliferating in response to interleukin-2. I. The effect of lectin on the proliferative frequency and cytotoxic activity of cultured lymphoid cells, *J. Immunol.*, 130, 687, 1983.
31. **Lutz, C. T., Glasebrook, A. L., and Fitch, F. W.,** Alloreactive cloned T cell lines. I. Accessory cell requirements for the growth of cloned cytolytic T lymphocytes, *J. Immunol.*, 126, 1404, 1981.
32. **Wagner, H., Hardt, C., Rouse, B. T., Rollinghoff, M., Scheurich, R., and Pfizenmeier, K.,** Dissection of the proliferative and differentiation signals controlling murine cytotoxic T lymphocyte responses, *J. Exp. Med.*, 155, 1876, 1982.
33. **Raulet, D. H. and Bevan, M. J.,** A differentiation factor required for the expression of cytotoxic T cell function, *Nature (London)*, 296, 754, 1982.
34. **Pawelec, G. P., Hadam, M. R., Ziegler, A., Lohmeyer, J., Rehbein, A., Kumbier, I., and Wernet, P.,** Long-term culture, cloning, and surface markers of mixed leukocyte culture-derived human T lymphocytes with natural killer-like cytotoxicity, *J. Immunol.*, 129, 1892, 1982.
35. **Hercend, T., Meuer, S., Reinherz, E. L., Schlossman, S. F., and Ritz, J.,** Generation of a cloned NK cell line derived from the "null cell" fraction of human peripheral blood, *J. Immunol.*, 129, 1299, 1982.
36. **Kornbluth, J., Flomenberg, N., and Dupont, B.,** Cell surface phenotype of a cloned line of human natural killer cells, *J. Immunol.*, 129, 2837, 1982.

37. **Bach, F.,** On getting a T-cell clone and being assured you have one, *Immunol. Today*, 4, 243, 1983.
38. **Brooks, C. G., Kuribayashi, K., Olabuenaga, S., Feng, M. F., and Henney, C. S.,** Characterization of cloned murine cell lines having high cytolytic activity against YAC-1 targets, in *NK Cells and Other Natural Effector Cells*, Herberman, R. B., Ed., Academic Press, New York, 1982, 851.
39. **Biron, C. A. and Welsh, R. M.,** Blastogenesis of natural killer cells during viral infection *in vivo*, *J. Immunol.*, 129, 2788, 1982.
40. **Brooks, C. G. and Henney, C. S.,** Interleukin-2 and the regulation of natural killer activity in cultured cell populations, in *The Interleukins. Contemporary Topics in Molecular Immunology*, Gillis, S. and Inman, F. P., Eds., Plenum Press, New York, 1984.
41. **Kawase, I., Brooks, C. G., Kuribayashi, K., Olabuenaga, S., Newman, W., Gillis, S., and Henney, C. S.,** Interleukin 2 induces γ-interferon production: participation of macrophages and NK-like cells, *J. Immunol.*, 131, 288, 1983.
42. **Welsh, R. M.,** Natural killer cells and interferon, *CRC Crit. Rev. Immunol.*, 5(1), 55, 1984.
43. **Yamamoto, J. K., Farrar, W. L., and Johnson, H. M.,** Interleukin 2 regulation of mitogen induction of immune interferon (IFNγ) production by human T cells and T cell subsets, *J. Immunol.*, 130, 1784, 1983.
44. **Kasahara, T., Hooks, J. J., Dougherty, S. F., and Oppenheim, J. J.,** Interleukin-2-mediated immune interferon (IFNγ) production by human T cells and T cell subsets, *J. Immunol.*, 130, 1784, 1983.
45. **Weigent, D. A., Stanton, G. J., and Johnson, H. M.,** Interleukin-2 enhances natural killer cell activity through induction of γ interferon, *Fed. Proc., Fed. Am. Soc. Exp. Biol.*, 42, 1072, 1983.
46. **Leonard, W. J., Depper, J. M., Uchiyama, T., Smith, K. A., Waldman, T. A., and Greene, W. C.,** A monoclonal antibody that appears to recognize the receptor for human T cell growth factor: partial characterization of the receptor, *Nature (London)*, 300, 267, 1982.
47. **Robb, R. J. and Greene, W. C.,** Direct demonstration of the identity of T cell growth factor binding protein and the Tac antigen, *J. Exp. Med.*, 158, 1332, 1983.
48. **Abo, T. and Balch, C. M.,** Characterization of HNK-1$^+$ (Leu-7) human lymphocytes. II. Distinguishing phenotypic and functional properties of natural killer cells from activated NK-like cells, *J. Immunol.*, 129, 1758, 1982.
49. **Timonen, T., Ortaldo, J. R., Stadler, B. M., Bonnard, G. D., Sharrow, S. O., and Herberman, R. B.,** Culture of purified human natural killer cells: growth in the presence of interleukin-2, *Cell. Immunol.*, 72, 178, 1982.
50. **Riccardi, C., Vose, B. M., and Herberman, R. B.,** Modulation of the Il-2-dependent growth of mouse NK cells by interferon and T lymphocytes, *J. Immunol.*, 130, 228, 1983.
51. **Riccardi, C., Vose, B. M., and Herberman, R. B.,** Regulation by interferon and T cells of IL-2-dependent growth of NK progenitor cells: a limiting dilution analysis, in *NK Cells and Other Natural Effector Cells*, Herberman, R. B., Ed., Academic Press, New York, 1982, 909.
52. **Vose, B. M., Riccardi, R. C., Bonnard, G. D., and Herberman, R. B.,** Limiting dilution analysis of the frequency of human T cells and large granular lynphocytes proliferating in response to interleukin 2. II. Regulatory role of interferon on proliferative and cytotoxic precursors, *J. Immunol.*, 130, 768, 1983.
53. **Grimm, E. A., Mazumder, A., Strausser, J. L., and Rozenberg, S. A.,** Lymphokine-activated killer cell phenomenon. Lysis of natural killer-resistant frest solid tumor cells by interleukin 2-activated autologous human peripheral blood lymphocytes, *J. Exp. Med.*, 155, 1823, 1982.

53a. **Timonen, T., Ortaldo, J. R., and Herberman, R. B.,** Analysis by a single cell cytoxicity assay of natural killer (NK) cell frequencies among human large granular lymphocytes and of the effects of interferon on their activity, *J. Immunol.*, 128, 2514, 1982.

54. **Moretta, L., Mingari, M. C., Sekaly, P. R., Moretta, A., Chapius, B., and Cerottini, J.-C.,** Surface markers of cloned human T cells with various cytolytic activities, *J. Exp. Med.*, 154, 569, 1981.
55. **Sugamura, K., Tanaka, Y., and Hinuma, Y.,** Two distinct human cloned T cell lines that express natural killer-like and anti-human effector activities, *J. Immunol.*, 128, 1749, 1982.
56. **Hercend, T., Reinherz, E. L., Meuer, S., Schlossman, S. F., and Ritz, J.,** Phenotypic and functional heterogeneity of human cloned natural killer cell lines, *Nature (London)*, 301, 158, 1983.
57. **Flomenberg, N., Welte, K., Mertelsmann, R., O'Reilly, R., and Dupont, B.,** Interleukin-2-dependent natural killer (NK) cell lines from patients with primary T cell immunodeficiencies, *J. Immunol.*, 130, 2635, 1983.
58. **Sheehy, M. J., Quintieri, F. B., Leung, D. Y. M., Geha, R. S., Dubey, D. P., Limmer, C. E., and Yunis, E. J.,** A human large granular lymphocyte clone with natural killer-like activity and T cell-like surface markers, *J. Immunol.*, 130, 524, 1983.
59. **Perussia, B., Fanning, V., and Trinchieri, G.,** A human NK and K cell subset shares with cytotoxic T cells expression of the antigen recognized by antibody OKT8, *J. Immunol.*, 131, 223, 1983.

59a. **Zugury, D., Bernard, J., Morgan, D. A., Fouchard, M., and Feldman, M.,** Phenotypic diversity within clones of normal T cells, *Int. J. Cancer*, 31, 705, 1983.

60. **Lagarde, A. E., Florian, M., and Longhurst, W.,** Spleen- and bone-marrow-derived murine cloned cell lines mediating natural killer activity. II. Morphology and analysis of cytochemical and cell surface markers, submitted.
61. **Dialynas, D. P., Loken, M. R., Glasebrook, A. L., and Fitch, F. W.,** Lyt-2$^-$/Lyt-3$^-$ variants of a cloned cytolytic T cell line lack an antigen receptor functional in cytolysis, *J. Exp. Med.*, 153, 595, 1981.
62. **Giorgi, J. V., Zawadzki, J. A., and Warner, N. L.,** Cytotoxic T lymphocyte lines reactive against murine plasmacytoma antigens: dissociation of cytotoxicity and Lyt-2 expression, *Eur. J. Immunol.*, 12, 825, 1982.
63. **Brooks, C. G., Urdal, D., and Henney, C. S.,** Lymphokine-driven "differentiation" of cytotoxic T cell clones into cells with NK-like specificity: correlation with display of membrane macromolecules, *Immunol. Rev.*, 72, 43, 1983.
64. **Brooks, C. G.,** Reversible induction of natural killer cell activity in cloned murine cytotoxic T lymphocytes, *Nature (London)*, 305, 155, 1983.
65. **Brooks, C. G., Burton, R. C., Pollack, S. B., and Henney, C. S.,** The presence of NK alloantigens on cloned cytotoxic T lymphocytes, *J. Immunol.*, 131, 1391, 1983.
66. **Klein, E.,** Natural and activated cytotoxic T lymphocytes, *Immunol. Today*, 1, iv, 1980.
67. **Vanky, F. and Klein, E.,** Alloreactive cytotoxicity of interferon-triggered human lymphoblasts detected with tumor biopsy targets, *Immunogenetics*, 15, 31, 1982.
68. **Acha-Orbea, H., Groscurth, P., Lang, R., Stitz, L., and Hengartner, H.,** Characterization of cloned cytotoxic lymphocytes with NK-like activity, *J. Immunol.*, 130, 2952, 1983.
69. **Binz, H., Fenner, M., Drei, D., and Wigzell, H.,** Two independent receptors allow selective target-lysis by T cell clones, *J. Exp. Med.*
70. **Heuer, J., Opalka, B., Rassat, J., Themann, H., and Kolsch, E.,** Characterization of the cytolytic activity of a cloned antigen-specific T suppressor cell derived from a tolerant CBA/J mouse, *Eur. J. Immunol.*, 13, 551, 1983.
71. **Moretta, A., Pantaleo, G., Morelta, L., Cerottini, J. C., and Mingari, M. C.,** Direct demonstration of the clonogenic potential of every human peripheral blood T cell. Clonal analysis of HLA-DR expression and cytolytic activity, *J. Exp. Med.*, 157, 743, 1983.
72. **Shortman, K., Wilson, A., Scollay, R., and Chen, W. F.,** Development of large granular lymphocytes with anomalous, nonspecific cytotoxicity in clones derived from Ly-1$^+$ cells, *Proc. Natl. Acad. Sci. U.S.A.*, 80, 2728, 1983.
73. **Galili, V., Galili, N., Vanky, F., and Klein, E.,** Natural species-restricted attachment of human and murine T lymphcotyes to various cells, *Proc. Natl. Acad. Sci. U.S.A.*, 75, 2396, 1978.
74. **Welsh, R. M., Zinkernagel, R. M., and Hallenbeck, L. A.,** Cytotoxic cells induced during lymphocytic choriomeningitis virus infection of mice. II. "Specificities" of the natural killer cells, *J. Immunol.*, 122, 475, 1979.
75. **Silver, R. M., Redelman, D., Zvaifler, N. J., and Naides, S.,** Studies of rheumatoid synovial fluid lymphocytes. I. Evidence for activated natural killer (NK) cells, *J. Immunol.*, 128, 1758, 1982.
76. **Piontek, G. E., Gronberg, A., Ahrlund-Richter, L., Kiessling, R., and Hengartner, H.,** NK-patterned binding expressed by non-NK mouse leukocytes, *Int. J. Cancer*, 30, 225, 1982.
77. **Dennert, G., Yogeeswaran, G., and Yamagata, S.,** Cloned cell lines with natural killer activity. Specificity, function, and cell surface markers, *J. Exp. Med.*, 153, 545, 1981.
78. **Pawelec, G. P., Hadam, M. R., Schneider, E. M., and Wernet, P.,** Clonally-restricted natural killer-like cytotoxicity displayed by cloned human T cell lines, *J. Immunol.*, 129, 2271, 1982.
79. **Spits, H., Ijssel, H., Terhorst, C., and deVries, J. E.,** Establishment of human T lymphocyte clones highly cytotoxic for an EBV-transformed B cell line in serum-free medium: isolation of clones that differ in phenotype and specificity, *J. Immunol.*, 128, 95, 1982.
80. **Galli, S. J., Dvorak, A. M., Ishizaka, T., Nabel, G., Der Simonian, H., Cantor, H., and Dvorak, H. F.,** A cloned cell with NK function resembles basophils by ultrastructure and expresses IgE receptors, *Nature (London)*, 298, 288, 1982.
81. **Dvorak, A. M., Galli, S. J., Marcum, J. A., Nabel, G., Der Simonian, H., Goldin, J., Monahan, R. A., Pyne, K., Cantor, H., Rosenberg, R. D., and Dvorak, H. F.,** Cloned mouse cells with natural killer function and cloned suppressor T cells express ultrastructural and biochemical features not shared by cloned inducer T cells, *J. Exp. Med.*
82. **Dvorak, A. M., Tyler, J. D., Malek, T. R., Pyne, K. E., Shevach, E. M., Steinmuller, D., and Galli, S. J.,** Ulstructure of antigen-specific cytolytic T cell lines in the mouse and guinea pig, submitted.
83. **Davey, F. R., Lock, N. L., and MacCallum, J.,** Cytochemical reactions in resting and activated T-lymphocytes, *Am. J. Clin. Pathol.*, 74, 174, 1980.
84. **Olabuenaga, S., Brooks, C. G., Gillis, S., and Henney, C. S.,** Interleukin 2 is not sufficient for the continuous growth of cloned NK-like cytotoxic cell lines, *J. Immunol.*, 131, 2386, 1983.
85. **Moller, G., Ed.,** Effects of anti-membrane antibodies on killer T cells, *Immunol. Rev.*, 68, 1982.

86. **Minato, N., Reid, L., Cantor, H., Lengyel, R., and Bloom, B. R.,** Mode of regulation of natural killer cell activity by interferon, *J. Exp. Med.*, 152, 124, 1980.
87. **Seaman, W. E., Talal, N., Herzenberg, L. A., Herzenberg, L. A., and Ledbetter, J. A.,** Surface antigens on mouse natural killer cells: use of monoclonal antibodies to inhibit or enrich cytotoxic activity, *J. Immunol.*, 127, 982, 1981.
88. **Krensky, A. M., Ault, K. A., Reiss, C. S., Strominger, J. L., and Burakoff, S. J.,** Generation of long-term human cytolytic cell lines with persistent natural killer activity, *J. Immunol.*, 129, 1748, 1982.
89. **Podack, E. R. and Dennert, G.,** Assembly of two types of tubules with putative cytolytic function by cloned natural killer cells, *Nature (London)*, 302, 442, 1983.
90. **Lachman, P. J.,** Are complement lysis and lymphocytotoxicity analogous?, *Nature (London)*, 305, 473, 1983.
91. **Russell, J. M.,** Internal disintegration model of cytotoxic lymphocyte-induced target damage, *Immunol. Rev.*, 72, 97, 1983.
92. **Wayner, E. A. and Brooks, C. G.,** NKCF production in mixed lymphocyte-tumor cell culture: direct involvement of mycoplasma infection of tumor cells, submitted.
93. **Nabel, G., Allard, W. J., and Cantor, H.,** A cloned cell line mediating natural killer cell function inhibits immunoglobulin secretion, *J. Exp. Med.*, 156, 658, 1982.
94. **Warner, J. F. and Dennert, G.,** Effects of a cloned cell line with NK activity on bone-marrow transplants, tumour development and metastasis *in vivo*, *Nature (London)*, 300, 31, 1982.
95. **Ortaldo, J. R.,** personal communication.
96. **Brooks, C. G. et al.,** in preparation.
97. **Brooks, C. G.,** unpublished.
98. **Wayner, E. A. and Brooks, C. G.,** unpublished.

Chapter 12

A COMPARISON OF ANTIBODY-DEPENDENT CELLULAR CYTOTOXICITY AND NK ACTIVITY

Andrew V. Muchmore

TABLE OF CONTENTS

I. INTRODUCTION

In this chapter we will discuss models of antibody-dependent cellular cytotoxicity (ADCC) and their relationship to natural killer (NK) activity. Such a discussion immediately becomes complex because ADCC may be mediated by many different types of cells; furthermore, these antibody-directed killer cells can lyse a varied spectrum of targets. Because of this heterogeneity, it is apparent that any attempt to compare and contrast NK activity and ADCC must start with a definition of what is meant by each term. In fact, the lack of any generally accepted rigorous definition for either of these activities, coupled with the fact that a variety of cell types mediate similar functions, has led to a confusing array of claims.

From a historical perspective each activity was defined operationally using in vitro models which appeared to measure unique forms of cell-mediated cytolysis. Initial characterization of such models emphasized differences from previously characterized forms of in vitro cell-mediated cytolysis.[1] For example, ADCC was originally characterized by measuring non-immune cell-mediated target cell cytolysis which depended upon the presence of target-specific antibody. This operational definition was then shown to differ from known mechanisms of cell-mediated lysis. A large number of studies were undertaken to characterize the nature of the effector cell capable of interacting with target-specific antibody leading to target cytolysis. Table 1 gives some idea of the different cells which can mediate such an effect. It would indeed be surprising if polymorphonuclear leukocytes, lymphocytes, monocytes, eosinophils, and even malignant cells were capable of killing tumor cells, intracellular parasites, extracellular parasites, and red blood cells (RBCs) via a common final pathway. Thus, the original operational definition of ADCC is inadequate if one desires to characterize any one specific model, sine ADCC as defined both historically and operationally represents a family of related models each capable of mediating antibody-dependent cell-mediated target cell destruction. Similar problems arise with NK activity. As originally described, nonimmune spleen cells were noted to spontaneously lyse certain malignant cell lines.[3,4] Investigation of this phenomenon demonstrated that neither target-specific, naturally occurring antibody nor prior antigen exposure were required. Thus, NK activity came to mean the presence of cytolytic cells which appeared to naturally reside in lymphoid tissue and exhibited target cell cytolysis in the absence of prior immunity, exogenous antibody, lectin, or other known stimuli. It soon became apparent that certain tumor cell lines were exquisitely sensitive to this form of killing, most notably the mouse cell line YAC-1 and the human myeloid cell line K562. Originally, this target specificity was felt to be the result of target cell infection with C-type RNA tumor viruses or Moloney leukemia virus, but further studies have failed to support this generalization.[5,6] This apparent target preference led to a host of studies using different malignant and cell line targets. Such studies showed that many freshly obtained tumor cells were "NK resistant". Furthermore, certain tumors seemed to be lysed by a different population of effector cells and the name NC for natural cytotoxicity was proposed.[7] It had also been appreciated for some time that macrophages could lyse targets in an analogous fashion. Similar models of spontaneous cytotoxicity have been developed which involve prolonged in vitro culture or the addition of exogenous nonspecific stimuli such as interferon (IFN) or interleukin-2 (IL-2) and these activities have been termed NK or NK-like.[8] Thus, NK activity, like ADCC, has frequently come to mean a variety of things to different investigators. Eva-Lotta Larson,[9] addressing similar kinds of nomenclature problems in the lymphokine field, chose an admirable quote from Lewis Carroll's, *Through the Looking Glass and What Alice Found There,* which whimsically summarizes such linguistic frailities:

> "Must a name mean something? Alice asked doubtfully . . .
> "When I use a word," Humpty Dumpty said in a rather scornful tone,
> "It means just what I choose it to mean, neither more nor less."
> "The question," said Alice, "is whether you can make words mean so many different things?"

Table 1
HUMAN CELLS CAPABLE OF MEDIATING ADCC

Cell type	Target
K cells	Cell lines, tumor cells, RBCs
Monocytes	Cell lines, tumor cells, RBCs, bacteria
Polymorphonuclear leukocytes	RBCs, tumor cells, bacteria, yeast
Eosinophils	Tumor cells, extracellular parasites
Malignant cell lines, e.g., mastocytoma (P815Y) (see Reference 2)	RBCs

Note: Summary of cells capable of mediating target cell lysis in the presence of target specific antibody. The majority of "K" cells express SRBC receptors and express IgG FcR (see text).

This raises the question of how we should define ADCC and NK activity. It seems that for purposes of comparison such definitions should be rather restrictive. Recent discussions seem to support a general consensus that narrowly defines NK activity. It is (1) mediated by nonadherent lymphocytes, (2) does not require in vitro or in vivo stimulation, and (3) target specificity is neither defined by antibody nor major histocompatibility-restricted T cell recognition structures. Attempts to define these cells morphologically have not been entirely successful and this led Eva Klein[10] to suggest that such a lack of unanimity is in itself a good indication that the lytic cells are in fact a heterogeneous lot.

For this chapter we will start with a somewhat arbitrary definition of ADCC. Initially we will restrict ADCC to target cell lysis mediated by nonadherent lymphocytes which require an intact Fc IgG receptor, and target specificity is conferred by the combining site of the particular antibody employed.

It is important to realize at the outset that these are very restrictive definitions and, as such, we will initially be examining only one part of a continuum of cell-mediated lytic activity. Such caveats apply especially to any discussion of ADCC since this definition is unduly restrictive and is only being used at the outset of this discussion as a mechanism by which we can compare similar cells.

Utilizing these definitions we will discuss phenotypic markers found on cells responsible for ADCC and NK activity. Next, the development and tissue distribution of these two cell types will be reviewed. Then we will compare the mechanisms of target cell damage for each form of cytolysis. After examining these activities using our restricted definitions an attempt will be made to place ADCC and NK activity in perspective with respect to other similar models.

II. PHENOTYPE OF THE CELLS RESPONSIBLE FOR NK AND ADCC

By our previous definition, NK cells do not encompass monocytes which may exhibit similar functional activity. Therefore, by definition, NK cells are nonadherent lymphocytes. Attempts to isolate NK activity in a homogeneous population have resulted in cells greatly enriched for large granular lymphocytes (LGLs). However, since some non-LGLs bind to NK-sensitive targets, it has been very difficult to completely exclude small amounts of NK activity in lymphocytes without these characteristic large granules.[11] The granules themselves appear to be lysosomal in origin. Using cytochemical techniques these granules were shown

Table 2
SURFACE PHENOTYPE OF THE NK CELL IN MOUSE AND MAN

	Man	Mouse
Nonadherent	Yes	Yes
IgG FcR	Yes	Yes
T cell markers	SRBC receptor	Thy-1
	OKT11	Qa 5
	OKT10	Ly-5
Markers more specific for NK cells	HNK-1 (Leu 7)	NK1
	Asialo-GM1	asialo-GM1
	Leu-11A	Ly-6
Myeloid/macrophage Specific reagents	Mac1	Mac1
	OKM1	

Note: Summary of major surface phenotypic markers of NK cells. See text for discussion.

to contain α-naphthyl-acetate esterase, acid phosphatase, and β-glucuronidase.[12] In marked contrast to lysosomes found in granulocytes and monocytes, LGLs do not stain for peroxidase. Despite the apparent morphologic homogeneity of these LGLs, approximately 20 to 30% of LGL cells apparently fail to lyse appropriate targets. Early work also established that NK cells expressed Fc receptors (FcR). Multiple groups have attempted to further characterize both human and murine NK cells using monoclonal antibodies (MoAbs) and rosetting techniques.

As can be seen in Table 2, NK cells have a heterogeneous surface phenotype. These data presented in this table are derived from three major types of experiments. The first is a functional approach. Cell populations with putative NK activity are depleted with a particular reagent and then tested for inhibition of function. For example, using these techniques a majority of human NK cells appear to have a low-affinity sheep red blood cell (SRBC) receptor and express an antigen defined by the monoclonal HNK-1 (Leu-7).[13] By contrast, depletion of cells which bear the markers OKT3, OKT4, or OKT8 have little effect on in vitro function. Depletion of cells bearing either the marker OKM1 or OKT11, however, reduces functional activity. Using the two together leads to even greater inhibition suggesting the presence of two partially nonoverlapping cell populations.[14]

A second approach involves enrichment of NK activity. These approaches frequently use density sedimentation to enrich for LGLs. Another strategy uses positive or negative selection with specific monoclonal antisera to enrich for function. Using such techniques, both T cell and myeloid cell surface markers are expressed in various quantities. For example, enrichment of LGLs by density sedimentation markedly enriches for the marker OKM1. Cells enriched for LGLs are also positive for OKT10 (60%), 3A1, a T cell marker (50%) and asialo-GM1 (70%).[15] In contrast, these enriched populations of human NK cells tend to express rather small quantities of the surface markers OKT3, OKT4, and OKT8. Using two-color immunofluorescence, HNK-1 (Leu-7) positive cells were found to coexpress the markers 3A1, T1, and T3 on 20 to 50% of the cells. Between 10 to 20% of cells coexpressed HNK-1 in association with T4, T5, or T8 whereas 60 to 70% of HNK-1 positive cells coexpressed the myeloid marker M1.[16]

Finally, single cell assays in agar have been employed. Using these techniques, targets and effectors are mixed. Targets are lysed and then individual lytic cell are typed microscopically with various monoclonal reagents. Using this approach, pretreatment with OKT10 dramatically inhibited cytolysis.[17]

Similar kinds of studies have been employed using murine cells. For example, cells enriched for the cell marker defined by the monoclonal NK1.1 were capable of both binding and lysing the NK-sensitive cell line YAC-1.[18] Another monoclonal Ly 5.2 blocks NK-mediated lysis even in the absence of complement.[19] In this same study, Thy-1.2, Ly-1.2, Ly-2.2, and Ly-3.2 did not decrease NK cell activity. Under the appropriate conditions it is believed that murine NK cells express low densities of the Thy-1 marker.[20] An interesting marker was discovered when NK cells were screened with antibrain antibodies. It was found that the majority of cells expressing NK activity also bound antibodies specific for the gluco-cerebroside, asialo-GM1.[21] Using flotation centrifugation on BSA gradients in combination with immune elimination, Koo et al.[22] estimated that murine splenic cells capable of lysing the tumor RL♂, were 80 to 90% positive for the antigens NK1, Qa 4, Qa 5, and Ly-5.

Unfortunately, all of these studies have generally used a single tissue source, either human peripheral blood or mouse spleen, and have generally looked only at lysis of certain "NK"-sensitive targets namely K562, YAC-1, and occasionally RL♂. As pointed out in other systems, different targets frequently lead to entirely different conclusions.[23] Identical problems occur with natural cytotoxicity. Thus, Stutman et al.[7] suggested that NC cells rather than NK cells were responsible for lysis of certain Meth A tumor cell targets. One can only conclude that no single cell marker is capable of defining an NK cell. In summary, human NK activity is strongly associated with the following phenotype: (1) large cytoplasmic granules, (2) IgG FcR, (3) Leu-11A, (4) OKT10, (5) OKM1, (6) 3A1, (7) asialo-GM1, and (8) HNK-1. Cells expressing OKT4, OKT8, and OKT3 do not appear to have much activity.

It is unlikely that these markers are describing a single population of cells, but rather a cell function associated with a heterogenous surface phenotype. Similar problems arise with murine NK cells. A majority of studies would suggest that such cells probably have low densities of Thy-1, express IgG FcR and are positive for antiasialo-GM1, express NK1, Mac1, Ly-5, Ly-6, and also are Qa 5 positive. Again, no known single population of cells expresses these diverse markers.[24-26]

The phenotype of the cell responsible for mediating ADCC is not as well characterized and confusion has been added when authors have failed to distinguish between ADCC mediated by monocytes and that mediated by lymphocytes. For example, in both mouse and man, cells capable of mediating ADCC of chicken RBC targets are found in more buoyant and slower-sedimenting fraction of cells than cells with NK activity. However, these fractions contain mostly monocytes and their precursors. Few would argue that monocytes are not potent mediators of ADCC towards erythrocyte targets. For the purposes of comparison it is necessary to compare monocyte ADCC with spontaneous monocyte-mediated cytotoxicity and lymphocyte ADCC with lymphocyte NK activity. Furthermore, most authors have only examined ADCC mediated through IgG FcR.

ADCC mediated by IgG FcR was originally found in a population of cells which lacked both high-avidity SRBC receptors and surface immunoglobulin. These cells were shown to have FcR for IgG and were at first termed "null cells", but the inappropriateness of this term was soon evident and such cells have become known as K cells.[27,28] It was noted by Perlmann et al.[29] that C3bi-coated target cells bound to C3bi receptors on effector cells and that this treatment markedly enhanced ADCC. Later work has characterized this as a type-3 complement receptor. Recently it was shown that Mac1 (a rat antimouse macrophage MoAB) in the presence of complement is capable of depleting cells of ADCC activity as well as NK activity. Conversely, cells enriched for Mac1 are enriched for NK and ADCC activity. Interestingly, recent evidence suggests that Mac1 preferentially binds either the type-3 complement receptor itself or a molecule in close association with it.[30]

With the realization that T cells expressed FcR, K cell activity was reexamined and it was found that ADCC activity, just like NK activity, could be found in both T-γ positive and T-γ negative fractions.[31] Further characterization of LGLs has shown that they not only mediate NK activity but also are potent mediators of ADCC activity.[15] OKM1, a myeloid marker, also is found on cells capable of mediating ADCC. Cells which coexpress IgG FcR and the SRBC receptor as assayed by the MoAb OKT11 also appear to mediate ADCC. Recently it has also been suggested that Leu-11A is another marker of ADCC as well as NK function. These investigators felt that Leu-11A was actually binding to the FcR itself since treatment with Leu-11A completely blocked the ability of cells to bind aggregated rabbit immunoglobulin. However, under saturating conditions, Leu-11A positive cells were still efficient mediators of ADCC. Thus, if Leu-11A binds to the FcR, it either binds in such a way as not to interfere with ADCC or it binds to only a subset of such receptors.[32] The FcR responsible for mediating ADCC is sensitive to treatment with proteolytic enzymes such as trypsin whereas NK activity is resistant to similar treatment.[4] In fact, this was a major piece of evidence used by earlier researchers to argue that NK did not simply represent ADCC mediated by naturally occurring cross-reactive antibodies. HNK-1 (Leu-7), originally proposed as a unique marker for NK activity as well as cells capable of mediating ADCC, has recently been shown to represent a subset of Leu-11A positive cells.[32,33] Cells capable of mediating ADCC are also characterized by binding to antiasialo-GM1. As mentioned previously, asialo-GM1 is found in the central nervous system. Interestingly, it has recently been reported that HNK-1 binds avidly to myelin sheaths in human and rodent central nervous tissue.[34] In summary, lymphocytes capable of mediating ADCC express FcR, C3bi receptors, bind to OKT11, HNK-1 (Leu-7), Leu 11A, asialo-GM1, OKM1, and Mac1.

Thus, using our narrow definition of the cells responsible for ADCC and NK, with the exception of a differential sensitivity to proteolytic enzymes, it is impossible to draw meaningful distinctions based on surface phenotype between NK cells and lymphocytes capable of mediating ADCC.

However, as mentioned earlier, our restricted definition is only for convenience and comparison since it is quite clear that many cells are capable of lysing targets through NK-like as well as ADCC types of mechanisms. The restricted definition that we have employed for ADCC is perhaps the more artificial since, in contradistinction to NK-like activity, the accepted definition of ADCC has focused on the functional presence of FcR and the ability to specifically direct lysis through the use of target-specific immunoglobulin. Through the judicious use of different targets and different sources of antibody, investigators have found that a whole family of ADCC activity exists. For example, using chicken RBCs and hyperimmune rabbit antibody we have found that T cells, monocytes, polymorphonuclear leukocytes, and even certain malignant cell lines such as P815Y mastocytoma are capable of efficient target cell lysis.[2] If, however, human ABO-typing antisera is screened for the ability to mediate ADCC of the appropriate human RBC targets, it is possible to select batches that are capable of selectively activating only monocyte-mediated target cell damage.[35] Furthermore, FcR for IgM as well as IgA may be able to mediate target lysis via an ADCC type of mechanism towards a variety of targets including bacteria, RBCs, and tumor cells.[36-39] Using SRBC targets, Fuson and co-workers[40] found that IgM as well as IgG could mediate ADCC towards modified SRBC targets. To control for trace contaminants of the other class of antibody these investigators showed that DEAE removed all of the ADCC reactivity in the IgM preparation while not affecting their IgG fraction. Conversely, protein A Sepharose removed activity in the IgG fraction while not affecting the IgM activity. Recent reports have questioned whether IgM by itself can mediate ADCC or whether it merely acts to enhance ADCC mediated by IgG. Using IgM depleted of contaminating IgG by passage over an anti-IgG column, Öhlander[41] was unable to demonstrate IgM-mediated ADCC towards bovine RBC targets.[42] Addition of trace quantities of IgG to the IgM preparation induced enhanced ADCC. These investigators argued that a T cell with both IgG and IgM FcR was responsible for ADCC in their experimental system. One potential difference between these two studies is the choice of targets. SRBCs already have an affinity for T cells and it may be that this by-passed a need for IgG.

Similarly, if IgA instead of IgG or IgM is utilized then one finds that human leukocytes are capable of mediating target cell damage. A recent study of IgA-directed ADCC mediated by gut-associated lymphoid tissue suggests that these gut-associated effector cells may share many phenotypic characteristics with LGLs.[43] It is clear from these studies that the source and class of antibody employed has an important effect on the type of cell capable of mediating ADCC.

Similar differences are found if different targets are employed. For example, using tumor cell targets and a rabbit antibody, both polymorphonuclear leukocytes and eosinophils were able to lyse murine tumor cells targets.[44] In this same study, if helminth targets in the form of schistosomula was employed instead of tumor targets then only eosinophils were able to mediate ADCC. Thus, the selection of the type of target as well as the source and class of antibody dramatically affects the type of effector cell being measured. Similarly, selection of different targets will dramatically alter NK-like activity. For example, precultured human mononuclear cells will spontaneously lyse chicken RBC targets.[45,46] Like NK activity, the cytotoxic cell is not dependent upon prior exposure to antigen nor does it require the exogenous addition of antibody or lectin. Unlike NK activity, however, the cell responsible for cytolysis is an adherent, Fc positive, phagocytic human monocyte/macrophage under the control of lymphocyte suppressors. Similar effector cell differences have already been alluded to with NC cells when "NK-resistant" targets are utilized.[6] Thus, NK-like activity, in a manner exactly analogous to ADCC activity, represents a spectrum of cell-mediated cytolysis.

III. EVIDENCE THAT NK AND ADCC DIFFER

Despite the inability to physically or morphologically separate cells with NK activity from cells with ADCC activity, some available evidence suggests that these activities may represent distinct cell types. For example, Koren and Williams[47] have presented evidence based on competitive inhibition assays which suggests that cells exhibiting NK and ADCC activity represent distinct subsets. Using K562 targets they found that unlabeled K562 as well as Molt 4 (an unrelated NK-sensitive T cell line) could compete in a cold target inhibition assay. Interestingly, the NK-resistant line SB (modified with TNP) failed to compete in the same experiment, but SB modified with TNP and coated with anti-TNP and chicken RBCs similarly coated did compete. These authors argued that TNP anti-TNP coated cells were sterically hindering NK activity, although the data was also consistent with cold target inhibition. They also went on to show that Molt 4 failed to compete in an ADCC assay. Thus, they argue that if NK and ADCC were mediated by the same effector cell, then Molt 4 should inhibit NK and ADCC equally. Other investigators using similar techniques have not reached the same conclusions.[48] These differences may be explained due to species differences or due to target selection.

Other lines of evidence also suggest that under certain circumstances NK cells may lack ADCC activity. Thus, Dennert et al.[49] were able to clone several lines obtained from nude mouse spleen cells. These cells exhibited good NK activity but convincingly failed to express ADCC activity. These cells, however, had a somewhat unusual phenotype in that besides reactivity with antiasialo-GM1, these cells reacted strongly with other ganglioside markers not usually associated with murine NK cells. Further evidence that NK and ADCC represent different activities comes from studies of the ontogeny of ADCC.

When murine NK systems were originally described perhaps the most difficult criticism to defend was that NK activity simply represented "natural" antibodies "occurring" K cells resulting in ADCC. Although this original criticism has been successfully dispatched, difficulty does arise with studies examining the ontogeny of NK and K cells since "naturally"

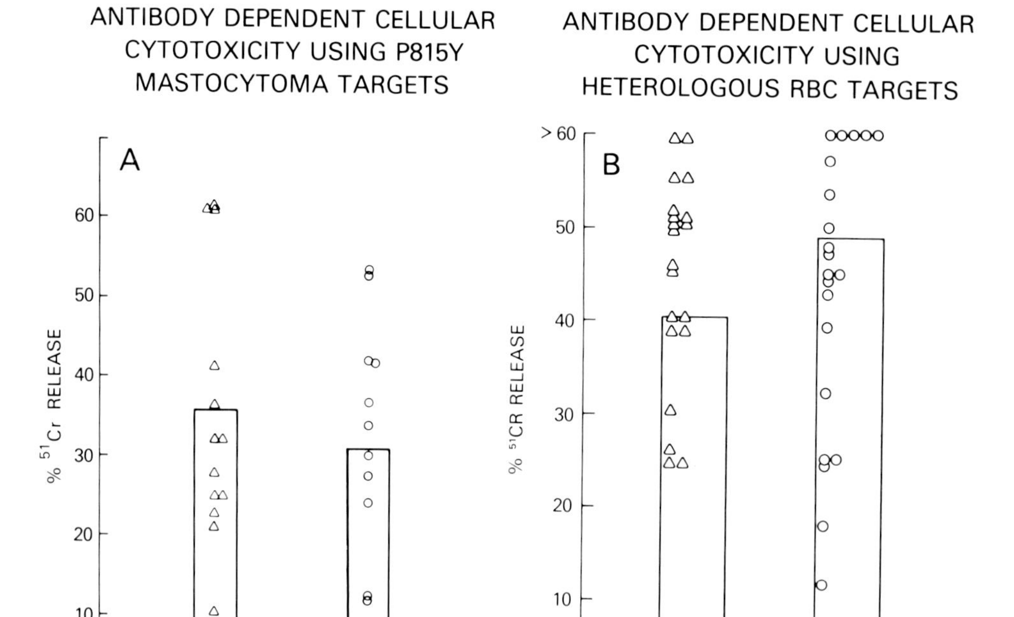

FIGURE 1. Patients with agammaglobulinemia were tested for their ability to lyse either P815-Y mastocytoma targets or chicken RBC targets. In both cases a rabbit heteroantibody with the appropriate specificity was employed. Background lysis was subtracted and results are expressed as percent ^{51}Cr released.

occurring antibody could arm "K" cells in vivo. With this dilemma in mind, Kim and co-workers[50] have performed elegant studies on NK and K cell development utilizing gnotobiotic miniature swine — exploiting the fact that immunologic virgin piglets should not have any "natural" antibodies. Using this model, these investigators have examined the tissue distribution, time of appearance, and differential susceptibility to several hetero-anti-NK antisera.[51,52] By 2 weeks, ADCC against an NK-resistant target is fully expressed in germ-free piglets whereas comparable NK activity against K562 is not seen until 6 weeks in these same animals. These data argue either that these activities are mediated by different cells or alternatively by the same cell at differing stages of maturation. These same authors found a different tissue distribution with ADCC activity found prominently in the bone marrow while NK activity was absent in the bone marrow. Finally, using appropriate dilutions of a hetero-"anti-NK" antisera and complement, these investigators have shown that NK activity could be inhibited leaving ADCC relatively intact. Unfortunately, it was not clear whether complement was required, thus leaving open the possibility that this antisera, rather than eliminating a population of cells, was simply blocking one activity (NK) while leaving another activity intact (ADCC).[51]

The final line of evidence that NK and ADCC represent distinct subsets of cells comes from studies of immunodeficiencies.[53] Koren and co-workers[53] found that four of five patients with sex-linked agammaglobulinemia lacked ADCC while retaining NK activity. However, we have found that neonatally bursectomized agammaglobulinemic chickens exhibit completely normal levels of ADCC in vitro when exogenous, target-specific immunoglobulin is supplied. Similarly, we have found that patients with agammaglobulinemia frequently exhibit normal levels of ADCC despite their inability to synthesize normal levels of antibody (Figure 1). Differences between these two studies may be the result of target selection. For example, the recessive beige mutation bg/bg has been reported to lack NK activity. Saxena et al.,[54] however, examined this phenomena and confirmed an inability to kill YAC-1 but found significant NK activity towards K562 targets.

In summary, it would appear that under certain circumstances NK and ADCC reactivity can be separated based on (1) differential enzyme sensitivity, (2) cold target inhibition studies, (3) certain cloned lines with NK activity, (4) temporal differences during ontogeny, and (5) differences seen in certain cases of agammaglobulinemia.

Although organisms lacking the ability to synthesize antibody may still express ADCC if exogenous target-specific antibody is employed, ADCC is absolutely dependent upon the expression of functional FcR. Interestingly, the appearance of FcR phylogenetically far antedates the appearance of ADCC. For example, FcR exist on several unicellular organisms, including *Staphylococcus* (staph protein A), group A streptococci, and the intestinal parasite *Entamoeba histolytica*.[55,56] The functional significance of such FcR remains speculative, although it may represent an interesting example of convergent evolution.

IV. MECHANISM OF TARGET CELL LYSIS

NK-mediated cytolysis can be viewed as occurring in several distint stages. The first stage involves target and effector approximation and can be measured in assays of target cell/effector cell adherence. This step is dependent upon the presence of divalent cations. After this step is completed, it is likely that contents from the large granules are released in the vicinity of the target cell. There is some controversy as to what happens next. Early reports of increased chemiluminescence, suggesting that cytolysis was dependent upon peroxide and superoxide formation, remains controversial.[57] More recent work suggests that perhaps these original observations may have been the result of contamination with monocytes. Other investigators have found that release of granules produces pores in the target cell membrane in a fashion exactly analogous to complement-mediated target cell damage. The size of the hole, however, clearly distinguishes NK lesions from complement-induced lesions.[58] ADCC-driven effector cells induce identical lesions in targets.[59] Morphologically, both ADCC and NK forms of cytolysis may produce identical types of target membrane holes, suggesting a common mechanism of target cell damage. In support of these observations is the recent description of a MoAb termed RH-1 which blocks cytolysis even after target cell binding has occurred.[60] Pretreatment of effector cells with RH-1 or addition in single cell assays of preformed, lymphocyte-target conjugates blocked lysis. These data suggested that this antibody blocked NK activity at a postbinding effector level. Not only was NK activity blocked but also ADCC of nucleated targets was inhibited, arguing for a similar final mechanism of target cell damage for both NK and ADCC of nucleated targets. Thus, for both NK activity and one form of lymphocyte-mediated ADCC, target cell damage appears to share a final common pathway. Other models of ADCC, however, strongly suggest that several other mechanisms of target cell damage exist. For example, both neutral proteases as well as arginase have been implicated in some forms of cytolysis.[61] Oxygen intermediates also play a role in some forms of ADCC.[61] For example, normal human polymorphonuclear leukocytes can lyse antibody-coated LSTRA targets, but polymorphonuclear leukocytes from patients with chronic granulomatous disease fail to lyse these targets, arguing for the necessity of a respiratory burst with the production of reactive oxygen intermediates.[62] In a similar study extending these observations to lymphocyte-mediated ADCC, patients with chronic granulomatous disease who lack the enzyme NADPH oxidase and thus fail to make hydrogen peroxide and superoxide also fail to mediate lysis of antibody-coated RBCs in suspension.[63] Interestingly, if targets were attached to surfaces so as to block phagocytosis, then chronic granulomatous disease lymphocytes effectively lysed human red cell targets. Furthermore, lymphocyte-mediated lysis of antibody-coated autologous lymphoid cells proceeded normally. This is in contrast to the defective ADCC seen with chronic granulomatous-diseased polymorphonuclear leukocytes previously described. These data argue that ADCC mediated by polymorphonuclear leukocytes in these systems require reactive oxygen intermediates while lysis mediated by lymphocytes does not. Similar results are seen with NK-like systems. For example, the spontaneous generation of monocyte-mediated cytotoxicity directed towards chicken RBC targets previously alluded to appears to be substantially mediated by oxygen intermediates since both catalase and superoxide dismutase block lysis of chicken RBC targets.[64]

Other more specialized types of targets require more specific effector mechanisms. For example, both lymphocytes and polymorphonuclear leukocytes fail to kill antibody-coated schistosomula. Eosinophils, however, were found to be efficient killers. Further study demonstrated that major basic protein, an arginine-rich material which comprises almost 50% of the granules of eosinophils, played an important role in schistosomula killing. Major basic protein was found to directly bind and damage isolated schistosomula and, furthermore, morphologic examination of the interaction between eosinophils and the worms showed that major basic protein was released directly onto the surface of the worms. In conclusion, if a limited array of tumor targets are examined and lysis is restricted to phenotypic NK-like cells, then both ADCC and NK appear to be mediated by an oxygen-independent form of killing. A MoAb has been described which appears to interfere with this post-target binding step in lysis and is likely directly interfering with the lytic molecule(s) itself. However, as different targets and different conditions are examined, it is clear that ADCC represents an array of cytolytic capabilities ranging from peroxide and superoxide formation to protease release and even specialized proteins like major basic protein.

V. SUMMARY

Phylogenetically, it is likely that NK-like forms of cytolysis pre-aged the development of ADCC. Invertebrates exhibit a large array of cytotoxic cells capable of target cell cytolysis in the absence of antibody or T-cell recognition.[65] However, with the appearance of antibody as a vector to direct target specificity, mammals have developed an impressive array of different forms of ADCC. Different targets, not surprisingly, have different weaknesses and it would appear that mammals have produced a panoply of cytotoxic capabilities. Not only do different targets elicit killing from different cell types but also each cell type appears to possess several mechanisms which can be utilized to damage target cells. Only if one restricts the type of target employed, the phenotype of the cell responsible for killing, and the class of antibody employed does one begin to limit the kind of cytolysis that can be evoked with antibody. Under these conditions, the cell type responsible for NK- and K cell-mediated ADCC exhibits a somewhat heterogeneous surface phenotype, and it has been difficult to physically separate cells capable of mediating ADCC from those capable of mediating NK activity. Furthermore, both NK cells and ADCC under such restricted circumstances appear to be mediated by a common final mechanism of cytolysis involving the release of granules in the immediate vicinity of the target cell membrane with subsequent target cell death. It would appear under certain circumstances that both ADCC and NK activity reside in the same effector cell. Such a cell can either be directed by specific antibody or directed in an as yet incompletely understood fashion to lyse tumor targets. However, evidence from (1) the study of the ontogeny of NK and ADCC activity in miniature swine, (2) differences in NK and ADCC activity in some cases of agammaglobulinemia, (3) differences in enzyme susceptibility, (4) studies of cold target inhibition, and (5) characterization of certain cloned lines suggest that NK and ADCC reactivity is clearly separable by functional criteria. However, these studies fail to differentiate between the possibility that NK and ADCC are mediated by the same cell at different stages of maturation or by physically separable cells.

In the same way that ADCC represent a spectrum of activity, cell lysis in the absence of antibody can be peformed by various effector cells exhibiting different cytolytic capabilities. When one imagines the enormous number of potential pathogens each with its own weaknesses and strengths, it is not surprising that host defenses have evolved into a complex interplay of factors involving specific and "nonspecific" forms of recognition as well as a large and varied arsenal of cytolytic mechanism to effect target cell damage and, thus, protect the host.

REFERENCES

1. **Perlmann, P. and Holm, G.,** Cytotoxic effects of lymphoid cells *in vitro, Adv. Immunol.*, 2, 1972.
2. **Muchmore, A. V., Nelson, D. L., and Blaese, R. M.,** The cytotoxic effector potential of some common non-lymphoid tumors and cultured cell lines with phytohemagglutinin and heterologous anti-erythrocyte antisera, *J. Immunol.*, 114, 3, 1975.
3. **Kiessling, R., Klein, E., and Wigzell, H.,** Natural killer cells in the mouse. I. Cytotoxic cells with specificity for mouse Moloney leukemia cells. Specificity and distribution according to genotype, *Eur. J. Immunol.*, 5, 112, 1975.
4. **Herberman, R. B., Nunn, M. E., and Lavrin, D. H.,** Natural cytotoxic reactivity of mouse lymphoid cells against syngeneic and allogeneic tumors. I. Distribution of reactivity and specificity, *Int. J. Cancer*, 15, 216, 1975.
5. **Herberman, R. B., Nunn, M. E., Holden, H. T., and Lavrin, D. H.,** Natural cytotoxic reactivity of mouse lymphoid cells against syngeneic and allogeneic tumors. II. Characterization of effector cells, *Int. J. Cancer*, 16, 230, 1975.
6. **Kiessling, R., Klein, E., Pross, H., and Wigzell, H.,** "Natural" killer cells in the mouse. II. Cytotoxic cells with specificity for mouse Moloney leukemia-cells characteristic of the killer cell, *Eur. J. Immunol.*, 5, 117, 1975.
7. **Stutman, O., Paige, C. J., and Figarella, E. F.,** Natural cytotoxicity of methylchloranthrene tumor targets, *J. Immunol.*, 121, 1819, 1978.
8. **Rosenberg, S., Grimm, E. A., Mazunder, A., Zhang, H. Z., and Rosenberg, S. A.,** The lymphokine activated killer cell phenomenon: lysis of NK resistant fresh solid tumor cells by IL-2 activated autologous human peripheral blood lymphocytes, *J. Exp. Med.*, 155, 1823, 1982.
9. **Larson, E.-L.,** Naming lymphocyte-specific growth and differentiation factors, *Immunol. Today*, 3, 81, 1982.
10. **Klein, E.,** Naming in clonal terms, *Immunol. Today*, 4, 97, 1983.
11. **Timonen, T., Ortaldo, J. R., and Herberman, R. B.,** Characteristics of human large granular lymphocytes and relationship to NK and K cells, *J. Exp. Med.*, 153, 569, 1981.
12. **Grossi, C. E. and Ferrarini, M.,** Morphology and cytochemistry of human L.G.L. in *NK Cells and Other Natural Effector Cells*, Herberman, R. B., Ed., Academic Press, New York, 1982, 1.
13. **Abo, T. and Balch, C. M.,** A differentiation antigen of human NK and K cells identified by a monoclonal antibody HNK-1, *J. Immunol.*, 127, 1024, 1981.
14. **Zarling, J. M., Clouse, K. A., Biddison, W. E., and Kung, P. C.,** Phenotypes of human natural killer cell populations detected with monoclonal antibodies, *J. Immunol.*, 127, 7575, 1981.
15. **Ortaldo, J. R., Sharrow, S. O., Timonen, T., and Herberman, R. B.,** Determination of surface antigens on highly purified human NK cells by flow cytometry with monoclonal antibodies, *J. Immunol.*, 127, 2401, 1981.
16. **Abo, T., Cooper, M. D., and Balch, C. M.,** Characterization of human NK cells identified by the monoclonal HNK-1 antibody, in *NK Cells and Other Natural Effector Cells*, Herberman, R. B., Ed., Academic Press, 1982, 31.
17. **Brandt, C. P. and Koren, H. S.,** Phenotypic and functional characteristics of natural killer cells by monoclonal antibodies, in *NK Cells and Other Natural Effector Cells*, Herberman, R. B., Eds., Academic Press, 1982, 79.
18. **Lust, J. A., Kumar, V., Burton, R. C., Bartlett, S. P., and Bennett, M.,** Heterogeneity of natural killer cells in the mouse, *J. Exp. Med.*, 154, 306, 1981.
19. **Pollack, S. B., Tamm, M. R., Emmons, S. L., and Nowinski, R. C.,** Presence of T-cell associated antigens on immune NK cells, *J. Immunol.*, 123, 1818, 1979.
20. **Herberman, R. B., Nunn, M. E., and Holden, H. T.,** Low density of Thy-1 antigen on mouse effector cells mediating natural cytotoxicity against tumor cells, *J. Immunol.*, 121, 304, 1978.

21. **Habu, S., Fukui, H., Shimamaro, K., Kasai, M., Nagel, Y., Okumura, K., and Tamaoki, N.,** *In vivo* effects of anti-asialo GM-1: reduction of NK activity and enhancement of tumor growth in nude mice, *J. Immunol.*, 127, 34, 1981.
22. **Koo, G., Jacobson, J. B., Hammerling, G., and Hammerling, U.,** Antigenic profile of murine NK cells, *J. Immunol.*, 125, 1003, 1980.
23. **Muchmore, A. V., Nelson, D. L., Kirchner, H., and Blaese, R. M.,** A reappraisal of the effector cells mediating mitogen induced cellular cytotoxicity, *Cell. Immunol.*, 19, 78, 1975.
24. **Tam, M. R., Emmons, S. L., and Pollack, S. B.,** Analysis and enrichment of mouse natural killer cells with the fluorescence activator cell sorter, *J. Immunol.*, 124, 650, 1980.
25. **Burton, R. C., Bartlett, S. P., and Winn, H. G.,** Alloantigens specific for natural killer cells, in *NK Cells and Other Natural Effector Cells*, Herberman, R. B., Ed., Academic Press, New York, 1982, 105.
26. **Glimcher, L. F., Shen, W., and Cantor, H.,** Identification of a cell surface antigen expressed on the natural killer cell, *J. Exp. Med.*, 145, 1, 1977.
27. **Nelson, D. L., Bundy, B. M., Pitchon, H. E., Blaese, R. M., and Strober, W.,** The effector cells in human peripheral blood mediating mitogen induced cellular cytotoxicity and antibody dependent cellular cytotoxicity, *J. Immunol.*, 117, 1472, 1976.
28. **MacDonald, H. R., Bonnard, G. D., Sordat, B., and Zawodnik, S. A.,** Antibody dependent cell-mediated cytotoxicity, heterogeneity of effector cells in human peripheral blood, *Scand. J. Immunol.*, 4, 487, 1975.
29. **Perlmann, H., Perlmann, P., Schreiber, R. D., and Muller-Eberhard, H. J.,** Interaction of target cell bound C3bi and C3d with human lymphocyte receptors: Enhancement of ADCC, *J. Exp. Med.*, 153, 1592, 1981.
30. **Beller, D. I., Springer, T. A., and Schreiber, R. D.,** Anti-Mac-1 selectively inhibits the mouse and human type three complement receptor, *J. Exp. Med.*, 156, 1000, 1982.
31. **Shaw, S., Pichler, W. J., and Nelson, D. L.,** Fc receptors on human T lymphocytes. III. Characterization of subpopulations involved in cell mediated lympholysis and ADCC, *J. Immunol.*, 122, 599, 1979.
32. **Lanier, L. L., Lee, A. M., Phillips, J. H., Warner, M. L., and Babcock, G. F.,** Subpopulations of human natural killer cells defined by expression of Leu 7 and Leu 11 antigens, *J. Immunol.*, 131, 1789, 1983.
33. **Abo, T., Cooper, M. D., and Balch, C. M.,** Characterization of human NK cells identified by the monoclonal HNK-1 antibody, in *NK Cells and Other Natural effector Cells*, Herberman, R. B., Ed., Academic Press, New York, 1982, 31.
34. **Schuller-Petrovic, S., Berhart, W., Lassmann, H., Rumpold, H., and Kraft, D.,** A shared antigenic determinant between natural killer cells and nervous tissue, *Nature (London)*, 306, 179, 1983.
35. **Poplack, D. G., Bonnard, G. D., Holiman, B. J., and Blaese, R. M.,** Monocyte mediated antibody dependent cellular cytotoxicity: a clinical test of monocyte function, *Blood*, 48, 110, 1976.
36. **Wahlin, B., Perlmann, H., and Perlmann, P.,** Analysis by a plaque assay of IgG and IgM-dependent cytolytic lymphocytes in human blood, *J. Exp. Med.*, 144, 1375, 1976.
37. **Lamon, E. W., Skurzak, H. M., Andersson, B., Witten, H. D., and Klein, E.,** Antibody dependent lymphocyte cytotoxicity in the murine sarcoma virus system: activity of IgM and IgG with specificity for MLV determined antigens, *J. Immunol.*, 114, 1171.
38. **Lowell, G. H., MacDermott, R. P., Summers, P. L., Reeder, A. A., Bertovich, M. J., and Fornal, S. B.,** Antibody-dependent cell mediated antibacterial activity: K lymphocytes, monocytes and granulocytes are effective against shigella, *J. Immunol.*, 125, 2778, 1980.
39. **Fuson, E. W. and Lamon, E. W.,** IgM-induced cell mediated cytotoxicity with antibody and affector cells of human origin, *J. Immunol.*, 118, 1907, 1977.
40. **Fuson, E. W., Whitten, H. D., Ayers, R. D., and Lamon, E. W.,** Antibody dependent cell mediated cytotoxicity by human lymphocytes. I. Comparison of IgM and IgG-induced cytotoxicity, *J. Immunol.*, 120, 1726, 1978.
41. **Öhlander, C., Perlmann, H., and Perlmann, P.,** Regulation of IgG-IgM interlay by antibody specificity in human K-cell-mediated cytotoxicity, *Scand. J. Immunol.*, 15, 409, 1982.
42. **Perlmann, H., Perlmann, P., Pape, G. R., and Halldén, G.,** Regulation of IgG antibody dependent cellular cytotoxicity *in vitro* by IgM antibodies mechanism and characterization of effector lymphocytes, *Scand. J. Immunol.*, 14, 47, 1981.
43. **Tagliabae, A., Nencioni, L., Villa, L., Keren, D. F., Lowell, G., and Boroschi, D.,** Antibody dependent cell mediated anti-bacterial activity of intestinal lymphocytes with secretory IgA, *Nature (London)*, 306, 184, 1983.
44. **Vadas, M. A., Nicola, N. A., and Metcalf, D.,** Activation of ADCC of human neutrophils and eosinophils by separate colony-stimulating factors, *J. Immunol.*, 130, 795, 1983.
45. **Muchmore, A. V., Decker, J. M., and Blaese, R. M.,** Spontaneous cytotoxicity of human peripheral blood mononuclear cells towards RBC targets, I. characterization of the killer cell, *J. Immunol.*, 119, 1680, 1977.

46. **Muchmore, A. V., Decker, J. M., and Blaese, R. M.,** Spontaneous cytotoxicity of human peripheral blood mononuclear cells towards RBC targets. II. Time dependent loss of suppressor cell activity, *J. Immunol.*, 119, 1686, 1977.
47. **Koren, H. S. and Williams, M. S.,** Natural killing and ADCC are mediated by different mechanisms and by different cells, *J. Immunol.*, 121, 1956, 1978.
48. **Ojo, E. and Wigzell, H.,** Natural killer cells may be the only cells in normal mouse lymphoid cell populations endowed with cytolytic ability for antibody-coated tumor target cells, *Scand. J. Immunol.*, 7, 297, 1978.
49. **Dennert, G., Yogeesworon, G., and Yamagota, S.,** Cloned cell lines with natural killer activity. Specificity function and cell surface markers, *J. Exp. Med.*, 153, 545, 1981.
50. **Kim, Y. B., Huh, N. D., Koren, H. S., and Amos, D. B.,** Natural killing and ADCC in specific pathogen free miniature swine and germ free piglets. I. Comparison of NK and ADCC, *J. Immunol.*, 125, 755, 1978.
51. **Huh, N. D., Kim, Y. B., and Amos, D. B.,** NK and ADCC in specific pathogen free miniature swine and germ free piglets. III. Two distinct effector cells for NK and ADCC, *J. Immunol.*, 127, 2190, 1981.
52. **Huh, N. D., Kim, Y. B., Koren, H. S., and Amos, D. B.,** Natural killing and ADCC in specific pathogen free miniature swine and germ free piglets. II. Ontogenetic development of NK and ADCC, *Int. J. Cancer*, 28, 175, 1981.
53. **Koren, H. S., Amos, D. B., and Buckley, R. H.,** Natural killing in immunodeficient patients, *J. Immunol.*, 120, 796, 1978.
54. **Saxena, R. K., Saxena, Q. B., and Adler, W. H.,** Decline of murine natural killer activity in response to starvation, hypophysectomy, tumor growth and beige mutation: a comparative study, in *NK Cells and Other Natural Effectors*, Herberman, R. B., Ed., Academic Press, New York, 1982, 645.
55. **Myhre, E. B. and Kronvall, G.,** Specific binding of bovine, ovine, caprine and equine IgG subclasses to defined types of Ig receptors in gram(+) cocci, *Comp. Immunol. Micro. Infect. Dis.*, 4, 317, 1981.
56. **Galatiuc, C., Cioanu, M., Ponaitescu, D., and Sulica, A.,** Identification of IgG binding site on *E. histolytica*, *Dev. Comp. Immunol.*, 5, 201, 1981.
57. **Koren, H. and Herberman, R. B.,** The cryptic orphan killer cells, *Immunol. Today*, 4, 97, 1983.
58. **Henkart, M. P. and Henkart, P. A.,** Lymphocyte mediated cytolysis as a secretory phenomenon, in *Mechanisms of Cell Mediated Cytotoxicity*, Clark, W. R. and Goldstein, P., Eds., Plenum Press, New York, 1982, 227.
59. **Dourmashkin, R. R., Deteix, P., Simone, C. B., and Henkart, P.,** Electron microscopic demonstration of lesions on target cell membranes associated with antibody-dependent cellular cytotoxicity, *Clin. Exp. Immunol.*, 43, 554, 1980.
60. **Neville, M. E. and Hiserodt, J. C.,** Inhibition of human antibody-dependent cellular cytotoxicity, cell mediated cytotoxicity and natural killing by xenogenic antiserum prepared against "activated" alloimmune human lymphocytes, *J. Immunol.*, 128, 1246, 1982.
61. **Nathan, C. F., Murray, H. W., and Cohn, Z.,** The macrophage as an effector cell, *N. Engl. J. Med.*, 303, 622, 1980.
62. **Clark, R. A. and Klebanoff, S. J.,** Studies on the mechanism of antibody dependent polymorphonuclear leukocyte mediated cytotoxicity, *J. Immunol.*, 119, 1413, 1980.
63. **Katz, P., Simone, C. B., Henkart, P. A., and Fauci, A. S.,** Mechanisms of antibody dependent cellular cytotoxicity, *J. Clin. Invest.*, 65, 55, 1980.
64. **Hall, R. E., Muchmore, A. V., and Blaese, R. M.,** Monocyte cytotoxicity: evidence for multiple mechanisms of *in vitro* target killing trypan blue can both inhibit and enhance target lysis, *J. Reticuloendothel. Soc.*, 32, 233, 1982.
65. **Assolima, L. S., Tridente, G., and Cooper, E. L.,** Proceedings of the Verona Workshop, *Suppl. Dev. Comp. Immunol.*, 5, 1981.

INDEX

A

B

C

D

E

F

G

H

J

K

L

M

N

O

P

R

S

T

U

V

W

X

Y